Genitourinary Cancer 1

Cancer Treatment and Research 6

WILLIAM L. MCGUIRE, *series editor*

1. R.B. Livingston, ed., Lung Cancer 1. 1981. ISBN 90-247-2394-9.
2. G. Bennett Humphrey, Louis P. Dehner, Gerald B. Grindey and Ronald T. Acton, eds., Pediatric Oncology 1. 1981. ISBN 90-247-2408-2.
3. Jerome J. DeCosse and Paul Sherlock, eds., Gastrointestinal Cancer 1. 1981. ISBN 90-247-2461-9.
4. John M. Bennett, ed., Lymphomas 1, including Hodgkin's Disease. 1981. ISBN 90-247-2479-1.
5. C.D. Bloomfield, ed., Adult Leukemias 1. 1982. ISBN 90-247-2478-3.

Genitourinary Cancer 1

edited by

DAVID F. PAULSON

Duke University Medical Center, Durham, NC

1982

MARTINUS NIJHOFF PUBLISHERS

THE HAGUE / BOSTON / LONDON

Distributors:

for the United States and Canada

Kluwer Boston, Inc.
190 Old Derby Street
Hingham, MA 02043
USA

for all other countries

Kluwer Academic Publishers Group
Distribution Center
P.O. Box 322
3300 AH Dordrecht
The Netherlands

Library of Congress Cataloging in Publication Data CIP
Main entry under title:

Genitourinary cancer.

(Cancer treatment and research ; v. 6-)
Includes index.
1. Genito-urinary organs--Cancer. I. Paulson, David F. II. Series. [DNLM: 1. Urogenital neoplasms. W1 CA693 v. 6 / WJ 160 G331]
RC280.G4G47 1982 616.99'46 81-18946

ISBN-13: 978-94-009-7438-8 e-ISBN-13: 978-94-009-7436-4
DOI: 10.1007/978-94-009-7436-4

Contents

Foreword vii

Preface ix

List of contributors xi

1. Carcinogenesis in urogenital tissues 1
   ROBERT A. BONAR

2. Marker proteins as a guide in clinical management of genitourinary cancer 45
   PAUL H. LANGE

3. Assessment of biologic hazard of urologic tumors 73
   DAVID F. PAULSON

4. Surgical management of high stage renal cell carcinoma 101
   JEAN B. DEKERNION

5. Health risk and management of localized prostate cancer . . . 121
   CARL A. OLSSON

6. Chemotherapy of superficial bladder carcinoma 143
   GEORGE R. PROUT, JR.

7. Immunology of genitourinary tumors 169
   WILLIAM J. CATALONA

8. Does radiotherapy alter the course of genitourinary cancer? . . 215
   M.V. PILEPICH and CARLOS A. PEREZ

9. Current status of androgen receptor measurements in prostatic cancer 239
   JOHN TRACHTENBERG

Subject Index 251

Foreword to the series

Where do you begin to look for a recent, authoritative article on the diagnosis or management of a particular malignancy? The few general oncology textbooks are generally out of date. Single papers in specialized journals are informative but seldom comprehensive; these are more often preliminary reports on a very limited number of patients. Certain general journals frequently publish good indepth reviews of cancer topics, and published symposium lectures are often the best overviews available. Unfortunately, these reviews and supplements appear sporadically, and the reader can never be sure when a topic of special interest will be covered.

Cancer Treatment and Research is a series of authoritative volumes which aims to meet this need. It is an attempt to establish a critical mass of oncology literature covering virtually all oncology topics, revised frequently to keep the coverage up to date, easily available on a single library shelf or by a single personal subscription.

We have approached the problem in the following fashion. First, by dividing the oncology literature into specific subdivisions such as lung cancer, genitourinary cancer, pediatric oncology, etc. Second, by asking eminent authorities in each of these areas to edit a volume on the specific topic on an annual or biannual basis. Each topic and tumor type is covered in a volume appearing frequently and predictably, discussing current diagnosis, staging markers, all forms of treatment modalities, basic biology, and more.

In *Cancer Treatment and Research,* we have an outstanding group of editors, each having made a major commitment to bring to this new series the very best literature in his or her field. Martinus Nijhoff Publishers has made an equally major commitment to the rapid publication of high quality books, and world-wide distribution.

Where can you go to find quickly a recent authoritative article on any major oncology problem? We hope that *Cancer Treatment and Research* provides an answer.

WILLIAM L. MCGUIRE
Series Editor

Preface

Malignant disease of the genitourinary tract continues to provide a major health hazard. The study of these disease processes has been hampered at the clinical level as there has been a serious lack of reasonably controlled treatment trials, and at the basic science level as many of the animal model systems do not compare favorably with the human tumor situation.

This volume defines current cancer treatment and research and its application to the control of human genitourinary malignancy. The authors have developed their chapters in such a way as to provide an up-to-date resource for the clinician who is involved in day-to-day patient care problems, for the clinician-investigator who is attempting to construct programs designed to evaluate the impact of current treatments, and for the clinician-scientist who is seeking to apply basic research technology and skills to understanding and control in this disease area.

This book does not attempt to cover the entire breadth of urinary malignant disease, but focuses in depth on specific problem areas. It provides the reader with sufficient background and understanding for him to be able to evaluate future studies in the areas addressed, or even to develop his own projects. A reasonable balance has been established between clinical and basic research problems, recognizing that the two disciplines truly are not separable. The book serves to define the state of the art and, as such, will provide a valuable resource for the student of urologic oncology.

List of Contributors

BONAR, Robert A., Ph.D., Associate Director, Urology Research Laboratories, Veterans Administration Medical Center, Durham, NC 27705, U.S.A.

CATALONA, William J., M.D., Associate Professor of Urology, Washington University Medical Center, 4960 Audubon Avenue, St. Louis, MO 63110, U.S.A.

DEKERNION, Jean B., M.D., Department of Urology, Tulane University Medical Center, New Orleans, LA 70112, U.S.A.

LANGE, Paul H., M.D., Chief, Urology Section, Veterans Administration Medical Center, 54th Street and 48th Avenue South, Minneapolis, MN 55417, U.S.A.

OLSSON, Carl A., M.D., Professor and Chairman, Department of Urology, College of Physicians and Surgeons, Columbia University, 630 West 168th Street, New York, NY 10032, U.S.A.

PAULSON, David F., M.D., Associate Professor of Urology, Post Office Box 2977, Duke University Medical Center, Durham, NC 27110, U.S.A.

PEREZ, Carlos A., M.D., Director of Radiation Oncology, Rhe Edward Mallinckrodt Institute of Radiology. 4511 Forest Park, St. Louis, MO 63108, U.S.A.

PILEPICH, Miljenko V., M.D., The Edward Mallinckrodt Institute of Radiology, 4511 Forest Park, St. Louis, MO 63108, U.S.A.

PROUT, George R., Jr., M.D., Professor and Chief, Department of Urology, Massachusetts General Hospital, Boston, MA 02114, U.S.A.

TRACHTENBERG, John, Department of Urology and Laboratory for Reproductive Medicine, Department of Obstetrics & Gynecology, McGill University, Montreal, Quebec, H3A 1A1, Canada.

1. Carcinogenesis in Urogenital Tissues

ROBERT A. BONAR

1. INTRODUCTION

Much has been learned about carcinogenesis in recent decades, although our ignorance still far exceeds our knowledge. The information already acquired is being used to reduce cancer risk, and further research offers substantial promise of additional understanding and, therefore, of additional ways of preventing some of our human cancer burden. This chapter will present a brief overview of what is known or suspected about carcinogenesis in general and, more specifically, deal with neoplasia in the urinary tract of both sexes and in the genital tissues of the male.

2. OVERVIEW OF CARCINOGENESIS

2.1. Carcinogenic Agents

A variety of kinds of agent is known to be carcinogenic in various tissues and species, including organic and inorganic chemicals, viruses, radiation, other physical factors, and elements of 'life-style' which probably consist, at least in part, of these other agents. Among those human tumors for which etiology is known or strongly suspected, organic chemicals are the most frequently implicated agents (Miller, 1978). Radiation is clearly important at certain sites, particularly in the induction of skin cancer by ultraviolet light. Viruses have been associated as causative agents with only a few kinds of human tumors (Rapp, 1980). It is important to note, however, that the specific causes of most human cancers remain unknown.

It appears likely that environmental factors play an important role (Miller, 1978) in the induction of a large proportion, perhaps 60–90%, of human cancer including urologic cancer. The term environment is used here in a very broad sense, meaning all those external factors which affect the organ-

D.F. Paulson (ed.), Genitourinary Cancer 1, 1-44.

ism. The principal basis for this estimate of the importance of environmental factors is the marked geographic and temporal variation in the occurrence of most kinds of cancer (Doll, 1972; Wynder and Gori, 1977). Mortality from prostate cancer, for example, is low in Japan and much higher in the United States. This is true of colon cancer as well. Stomach cancer, on the other hand is more common in Japan. There are many other striking examples of variation in neoplastic disease among countries. It is unlikely that these are due to hereditary differences, since migrant populations tend to acquire the cancer incidence patterns of the country to which they move (Kmet, 1970).

Changes in incidence with time also suggest environmental rather than hereditary factors. Lung cancer, for example, was a relatively rare disease before about 1930 when its incidence began to increase considerably. This phenomenon followed, by about 20 years, the period when cigarette smoking had begun its rise in popularity among men. The lung cancer rate in women began to increase in a similar way about 1960, again following by about 20 years the rise in cigarette smoking among women.

While temporal and geographic variations strongly suggest the importance of environmental factors in human cancer, the relationship between a particular factor and a specific neoplasm is rarely so clear as in the case of lung cancer and cigarette smoking. We are exposed to an enormous array of environmental agents, natural and man-made, brought to our individual microenvironments by natural processes, by the activities of others, and by our own actions, and introduced into our bodies by a variety of routes. Moreover, these factors interact with each other and with the individual in complex ways.

One major group of agents of much concern as potential carcinogens is that of organic and inorganic chemicals. The mere number of such compounds is impressive (Maugh, 1978). As of November, 1977, the Chemical Abstract Service's registry of chemicals listed 4 039 907 distinct entities, and new ones were accruing at about 6 000 per week. Of these compounds about 96% contained carbon. About 3.4 million compounds were fully defined and about 3 million contained at least one ring system. Of course, many of these chemicals never leave the laboratory, but some 63 000 were in 'common use'. The Environmental Protection Agency (EPA) estimated that there were about 50 000 chemicals in common use, not including pesticides, pharmaceuticals and food additives, and that about 1 500 different ingredients were used in pesticides. The Food and Drug Administration estimated that drugs included about 4 000 active ingredients and 2 000 excipients, while food additives included 2 500 used for nutritional value and flavoring, and 3 000 to promote product life.

These figures are important in emphasizing the magnitude of the task of testing and of toxicological evaluation, but it should be stressed that relatively few chemicals are known to be carcinogenic (Tomatis, 1979).

Much attention is being given to possible carcinogens in the workplace. The proportion of cancer incidence related to occupation varies greatly with site. Overall, the incidence ascribable to occupational exposure has been estimated to be about 5% of all cancer in the industrial countries (Higginson, 1979). The figure varies substantially with different populations and different tumors and cannot be determined precisely. For certain sites higher values are probable, and 20–30% of all bladder cancer in industrialized countries may be due to occupational exposure (Morrison & Cole, 1976).

Of the factors in the environment which may be involved in the induction or promotion of malignancy some are natural, such as sunlight, radiation from the decay of radioactive minerals, cosmic rays, and, possibly, certain food constituents. Other factors, such as the mycotoxins which can occur in a variety of grains and seeds in the field and in storage, are natural products whose occurrence depends in part on conditions of harvest and storage. Still others are formed as byproducts of our industrial society, reaching us through air, water or food. Elements which also appear to be important are a variety of customs and activities often called 'lifestyle'.

The effect of a potentially carcinogenic agent may be modulated by a number of factors. For example, the incidence of skin cancer as a result of ultraviolet exposure varies geographically, being higher in the middle latitudes where the amount of sunlight is greater. The incidence is also affected by inherited characteristics and is greater in light-skinned people than in those with more pigmentation. There is an occupational component, related to indoor vs. outdoor work and, also, an ingredient of 'life-style' such as the social desirability of a suntan, which encourages greater exposure.

While the emphasis in this chapter will be on carcinogenesis by extrinsic factors, it must be remembered that each individual may respond differently to a particular carcinogen. This individuality results both from genetic constitution and previous environmental influences. There is evidence of familial susceptibility to cancer in humans (Anderson, 1975, Knudson, 1979) and species and strain differences among experimental animals are well-known. A particularly striking example of genetic influence is provided by the platyfish-swordtail system (Anders and Anders, 1978). Inbreeding of wild-type populations produces normal offspring, but crossings produce progeny which spontaneously develops a variety of neoplasms.

2.2. The Carcinogenic Process

The development of urologic cancer, like that of cancer at other sites, appears to be a complex, multi-stage process. In an early demonstration that at least two stages were involved, it was shown (Berenblum and Shubik, 1949) that tumors could be induced in mouse skin by a single 'initiating' dose of polycyclic aromatic hydrocarbon followed by repeated treatment with a 'promoter', croton oil. Tumors did not develop after the single dose of initiator alone, or after promoter alone, or if the order of application was reversed. Another interesting feature of the system was that the first application of promoter could be delayed many months after initiation, and still be effective in eliciting tumor formation. These observations suggested that one or more cells responded to the application of initiator with an irreversible change, but that no additional progression to tumor occured until the further stimulation by the promoter. Similar results, in principle, have been reported in other systems (Van Duuren, 1976) including rat bladder (Cohen *et al.*, 1979; Hicks, 1980). A sufficiently large or repeated dose of 'initiator' may obviate the need for treatment with a separate promoter.

Another important factor in carcinogenesis by organic chemicals is the role of the host in metabolizing the compound. Most chemical carcinogens appear to be inactive in the form encountered in the environment. They must be metabolized to more reactive ultimate carcinogens (Miller, 1978), sometimes by several steps, before they can react with constituents of the susceptible cell. The potential carcinogen may instead be excreted or metabolized to harmless products. The competition among these pathways, and the resulting development of a tumor or sparing of the host, may be influenced by many factors, including genetic constitution, diet, and previous exposure to the carcinogen, or to other chemicals which can affect the activity of the enzyme systems involved.

After an ultimate carcinogen is formed in, or transported to a susceptible cell, the reaction(s) with cell constituents which lead to neoplasia must take place. Most well-studied chemical carcinogens have been found to react with deoxyribonucleic acid (DNA), ribonucleic acid (RNA) and protein. The fact that many carcinogens are also mutagens (Boyland, 1980) has suggested that a reaction with DNA leading to mispairing of bases, and thus to mutation, may be the key carcinogenic step. While the molecular mechanism of neoplastic change has not been established, the most widely held view seems to be that damage to DNA is the initiating event. Cells have means of repairing DNA damage (Roberts, 1980). If the repair is accurately carried out before cell division and the accompanying mutation, no harm is done to the cell. The effectiveness of DNA repair is thus another variable in the carcinogenic process, and it can be influenced by the genetic constitution of the host and by exogenous factors. It can also be influenced by the mitotic rate in the affected cell population and, thus, in turn influence the time available for repair.

It should be noted that while DNA modification and the resulting somatic mutations are probably the most widely accepted mechanism of the initiation of carcinogenesis, this has not been proved to be the only, or even the usual, mechanism (Sivak, 1979). Analogy with tissue differentiation during which there is development of a great variety of cells with widely varying properties but with, apparently, the same genome, has suggested that changes in epigenetic regulatory mechanisms may explain neoplastic alteration. It is quite possible that both genetic and epigenetic mechanisms are involved in different tumors, and even in the same tumor. Even if the initiating event is a genetic change, many other factors play a role in determining whether a tumor forms and how it behaves. We know little about the actual mechanisms or steps in the development of most tumors. We are learning, however, and the picture which is emerging is one of many factors, both endogenous and exogenous, interacting in complex ways.

3. BLADDER AND LOWER URINARY TRACT

Tumors of the lower urinary tract will be considered first because more is known about carcinogenesis in this site than in other genitourinary sites and, indeed, more than almost any other site in the body. Most tumors of the lower urinary tract arise in the transitional epithelium, the urothelium, which lines the tract. The most frequent specific site is the bladder and the term bladder tumor is often used for brevity for all urothelial tumors. The discussion will deal almost exclusively with transitional cell tumors, about which we have the most information concerning etiology. Tumors of the renal pelvis will be considered in this section rather than with other kidney tumors because most renal pelvic tumors arise in the urothelial lining.

There is substantial international variation in bladder cancer mortality rates, the highest being in Great Britain and the lowest in the Asian Countries (Staszewski, 1980). The worldwide trend has been upward (Parkes, 1976). There is a dramatic difference in incidence between men and women (Mason *et al.*, 1975). The higher incidence in males may be partly explained by differences in occupational exposure to carcinogens and in smoking habits. Silverberg (1980) estimated that there would be about 35 000 new bladder cancer cases in the U.S. in 1980 (26 000 in men and 9500 in women) and 10 300 bladder cancer deaths (7000 men and 3300 women).

A feature of urothelial tumors which is of importance to an understanding of etiology, as well as to treatment and prognosis, is their frequent association with abnormal epithelium (Koss, 1975) elsewhere in the bladder. These abnormal epithelial cells may represent stages in developing neoplasia (Koss, 1975), and suggest multiple sites of tumor origin. Such multiplicity is consistent with a chemical or viral etiology. The possibility of intraepithelial migration of tumor cells has also been suggested (Weinstein, 1979).

It appears likely that the majority of human bladder cancers are induced by chemical agents and that radiation plays a relatively minor role (Hueper, 1969). There is some suggestive evidence of an association of herpes viruses with bladder tumor (Rapp, 1980). Cancer of the bilharzial bladder is a special case (Chevien *et al.*, 1979). The strong geographic coincidence of common infection with Schistosoma haematobium and a high incidence of bladder cancer leaves little doubt of a causative relation, although the mechanism is not established. In Egypt, the bladder is the most common site of cancer and, in contrast to industrial countries, most are squamous cell tumors.

3.1. Occupational Exposure

Much of the work on bladder carcinogenesis has focused on induction by exposure to organic chemicals, particularly in the workplace. An observant clinician, L. Rehn (1895), first reported an unusually high incidence of bladder tumors in workers engaged in the production of fuchsin (magenta) in an aniline-dye works. Rehn's study led him to the conclusion that aniline vapors inhaled by the workers over many years induced the bladder cancer, and the disease became known as aniline tumor of the bladder. Later studies showed that aniline was not itself at fault, but that other arylamines, particularly 2-naphthylamine, were associated with the increased risk of bladder cancer in dye workers.

The bladder carcinogenicity of commercial 2-naphthylamine was confirmed by the induction of bladder tumors in dogs fed the compound (Hueper *et al.*, 1938). These early studies have led to a large amount of work on bladder carcinogenesis in various animals (Clayson and Cooper, 1970; Friedell and Cohen, 1979), as well as to continuing epidemiologic investigations. More than in most other cancers, studies in bladder cancer have seen correlation of epidemiologic and laboratory studies, resulting in better progress in understanding the disease.

The extensive study of British dye-workers by Case *et al.* (1954) showed that the induction period, the time from first exposure to risk to the recognition of the bladder tumor, was both long and variable. The distribution of induction times was approximately Gaussian, with a mean of 17.8 years and a standard deviation of 7.2 years, and the range was from less than 2 to more than 45 years. An even longer mean latent period was found by Hoover and Cole (1973) in a different population. An exposure time of as little as one year was sufficient to induce the disease. The short effective exposure time and the long and variable latent period indicate some of the difficulties in determining possible etiologic factors from personal histories.

Workers in several other industries have an increased incidence of bladder cancer. In Great Britain (Somerville *et al.*, 1980) most occupational bladder cancers have occurred following work in the manufacture of dyes, in the rubber and electric cable industries, and in the retort houses of gasworks producing coal gas. Industries implicated less often were paint and pigment manufacture, chemistry laboratories, textile printing shops, and the production of rodent poisons. Other studies (reviewed by Morrison and Cole, 1976; Wynder and Goldmsith, 1977) have added other occupations to this list: Pitch and coal-tar workers, leather workers (especially leather finishing), hairdressers, tailors, printers, and cooks and kitchen workers. In many of these occupations the specific cancer-causing agent is unknown.

The excess bladder cancer in rubber workers was due, apparently, to the use of 2-naphthylamine in rubber compounding. Waterhouse (1979) reported that workers employed in the British rubber industry after 1949, the year in which 2-naphthylamine was banned, show no excess bladder cancer.

In the United States clusters of excess bladder cancer in males were found (Mason *et al.*, 1975) in New Jersey, in New York City, and in urban areas around the Great Lakes, probably associated with industrial exposure. Rates were also elevated in some rural areas. Hoover and Fraumeni (1975) found a significantly elevated risk for bladder (and lung and liver) cancer in men in the U.S. countries with the highest concentrations of chemical industries.

Under some conditions carcinogenic arylamines may be formed or liberated in the gastrointestinal tract from ingested compounds. Yoshida and Miyakawa (1973) reported that Yuzen dye painters show an eleveated risk of bladder cancer arising from azo dyes ingested when the dye brushes are touched to their lips. The carcinogenic benzidine moiety is liberated from some of these dyes by the action of intestinal bacteria.

The development of cancer in an individual depends on many factors (Bryan 1979, Sivak, 1979) interacting in complex ways. One important factor is variation in susceptibility which may be partly genetic. Families whose members have experienced an unssually high incidence of bladder cancer have been described (Lynch *et al.*, 1979; Purtilo *et al.*, 1979). One aspect of susceptibility may be the way in which the individual metabolizes environmental procarcinogens. Studies by Lower *et al.* (1979) showed that the capacity to acetylate N-hydroxyarylamines varies in human populations and suggested that this capacity is related to susceptibility to bladder cancer. This phenotypic variation could have both genetic and environmental components.

Increasing dose levels of carcinogen (Frith *et al.*, 1979) or longer time of feeding (Jacobs *et al.*, 1977) have both been shown to increase bladder tumor incidence in experimental animals, as might be expected. In humans increased intensity or time of exposure can shorten the latent period of the disease (Case *et al.*, 1954; Hoover and Cole, 1973).

That a sufficient dose of a potent carcinogen can overwhelm individual differences in susceptibility was shown by the case studied by M. H. C. Williams (Parkes, 1976), of a group of 78 men who worked in a 2-naphthylamine distillation unit. All 18 of the men who worked there for more than 5 years developed bladder cancer.

3.2. Other Factors

In addition to the arylamines which have been particularly important in occupational bladder cancer, some N-nitroso compounds are potent bladder carcinogens in experimental animals and, therefore, suspect carcinogens in humans. They are of particular interest because they may be formed by the reaction of nitrite with certain amines. Their formation has been shown in the human achlorhydric stomach, infected urinary bladder, colon, and saliva (Hill, 1979). However, there was no relation of human bladder cancer incidence to estimated nitrate and nitrite consumption in cured meats (Howe *et al.*, 1980).

Following reports of the isolation of a RNA tumor virus from papillary transitional cell tumors of the human renal pelvis and bladder (Fraley *et al.*, 1974) we looked for evidence of such a virus in human bladder tumors (R. A. Bonar, Y. Sharief and C. F. Reich, unpublished observations). We examined fluids from cell cultures derived from 34 human bladder tumors for the presence of particulate RNA-dependent DNA polymerase activity, a property of the C-type RNA tumor viruses (oncornaviruses). Synthetic templates were used to increase the sensitivity of the assay. In no case did repeated testing reveal evidence of virus. In addition, RNA's were extracted from portions of 24 human bladder tumors and treated under hybridizing conditions with a DNA probe prepared from simian sarcoma virus (SSV-1) by the RNA-dependent DNA polymerase reaction. The hybridization products were fractionated on hydroxylapatite. There was no evidence of hybridization, which would have indicated the presence in the tumors of RNA's related to the primate oncornavirus. In summary, these experiments revealed no evidence for the association of oncornavirus or its RNA with human bladder tumors.

Several epidemiologic studies have implicated cigarette smoking as an important etiologic factor in bladder cancer. An elevated risk was found for cigarette smokers among both men and women (Cole *et al.*, 1971; Howe *et al.*, 1980; Morgan and Jain, 1974; Stevens and Moolgavkar, 1979; Wynder and Goldsmith, 1977). The relative risk (the ratio of the risk for users to that for non-users) was in the range of 2 to 6 and showed a dose-response effect. A smaller increased risk for pipe smokers was found by Howe *et al.* (1980), but no association was seen in the other studies. The carcinogenic (or cocarcinogenic) effect of smoking is much less potent than the more severe occupational exposures, but the number of people exposed is far greater. A possible pathway for smoking-induced carcinogenesis is by way of carcinogenic agents in the smoke, including polycyclic hydrocarbons, arylamines (Wynder and Goldsmith, 1977), and nitrosamines (Hecht *et al.*, 1979). The smoking hazard is not limited to tobacco. Opium users have also been reported to be at elevated risk for bladder neoplasia (Sadighi *et al.*, 1979).

There has been a great deal of interest and very long controversy with respect to the possible role of saccharin (Hoover, 1980) in bladder cancer. An increased incidence of bladder tumors was found (Taylor *et al.*, 1980) in male rats which had been fed sodium saccharin chronically at a dietary level of 7.5%, from weaning. The parents of these rats had also been fed the same diet from weaning through mating, gestation and lactation. It appeared that the exposure in utero was the critical factor. Female rats on the same diet showed an increased incidence of urinary bladder hyperplasia but not of tumor. Other work has shown that dietary sodium saccharin can act as a promoter of bladder tumorigenesis in the rat (Cohen *et al.*, 1979; Hicks, 1980). Saccharin feeding led to an increased incidence of bladder tumors following low initiating doses of known carcinogens. The saccharin feeding experiments have been criticized by Meneely (1979) who argued that the sodium in the sodium saccharin, which is used for solubility, added to the sodium chloride present in rat chow, gives sodium levels which are themselves frankly toxic in the rat. The high sodium levels may lead to hypertension, renal lesions, and, in the pregnant female, to teratogenic effects in the pups.

Epidemiologic studies have generally not shown a significant relationship between consumption of artificial sweeteners and human bladder cancer. A case-control study in Canada (Howe *et al.*, 1980) showed an increased risk in males (risk ratio of 1.6 for ever-used vs. never-used). This has not, however, been found in several other studies (Hoover and Strasser, 1980; Kessler and Clark, 1978; Morrision and Buring, 1980; Wynder and Stellman, 1980). There was also no elevation of urinary bladder cancer in diabetics (Wynder and Stellman, 1980) even though they generally have a higher consumption of artificial sweeteners. The controversy has been reviewed by Hoover (1980) who concluded that the use of artificial sweeteners by the diabetic or the occasional user carries little or no risk of bladder cancer. In view of the evidence of toxicity and the lack of objective evidence of benefit, he suggested that any use by nondiabetic children or pregnant women, heavy use by young women of childbearing age, and excessive use by anyone were ill-advised and should be actively discouraged by the medical community. From the various experimental and epidemiologic studies it seems clear that if saccharin is a carcinogenic agent in humans, it is a rather weak one, and an individual's judgement of the balance between risk and benefit will depend heavily on the perception of benefit.

Coffee drinking has attracted much attention for its possible association with bladder cancer. As Morrison and Cole (1976) note in their review, the results of epidemiologic studies on this association are mixed, but the exposure is so great that if a causal association is real it could account for about one-third of U.S. bladder cancer. Cole (1971) found a significantly increased risk of lower urinary tract cancer associated with coffee drinking among women (relative risk 2.58, $P<0.05$). Risk was not significantly elevated among men (r.r. = 1.24). No dose-response effect was seen. No association with coffee consumption was found by Morgan and Jain (1974) or Wynder and Goldsmith (1977), but Howe *et al.* (1980) reported a significantly elevated risk in males consuming all kinds of coffee, and in females drinking instant coffee. Again, no dose-response relationship was found. In a different approach to the question (Morrison, 1978), a weak correlation was found between the incidence of bladder cancer in ten countries and their *per capita* coffee imports. A comparison of the time trends of these variables in the U.S. and Denmark, however, gave mixed results. The question of the carcinogenic, or promoting, effect of coffee drinking must remain open, but warrants further study because of the great frequency of the custom.

Dunning *et al.* (1950) observed that added dietary tryptophan enhanced the induction of bladder tumors in rats by the carcinogen 2-acetylaminofluorene. Since some tryptophan metabolites are arylamines, as are some industrial bladder carcinogens, there was much interest in the possible role of this essential amino acid as a potential natural carcinogen (Bryan, 1971). Some bladder cancer patients showed an altered tryptophan metabolism, although this may be a consequence of the disease (Teulings *et al.*, 1978) rather than a cause. Tryptophan and its metabolites have not been shown to be carcinogenic. They could, however, be cocarcinogenic or promoting in humans, as they appear to be in dogs (Radomski *et al.*, 1977) and rats (Cohen *et al.*, 1979).

Several other dietary factors have been suggested as playing a role in urinary tract carcinogenesis. Consumption of bracken fern has been shown to induce bladder tumors in cattle and in laboratory animals (Evans, 1976; Pamukcu and Bryan, 1979). A carcinogenic factor was also found in the milk of the cows eating bracken fern. In addition to the potential human exposure via milk, fiddlehead greens, some of which are harvested from the bracken fern, are consumed directly by some human populations. There is no direct evidence, however, of induction of cancer in humans by bracken fern, and Howe *et al.* (1980) found no evidence of association with fiddlehead consumption.

An indication of a protective effect of carrots, milk, vitamin A, and, possibly, cruciferous vegetables was noted in a retrospective study by Mettlin and Graham (1979). Although the relation requires more study, it is consistent with the protective effect of retinoids against bladder tumorigenesis in the rat (Sporn *et al.*, 1977).

Several other factors have been reported to affect urinary tract neoplasia. The presence of a pellet or calculus in the bladder has an enhancing effect on carcinogenesis in experimental animals (Friedell and Cohen, 1979). This may be related to a stimulus of cell division in the urothelial cells which normally have a low mitotic index (Sharief *et al.*, 1980). Normal urine may also contain tumor promoters (Oyasu *et al.*, 1980) and may interact with implanted pellets in tumor promotion (Chapman *et al.*, 1973). The role of animal diets in affecting crystaluria and calculus formation could influence feeding trials of bladder carcinogens (Roe, 1979).

3.3. Renal Pelvis and Ureters

In general, the transitional cells of the renal pelvis and ureters are sensitive to the same agents as those of the bladder, but to a different degree. It seems likely that this is related to their difference in location and, thus, to their exposure to the flow of urine. Those factors which are excreted by the kidneys, but which have a relatively short lifetime in the urine might affect the cells of the renal pelvis but be inactivated before reaching the bladder. Longer-lived agents, on the other hand, would be more likely to affect the bladder during their longer residence there.

A number of reports have related abuse of the analgesic phenacetin to urinary tract tumors, especially in the renal pelvis and ureters (Fokkens, 1979; Mihatsch *et al.*, 1980; Orell *et al.*, 1979). The carcinogenicity of phenacetin has been challenged (Macklin *et al.*, 1979) and counter-arguments have been presented (Vaught and King, 1979) with a proposal that the compound be banned from non-prescription analgesics.

Tumors of the renal pelvis and ureters show a greatly elevated incidence in association with Balkan endemic nephropathy (Petkovic, 1975; Radovanovic and Krajinovic, 1979) in parts of Yugoslavia, Bulgaria and Romania. In Yugoslavia the incidence has increased substantially since about 1953. The frequency of tumors is about one hundred times greater in regions of endemic nephropathy than in other areas of Yugoslavia. The nephropathy is sharply limited geographically and appears to be familial, but not hereditary. The cause remains obscure.

3.4. Attributable Risk

The relative risk of bladder cancer associated with a hazardous exposure and the proportion of a population exposed to that hazard allow calculation of an attributable risk, the porportion of cases which can be ascribed to that exposure. Such estimates (Cole *et al.*, 1972; Howe *et al.*, 1980; Morrison and Cole, 1976; Wynder and Goldsmith, 1977) made for Great Britain and the U.S. indicate that cigarette smoking accounts for 39–61% of bladder cancer in males and 26–38% in females. Occupational exposure accounts for 18–33% in males and about 6% in females. Thus, the two established risk factors appear to account for about 60–80% of bladder cancer in males and 30–45% in females. Obviously, the proportions may vary substantially in different populations. Other possible risk factors remain to be established.

4. TUMORS OF THE KIDNEY

Primary kidney tumors may be of four types: 1) renal cell carcinoma (hypernephroma, renal adenocarcinoma), 2) nephroblastoma (Wilms tumor), 3) renal sarcoma, and 4) tumors of the transitional epithelium of the renal pelvis. Tumors of the transitional epithelium were considered with other tumors of the urinary tract because of their histological relationship. Renal cell carcinoma will be considered first in this section, and then, briefly, nephroblastoma. Kidney tumors constitute about 2–3% of all malignancies (Kantor, 1977) and renal cell carcinoma is the most common, about 89% (Bennington, 1973). Nephroblastomas make up about 9% and sarcomas 2%. Renal cancer shows substantial variation among countries (Wynder *et al.*, 1974) with death rates for males varying from about one per 100 000 (Japan, Venezuela) to more than four (Denmark, Sweden, Czechoslavakia). Rates for females are almost always less than for males, the ratio varying between 1:1 and 4.3:1 in different countries. Age-specific data from the Connecticut Tumor Registry (Kantor *et al.*, 1976) indicated an overall male:female incidence of renal cell carcinoma of 2:1. For persons under 15 years of age the ratio was about 1:1, rising to 3:1 for the 15- to 39-year-old age group, and then declining. The number of cases in persons under 40 was small, but the authors suggest that this apparent partial protection of women during their childbearing years warrants further study. Incidence was strongly age-dependent (Kantor *et al.*, 1976; Mason *et al.*, 1975). The Connecticut data showed an increase in age-adjusted incidence for males over the last several decades (Kantor *et al.*, 1976). There has been a similar increase in U.S. mortality in males (Wynder *et al.*, 1974). Rates for women have shown little change. Kantor *et al.* (1976) also noted a birth cohort effect among men but not among women. At a given age the incidence rate among men increased as the birth date became more recent.

Incidence rates for renal cell cancer in both males and females were positively associated with population density in Connecticut (Kantor *et al.*, 1976) and were higher in urban than in rural areas. U.S. mortality data also showed a higher rate for men in urban areas, but not for women (Blot and Fraumeni, 1979).

Within the U.S. there was a clustering of elevated rates of renal cell carcinoma in the north central states for both males and females and in the northeast for males (Blot and Fraumeni, 1979). The rates in the north central states were elevated in relation to the proportion of the population of German, Scandinavian or, especially, Russian descent. The ethnic associations appeared to account for about 40% of the elevated mortality among males and about 70% among females. Reported incidence of renal cancer was relatively high in Scandinavia, but not in Germany. The data for the Soviet Union were not available.

Studies of the association of renal cancer with socioeconomic factors have given mixed results (Wynder *et al.*, 1974). There was no significant association with the socioeconomic index of the town of residence in Connecticut (Kantor *et al.*, 1976), but a positive correlation was found with median income by U.S. county or state economic area (Blot and Fraumeni, 1979). Rates among U.S. whites and blacks were similar (Kantor, 1977; Wynder *et al.*, 1974). Wynder *et al.* (1974) reviewed briefly some other observations that may provide clues to renal cancer etiology. In a small study, rates in Japanese immigrants to the U.S. were higher than in Japan, but still lower than among U.S. whites. In New York City, mortality rates for Jews were higher than for Protestants or Catholics. Among Jews in Israel, rates for both men and women were higher for those born in Europe or America than for those born in Africa or Asia. The possible role of environmental factors such as diet is suggested by these studies.

Familial incidence of renal cell cancer is rare but the tumor is sometimes associated with von Hippel-Lindau's syndrome (Bennington, 1973; Wynder *et al.*, 1974). Cohen *et al.* (1979) recently reported a hereditary renal cell carcinoma associated with a balanced reciprocal translocation between chromosomes 3 and 8. An association between renal cancer and diabetes mellitus has been found in some studies, but not in others (reviewed by Kantor, 1977; Wynder *et al.*, 1974).

4.1. Etiologic Factors

In comparison to neoplasia of the lower urinary tract, evidence regarding etiologic factors in human renal cancer is sparse. Cigarette smoking appears to be a risk factor (Kantor, 1977; Wynder *et al.*, 1974), although in various studies the relative risk varied from no elevation (Armstrong *et al.*, 1976) to very high (Bennington and Laubscher, 1968). The increasing incidence rate with time and the appearance of a cohort effect among men in the Connecticut study (Kantor, 1976) are consistent with a relationship between cigarette smoking and renal cell cancer. A strong association was found, also, with other forms of tobacco use (Bennington and Laubscher, 1968).

Kolonel (1976) found no elevated risk associated with cigarette smoking alone, but did find a significantly increased risk among men with previous exposure to cadmium. Smoking increased the risk due to cadmium exposure. He noted that kidney is rich in zinc and also concentrates cadmium which can interfere with zinc-containing enzymes. In a study of malignancy in workers in the steel industry, an elevated mortality from kidney cancer was found in coke oven workers (Redmond *et al.*, 1972). However, Blot and Fraumeni (1979) did not find an association of renal cancer with geographic areas in the U.S. with primary metal manufacturing, where coke oven emissions would be greatest. A two-fold excess of deaths from cancer of the kidney due to asbestos exposure was found in insulation workers (Selikoff *et al.*, 1979). Unlike cancers of the respiratory tract, renal cancer mortality did not show a synergistic effect of smoking and asbestos exposure (Selikoff and Hammond, 1979). In a study of the association of cancer incidence with asbestos in drinking water (Kanarek, 1979), a marginally significant ($p<0.05$) increase in risk associated with the presence of asbestos was found for females but not for males.

In their case-control study of 202 patients and 394 controls, Wynder *et al.* (1974) found moderate correlations of renal adenocarcinoma with cigarette smoking, with prior myocardial infarction in males, and with obesity in females. No significant relation was found with coffee drinking, alcohol consumption, occupational exposure, or other disease history. They suggested, as a working hypothesis, that dietary factors, possibly fat and/or cholesterol, played a significant role. Internationally, there is a positive correlation between renal cancer mortality and *per capita* consumption of fat, milk, coffee, sugar, and animal protein (Armstrong and Doll, 1975). It is important to note that these dietary variables are correlated with each other to varying degrees and with economic and social variables. The associations, as Armstrong and Doll note, are valuable primarily as suggestions for further research. Armstrong *et al.* (1976), following these observations, conducted a retrospective study of 106 patients with renal adenocarcinoma, 33 patients with carcinoma of the renal pelvis and 139 matched controls. They concentrated their attention on consumption of coffee and of animal protein. The results did not support an association of renal adenocarcinoma with coffee drinking, or with consumption of animal protein or of different classes of animal protein (meat, seafood, eggs, milk, cheese).

There is little evidence for the induction of renal cell cancer in man by any specific chemical, although as Hard (1978) notes, more than fifty compounds have been shown to induce renal tumors in the rat, and these tumors have a range of histology resembling that in the human. There has been much interest in lead as a potential human kidney carcinogen (Moore and Meredith, 1979) as it has been known for many years to induce renal tumors in rats and mice. It has not, however, been shown to cause such tumors in dogs, hamsters, or primates. Studies of lead workers have not shown evidence of renal (or other) carcinogenicity of lead.

Cycasin, a glycoside occurring in some species of cycad plants (Hamilton, 1975; Matsumato, 1979) induced kidney (and liver) tumors when it or its aglycone, methylazoxymethanol, were fed to rats. When weanling rats were fed cycasin for only thirteen days before switching to a normal diet, a high proportion developed renal tumors. The compounds have recently been shown to induce renal and liver tumors in nonhuman primates (Sieber et al., 1980). They are of special interest because a flour prepared from the cycad plants is used as food by natives of Guam and some areas of Africa, especially when other foods are in short supply. There is no evidence of renal tumor induction in these people, perhaps because the carcinogen may be removed by the procedures used to prepare the flour.

Environmental agents of far more widespread distribution are the mycotoxins, of which the aflatoxins are the best known. These compounds are produced by molds (the aflatoxins by Aspergillus flavus) under certain environmental conditions in a wide variety of grains and other foodstuffs (Hamilton, 1975; Wogan, 1973). They are known primarily as liver carcinogens but induce kidney tumors as well. When aflatoxin B1 was fed to male Wistar rats (Epstein *et al.*, 1969) at 1.0, 0.5, or 0.25 parts per million in the diet for 147 days, followed by basal diet, kidney tumors developed in 57%, 28% and 23% of the animals, respectively. The tumors were similar to renal adenocarcinoma in the human. Malignant hepatomas were also induced. While aflatoxins have not been shown directly to cause human cancer, they have been epidemiologically associated with areas of high incidence of human liver cancer (Shank *et al.*, 1972). Aflatoxin contamination of agricultural products is found in many countries, including the U.S., and appears to be an important subject for further investigation as a potential human kidney and liver carcinogen. As noted by Stark and Demain (1980), few edible substances can be considered safe from mycotoxin contamination, and fungal invasion of foods can occur at any stage of the food processing chain. It should be noted, however, that on a worldwide scale, renal cell cancer mortality did not correlate positively with *per capita* consumption of grain (Armstrong and Doll, 1975), which might be expected to be a major source of aflatoxin in the human diet.

Some nitrosamines and nitrosamides (Hamilton, 1975) have been found to induce renal carcinoma. As discussed in relation to bladder tumors, these compounds occur in nature and can also be formed under some conditions from ingested nitrite and amines. A single oral dose of N-nitrosomorpholine was sufficient to induce kidney tumors in rats (Bannasch *et al.*, 1979). An interesting feature of nitrosamine carcinogenesis is the importance of the hormonal status of the animal. Carcinogenesis by dimethylnitrosamine in both kidney and liver in rats was enhanced by thyroidectomy (Noronha and Goodall, 1978). The authors suggested that the metabolism of the carcinogen was altered. Kidney tumor incidence after administration of N-butylnitrosourea to rats was reduced by prior gonadectomy and restored by hormone administration or ovarian grafts. There was no comparable affect on carcinogenesis by the more potent carcinogen, dimethylnitrosamine (Takizawa and Hirose, 1978). Nutritional status can also affect kidney carcinogenesis. Seven days on a protein-free diet increased the susceptibility of rats to the renal carcinogenicity of dimethylnitrosamine (DMN) (Swann *et al.*, 1980), apparently by altering DMN metabolism.

The renal carcinogenicity of a number of other compounds has been described in rats, including the flame retardant, tris(2,3-dibromopropyl) phosphate (Reznik *et al.*, 1979); the antischistosomal drug, niridazole, in rats (Bulay *et al.*, 1979); the hypolipidemic drug, ethyl chlorophenoxyisobutyrate (clofibrate) in male rats (Svoboda and Azarnoff, 1979), and chloroform in male rats (Reuber, 1979). Tumors can be induced in hamster kidney by estrogen (Li *et al.*, 1980), but this seems not to be general in other species.

Several virus-induced kidney tumors are known in experimental animals. The herpesvirus-associated Lucké kidney tumor of the North American leopard frog has been studied extensively (Hamilton, 1975). Kidney tumors have been induced in chickens by several virus strains of the avian leukosis complex. One, the BAI strain A, was shown to induce a nephroblastoma resembling the Wilms' tumor of man, with both epithelial and mesenchymal elements (Ishiguro *et al.*, 1962; Heine *et al.*, 1962). Another, strain MC29, induced wholly epithelial tumors (Mladenov *et al.*, 1967). These MC29 virus-induced renal carcinomas ranged from those which consisted largely of glomerular elements to some which were largely tubular. The largest tumors consisted entirely of tubular structures. With both strains the tumors appeared to originate from undifferentiated embryonal cell rests. Studies in chick embryo kidney cells in culture (Bonar and Paulson, 1974) confirmed the distinct biological effects of the two virus strains. Most MC29 virus-altered cell cultures were epithelial while BAI strain A virus treatment yielded predominantly spindle-shaped cells. In preliminary experiments, isolated chick kidney tubule cells could be transformed by the MC29 virus but not by BAI strain A, suggesting that the differentiated tubule cells could also be the origin of some of the adenocarcinomas seen *in vivo* (R. A. Bonar and C. F. Reich, unpublished observations). The original BAI strain A virus induced tumors in a variety of tissues. Recent work (Watts and Smith, 1980) has achieved a substantial separation of the nephroblastoma-inducing activity from the other tumorigenic activities of the original strain. The specificity shown by the BAI strain A and MC29 virus strains in the kind of renal tumor produced is paralleled, in part, by the induction of kidney tumors in the rat by certain chemicals (Hard, 1977, 1978). Here, also, some agents caused adenocarcinoma, and others nephroblastoma. Some compounds led to both types of tumor.

4.2. Nephroblastoma

Perhaps the most striking feature of nephroblastoma or Wilms' tumor is its early age of onset. Most patients are less than 7 years of age (Govan *et al.*, 1979), although the tumor also occurs very rarely in adults. In the U.S. there are about 6.8 kidney tumors per million children (under 15) per year. Most of these are nephroblastoma. It has been proposed (Knudson and Strong, 1972, Knudson, 1979) that about 38% of Wilms' tumor patients have an inherited predisposition to the tumor. According to this hypothesis, 2 mutations are required to produce a tumor cell. In the 'hereditary' form of the disease, the first mutation is prezygotic and may thus be transmitted to every cell. The second mutation is somatic. In the 'nonhereditary' form, both mutations are somatic. The individual with the germinal mutation thus has a large number of cells which require only one more 'hit' to become neoplastic. The number of daughter cells after a first somatic mutation will be very small by comparison. The chance of a second mutation is thus much higher in the hereditary form. The tumors arising from the genetic disorder are much more likely to be multifocal and bilateral, and to appear early. These two mutations would constitute the initiating event and the development (or not) of a tumor would still be subject to the usual promoting and restraining influences. The early age of onset of the tumor is also determined by its apparent origin in primitive cells of the metanephric blastema.

No chemical or other agents have been identified as being etiologic for the disease in humans. Nephroblastomas as well as other kidney tumors can be induced in rats by specific chemical carcinogens (Hard, 1977, 1978), and the viral induction of avian nephroblastoma was discussed above. Oral administration of citrulline and sodium nitrite to pregnant rats gave rise to Wilms'-type tumors in the offspring (Ivankovic, 1979). Jurgelski *et al.* (1979) induced nephroblastomas in neonatal opossums by inoculation of ethylnitrosourea. The period of susceptibility coincided with the presence in the kidney of stem cells (metanephric blastema) from birth to 6 or 8 weeks of age. The relative rarity of the tumor in humans makes the identification of etiologic factors by epidemiologic means very difficult.

5. PROSTATE

The prostate is by far the most frequent site of cancer in the male reproductive system. It is, indeed, the second most common site of cancer in U.S. males, behind lung (Silverberg, 1980), and the third in cancer deaths, behind lung and colorectal tumors. Silverberg (1980) estimated that there would be 66 000 new prostate cancer cases in the U.S. in 1980, and about 21 500 deaths from the disease. Mortality from prostate cancer is unusual under age 50, and increases markedly with age (Blair and Fraumeni, 1978; Franks, 1973).

5.1. Geographic Variation

Rates of death from prostate cancer show considerable international variation. The age-adjusted mortality rate in 1974-1975 ranged from 0.1 per 100 000 in Honduras to 22 in Sweden (Silverberg, 1980). Rates in the Asian countries were clustered at low values of 1–2, while countries of northern and western Europe showed middle to high rates. Eastern European and Latin American countries tended to have low to intermediate mortality. While some of this difference may be due to genetic factors (Doll, 1972), studies of migrant populations suggest that environmental factors probably account for most of the variation. Polish immigrants to the United States had a prostate cancer mortality rate higher than the low rate in Poland, but below that of U.S. native whites (Staszewski and Haenzel, 1965). Parallel results were obtained in a study of cancer mortality (1959-1962) among Japanese immigrants to the U.S. (Haenzel and Kurihara, 1968). The specific mortality ratio (SMR) of the immigrants was 40 compared to 100 among U.S. whites, and 380 compared to 100 among Japanese in Japan. Data from the San Francisco Bay area (Dunn, 1975) suggested that men of Japanese ancestry who were born in the U.S. had a prostatic cancer incidence even more like U.S. whites than did men who immigrated to the U.S. from Japan. Wynder *et al.* (1971) found that among Caucasians who were foreign-born, those who had been in the U.S. for less than 20 years, had significantly less prostatic cancer than those who had lived in the country for a longer time.

Carcinoma of the prostate often occurs as latent disease, defined as tumors which have not become manifest, i.e. tumors which are not clinically evident (Franks, 1973), but are found at autopsy or at surgery. The incidence of latent carcinoma is high and is age-related (Hutchison, 1976; Wynder *et al.*, 1971). In contrast to the higher mortality from prostate cancer among Japanese in Hawaii compared to those in Japan, Akazaki and Stemmermann (1973) found no significant difference in the incidence of latent cancer in prostates removed at autopsy from males over 50 years old in the two countries. The incidence of apparently proliferative lesions was, however, higher in the Japanese in Hawaii. In both countries, the incidence of latent cancer increased with age. In a study of latent carcinoma of the prostate in seven countries (Breslow *et al.*, 1977), there was no significant difference in the frequency of small carcinomas among the seven populations. There were, however, differences in incidence of the larger latent cancers, and the incidence rates approximately paralleled the international ranking by prostate cancer mortality. A marked increase in the frequency of latent cancer with age was seen in most of the studied populations.

The results of international studies suggest that factors leading to initiation and early promotion of prostate carcinoma, with the formation of small, recognizable, but latent tumors are common, worldwide and cumulative with age. The factors which enhance tumor growth, on the other hand, appear to be very different among cultures.

Within the U.S. there were clusters of elevated prostate cancer mortality in counties in the north-central and northeastern regions (Mason *et al.*, 1975). Blair and Fraumeni (1978) used the age-adjusted mortality rates for various combinations of counties stratified along regional, demographic and industrial lines to deterine the relation of the rates to several variables. There were significant regional differences, although the highest regional rate for whites in the north-central region (18.5 per 100 000) exceeded the lowest in the southeast (16.8) by only about 10%.

5.2. Demographic Factors

Rates for nonwhites were 50% higher or more than rates for whites in all areas where blacks made up most of the nonwhite population (Blair and Fraumeni, 1978). Over the period 1950-1969, rates for whites declined slightly in the U.S. as a whole and in most of its region, while rates for nonwhites rose about 29%. There was an increase in prostate cancer mortality among nonwhites with increased urbanization and population density, but no such pattern was observed among whites. Counties with high proportions of population of Scandinavian or German descent showed a significant elevation of prostate cancer mortality, and counties with a large proportion of people of Mexican or South American ancestry had lower rates. These patterns are consistent with international variations in the disease.

A striking feature of prostate cancer incidence in the U.S. is the high and rising rate among blacks, as noted above. Such high rates are not characteristic of blacks in Africa (Jackson *et al.*, 1977; Kovi and Heshmat, 1972; Wynder *et al.*, 1971). As with other populations, the rate of incidence of microscopic latent carcinoma of the prostate was similar in the high-risk black population of Washington, D.C., and the low-risk population of Ibadan, Nigeria (Jackson *et al.*, 1977). The age-adjusted incidence of invasive carcinoma, however, was higher in Washington. The overall pattern of prostate cancer experience of American blacks resembled that of American whites more closely than that of blacks in West Africa, (Kovi and Heshmat, 1972) the ancestral origin of most American blacks.

Another interesting feature of the difference between white and black prostatic cancer mortality rates is that before about 1945, the rates for nonwhites were lower (Ernster *et al.*, 1978a) and rates for both whites and nonwhites were rising. In most parts of the U.S., blacks constitute a large proportion of the nonwhite populatoin. The rate for whites peaked about 1940 and started a slight decline, while that for nonwhites continued to rise. While early underreporting may account for some of these effects, it seems unlikely to account for all of the rise, or the white-nonwhite difference. By analyzing the prostate cancer mortality data by birth cohort, Ernster *et al.* (1978a) were able to show that mortality for nonwhites rose to peak rates at every age in the 1896-1900 cohort and declined thereafter. If this trend among younger birth cohorts continues, the mortality rates among blacks will begin to decline. No such generational pattern was seen among whites, but the rate for whites has tended downward for several decades.

Some other racial and ethnic groups in the U.S. have prostate cancer mortality rates different from the national average. Rates are low for American Indians (Creagen and Fraumeni, 1972), for Mexican-Americans (Menck *et al.*, 1975), and for Chinese-Americans (Fraumeni and Mason, 1974). For Americans of Chinese and Mexican ancestry, the low rates are consistent with those for Asia and for Mexico. Whether this reflects genetic factors or continuing cultural practices remains for further study.

Another American population group, the Mormons, is interesting because, while its overall cancer incidence is low, its prostate cancer experience is little or no different from the U.S. as a whole. Lyon *et al.* (1977) reported that in Utah, where about 72% of the population is Mormon, there are 18% fewer cancer cases and 14% fewer deaths than expected from national rates. Prostate cancer incidence, however, was close to the national rate and mortality was somewhat elevated. Enstrom (1978) found that active Mormons in Utah and California had substantially reduced risks of cancer in smoking-related sites, as expected. They also had significantly reduced risks for many nonsmoking-related sites. For prostatic carcinoma, however, the risk was similar to that for the U.S. as a whole. These men abstained from tobacco, alcohol, coffee, tea, and cola, but appeared to be similar to other U.S. males in other aspects of diet and in socioeconomic status and urbanization.

The possibility that the higher prostate carcinoma rates among U.S. blacks might be explained, at least in part, by an effect of socioeconomic class, was examined by Ernster *et al.* (1978b). Using mortality and incidence data from Alameda County, California, they found no gradient of prostate cancer rates with socioeconomic status for either blacks or whites. Most other studies, chiefly among whites, have also shown weak or no association with social and economic status (Blair and Fraumeni, 1978; Hutchison, 1976; Wynder *et al.*, 1971). Ross *et al.* (1979), however, found higher rates in upper occupational and social class groupings in Los Angeles, while a strong upward trend of incidence with decreasing socioeconomic class was recently reported from England by Hakky *et al.* (1979). Hakky *et al.* also found a relatively high incidence in doctors and dentists.

Different studies of the relation of prostatic carcinoma to socioeconomic status have given results ranging from positive with increasing status, through no correlation, to positive with decreasing status. Whether this variation is random or artifactual, or a true reflection of different interactions of etiologic factors in different areas remains to be determined.

5.3. Occupation

No occupational exposures have been established as contributing to prostatic carcinoma. Studies of workers exposed to cadmium oxide suggested a carcinogenic role for cadmium (Potts, 1965; Kipling and Waterhouse, 1967). In a study of workers in a cadmium smelter Lemen *et al.* (1967) found an insignificant elevation of prostate cancer mortality except when the time interval since exposure was considered. There was a significant increase in workers first exposed 20 or more years earlier (4 observed v. 0.88 expected; $p<0.05$). In a case-control study of 176 prostate cancer patients, by Kolonel and Winkelstein (1977), the small elevation of risk in men with one or more years of job-related cadmium exposure was not significant. Ross *et al.* (1979) found no association between cadmium exposure and prostate cancer.

Since prostate tissue concentrates zinc, and since cadmium may interfere with zinc-containing enzymes, Habib *et al.* (1976) examined the zinc and cadmium contents of prostatic tissue: normal (autopsy), BPH (TUR), and carcinoma (TUR). Zinc content was similar in normal and BPH tissue (6.8 and 6.9 mmol/g, respectively) and reduced in carcinoma (2.6 mmol/g). Cadmium levels differed markedly: normal, 5.2; BPH, 23; and carcinoma, 130 μmol/g. The normal prostates were from younger men than the other two groups. Since cadmium was known to affect both testis and prostate tissue, Chandler and Timms (1977) addressed the question whether cadmium had a direct effect on prostate cells rather than affecting the prostate only indirectly by interfering with androgen production in the testis. Using rat lateral prostate in organ culture, they found that cadmium did have a direct effect, causing local necrosis and subsequent basal cell growth. Cadmium is widespread in the environment of developed countries and further study of its relation to prostate cancer is needed.

In a study possibly related to cadmium exposure, Winkelstein and Kantor (1969) found an elevation of prostatic cancer mortality associated with particulate air pollution. They discuss the possible relation to cadmium in the air particles.

In their study of prostate cancer mortality by county in the U.S., Blair and Fraumeni (1978) compared the rates, after adjustment for demographic and ethnic factors, to the proportion of the population employed in 19 manufacturing categories. Among whites there were small but significant elevations of risk in counties with textile, primary and fabricated metal products, and machinery industries. Among nonwhites, elevated rates were associated with the textile, apparel, and machinery industries.

No elevation of prostate (or bladder or kidney) cancer mortality was seen in 15 000 employees of Imperial Oil Ltd, of Canada (Hanis *et al.*, 1979). Other findings in several studies of the relation of occupational exposure to prostate cancer have been reviewed by Ernster *et al.* (1979a). These include an elevation of risk in rubber workers, persons exposed to fertilizer or automobile exhaust, farmers and managers on dairy farms, operatives in various manufacturing industries, blacksmiths, foremen (all industries combined), mechanics and repairmen, ministers, farm laborers, and plumbers. In their own study in two California counties, Ernster *et al.* (1979a) found indications of increased prostatic cancer mortality among bookkeepers, shipping and receiving clerks, compositors and typesetters, and shipfitters.

With the exception of the rather strong suspicion directed toward cadmium exposure, no carcinogenic agent is clearly implicated by any of these studies. The geographic variation, the time trends, and the experience of migrants, however, all suggest an important role for factors of environment or life style.

5.4. Experimental Studies

Carcinogenesis studies in experimental animals have been less extensive than with bladder or kidney tumor induction. 3-Methylcholanthrene applied directly to prostate tissue induced glandular carcinomas in mice (Horning, 1946) and squamous cell carcinomas in rats (Dunning *et al.*, 1946). This same compound induced precancerous changes in mouse prostate tissue in organ culture (Lasnitzki, 1963). Hyperplasia and anaplasia were induced in cells of mouse prostate in organ culture by benzo(a)pyrene and N-methyl-N′-nitro-N-nitrosoguanidine (MNNG) as well as by 3-methylcholanthrene (Chopra and Wilkoff, 1977). MNNG was also applied to explant cultures of human prostatic tissue obtained at immediate autopsy from young adults (Sanefuji *et al.*, 1979). There was a marked proliferation of basal cell derivatives leading to production of atypical polymorphic epithelial cells with premalignant and malignant characteristics. In a rather rare report of induction of experimental prostate cancer by systemic administration of a chemical, Pliss and Volfson (1979) found tumors in the prostate (and other sites) after giving dicarboxydine to rats. Prostatic adenocarcinoma was induced in mice by pelvic irradiation with X-rays (Hirose *et al.*, 1976).

Spontaneous cancer of the prostate is very rare in experimental animals (Wynder *et al.*, 1971). This may be related to the fact that such animals seldom survive to very old age. Spontaneous adenocarcinoma has been reported in aged rats (Pollard, 1973; Shain *et al.*, 1975) and the frequency appeared to correlate with age.

5.5. Hormones

Since hormones are known to play a role in the normal development of the prostate, and prepubertal eunuchs do not develop prostate cancer, there has been much interest in the possible role of hormones in prostatic cancer etiology. Franks (1973) suggested that their principal role may be to stimulate the development and maintenance of the prostatic epithelium so that a sufficient number of cells is present in which malignant change can occur. Prolonged administration of testosterone has induced adenocarcinoma in the dorsal lobe of the prostate in 18% of male rats (Noble, 1977). The latent period was shortened by combining the androgen with estrone. Prostatic carcinomas were also found in male rats parabiosed to castrated males or oophorectomized females (Brown *et al.*, 1979). The results suggested a correlation between serum androgen levels and the development of prostatic adenocarcinoma.

5.6. Sexuality

A number of studies have looked at aspects of male sexuality in relation to prostatic cancer. In a case-control study, Greenwald *et al.* (1974a) examined the experience of former Harvard students for whom various physical measurements as well as later marital and medical histories were available. There was no significant association of prostate cancer deaths with any of the anthropometric indeces (including somatotype, baldness, and pilosity) or with proportion married, or with various aspects of fertility. Several studies on the relation of prostate cancer incidence to marital status were reviewed by Wynder *et al.* (1971), and the results seem mixed with, perhaps, an elevation for divorced and widowed men. In their own study, no correlation with marital status or fertility was found. They also found no association with hair distribution, height, weight, or circumcision. In his review, Hutchison (1976) comments that mortality from carcinoma of the prostate in U.S. whites is strongly associated with marital status, and increases in the order single, married, widowed, and divorced, at all ages above 64. There are indications of increased incidence among married men whose wives have had more pregnancies (Armenian *et al.*, 1975). From a study of widowers in New York State in 1958-1967, Greenwald *et al.* (1979) concluded that the high rates of prostatic cancer reported among widowers are probably artifactual. The question of the relation of marital status was examined by Ernster *et al.* (1979) using the data of the U.S. Third National Cancer Survey. They found prostate cancer incidence was related to marital status in whites, with widowed males at the greatest risk. The pattern was not significant for black men, and black widowers had a low to intermediate incidence. The variation of pattern with race makes interpretation of the role of marital status difficult.

The association with sexual activity has been examined and is reviewed by Hutchison (1976). In a case-control study patients reported no unusual frequency of coitus (high or low), but indicated an interest in greater frequency than they had experienced. Rotkin (1977) reported that prostate cancer patients differed from controls in three tendencies: delayed sexual drive and develoment, early repression of sexuality, and premature cessation of sexuality. There was no difference in the frequency of multiple marriages or multiple sex partners.

5.7. Veneral Disease

The possible association of prostate cancer incidence with sexuality has directed attention, too, to the possible relevance of venereal disease. Wynder *et al.* (1971) found no significant difference between patients and controls with regard to previous history of gonorrhea, but such an association has been seen by others (reviewed by Heshmat *et al.*, 1975). An epidemiologic study by Heshmat *et al.* (1975) using Danish data on gonorrhea incidence (1891-1940) and prostatic cancer mortality (1941-1970) showed a remarkable match between the two curves, with a lag period of 42–45 years. In a case-control study in two predominantly black hospitals in Washington, D.C., a significant association was found between prostatic carcinoma and prior gonorrhea. Of the cancer patients with a history of gonorrhea, 85% had had it before 1942, in the pre-penicillin era. The authors suggest two possible mechanisms for the association of prostatic cancer with prior gonorrhea, the viral-venereal and the chronic prostatitis theories. In the first case they postulate a greater early sexual activity with more partners on the part of the prostate cancer patient with a resulting greater opportunity for exposure to gonorrhea and to a hypothetical prostate cancer virus. The gonococcal infection might also facilitate viral infection and cancer development. The other hypothesis suggests that a chronic gonorrheal infection together with iatrogenic damage from the treatments of the pre-penicillin era would lead to prostatitis, tissue damage, atrophy, and recurrent regeneration, providing a favorable milieu for neoplastic change. The two theories lead to different forecasts for the future. If the viral -venereal theory is correct, the gonorrhea epidemics of the mid-forties and the present may presage large new increases in the incidence of prostatic carcinoma. If, on the other hand, the chronic prostatitis theory is correct, we should expect a decline in prostatic carcinoma as the older cohorts treated in the pre-penicillin era decrease in numbers. Hopefully, the declines in mortality in U.S. whites and in the more recent birth cohorts of U.S. blacks (Ernster *et al.*, 1978) indicate the latter alternative.

5.8. Viruses

The possible role of viruses in prostatic cancer has attracted much attention. Paulson *et al.* (1968) showed that hamster prostate cells in vitro could be transformed with SV40 virus and that the transformed cells, when inoculated into adult male hamsters, produced nodules whose architecture resembled human prostatic adenocarcinoma. A recent series of papers (Rapp *et al.*, 1975; Sanford *et al.*, 1977; Geder and Rapp, 1980) has reported interesting findings which suggest the possible association of cytomegalovirus (CMV), a herpesvirus, with prostate carcinogenesis. These authors have reported evidence for isolation of a CMV from human prostate, for persistant infection of prostate cells, for the capacity of the CMV isolate to transform normal human cells, and for the frequent presence of CMV-antibody and specific cell-dependent cytotoxic response in prostate cancer patients. While much remains to be done, the results suggest that the association of CMV with prostatic carcinoma may be more than coincidental.

5.9. Benign Prostatic Hyperplasia

The possible relation of benign enlargement of the prostate to prostatic cancer is an obvious consideration, even though the two diseases appear to arise in different parts of the gland, the inner and outer, respectively (Franks, 1973). Greenwald *et al.* (1974b) followed 838 patients who had undergone subtotal prostatectomy for benign prostatic hyperplasia (BPH) and 802 age-matched controls. Twenty-four patients and twenty-six controls developed prostatic cancer and the difference was not significant. Armenian *et al.* (1974), however, reported that the age-adjusted death rate from prostatic cancer was significantly elevated in BPH patients with respect to controls. Their BPH patients had been studied clinically (48%), by biopsy (27%), or were operated on (26%). They suggested that the lack of elevated incidence of later prostatic cancer in the BPH patients who had undergone subtotal prostatectomy (Greenwald *et al.*, 1974b), as compared to their patients, warranted consideration of a study of prostatectomy as a possible prophylactic measure for BPH patients who have other characteristics associated with a high risk of prostatic cancer. Unfortunately, the ability to identify such characteristics is still rather weak.

5.10. Immunology

The possible role of immunologic factors has been studied by several workers. Ablin *et al.* (1974) found evidence of circulating autoantibodies reactive with interepithelial consituents of prostatic secretory epithelial cells in a patient with metastatic prostatic adenocarcinoma. Stein-Werblowsky (1978) was able to induce metastatic cancer by inoculation of homologous sperm into the prostate in 2 of 20 rats. She suggested that autoimmune processes might play a role. Ablin *et al.* (1979) measured the reaction of peripheral blood leucocytes from patients with prostatic carcinoma with extracts of allogeneic malignant prostate. The reaction was significantly suppressed by treatment of the cells with human seminal plasma obtained from healthy donors. They suggested that, under some conditions, unejaculated spermatozoa might penetrate the prostate and induce the neoplastic process which leads to tumor foci, while the host immune response was suppressed by the presence of seminal plasma. The impairment of immune mechanisms in prostatic cancer patients has recently been discussed by Catalona (1980) in a review of several aspects of the immunobiology of carcinoma of the prostate.

5.11. Diet

As noted earlier, there is a substantial international variation in prostate cancer mortality and a tendency for migrant populations to acquire prostate cancer mortality rates characteristic of their host countries. These observations suggest an important role for environmental factors, and diet is clearly a possibility. Among various countries, the age-adjusted death rates for prostate cancer showed a correlation with *per capita* consumption of fat (Reddy *et al.*, 1980). Also, in international comparison, prostate cancer correlated with colon cancer (Berg, 1975), for which there is better evidence of the importance of dietary factors. However, the correlation of prostate cancer with colon cancer was not apparent in U.S. white men. Among regions of the U.S., an association was noted between rankings for prostatic cancer mortality and consumption of five 'high-fat foods' (Blair and Fraumeni, 1978). However, if the weight of fat in these foods (Watt and Merrill, 1963) is used rather than total food weight, the correlation no longer holds. Reddy *et al.* (1980) suggested that if diet influences prostatic cancer development, it may be by means of an effect on the hormonal status of the individual or on the hormone-sensitivity of the target organ. Diet can influence sex hormone levels (Hill and Wynder, 1979). Hill *et al.* (1979) found in a study of rural black South African men and black and white North American men, that urinary excretion of estrogens and androgens was lower in men on the customary rural South African diet (largely vegetarian). When the black South African men were fed a western diet their hormone excretion increased, while the reverse was true for North American black men changed from a western to a vegetarian diet.

Hirayama (1977) suggested that an increase in prostate cancer seen in Japan between 1950 and 1975 was due in part to a considerable change among Japanese to a western-type diet. It is likely, of course, that many other aspects of Japanese life-style underwent changes between 1950 and 1975, and some of the increase was thought to be due to smoking and to occupation. In a prospective study, however, those Japanese who continued a predominantly vegetarian diet had significantly less prostatic cancer, although they may, too, have been more conservative in other respects. On the other hand, Phillips (1975) found that Seventh-Day Adventists, about one-half of whom are ovo-lacto-vegetarians, showed no significant decrease in prostatic cancer compared to the general California population. The cancer mortality rates for most sites were much reduced. In another possibly related observation, Wynder *et al.* (1971) found no association of prostatic cancer with body weight. The role of diet in the etiology of prostatic cancer remains unresolved, with opinions of workers in the field ranging from 'perhaps yes' (Reddy *et al.*, 1980) to 'probably no' (Cole and Cramer, 1977).

It is striking that we should know so little about the etiology of a disease of such frequency and importance. It seems fair to say that the great range of studies described above has provided a number of important leads for further investigation, but nothing has been sufficiently well established to provide the basis for preventive action.

6. CANCER OF THE TESTIS

Germ cell tumors constitute more than 94% of testicular tumors (Mostofi, 1973), and interstitial (Leydig) cell tumors perhaps half of the remainder. Incidence and mortality rates are relatively low, but the former has been rising. Age-specific rates show three peaks: a small one in infants (predominantly embryonal carcinoma and teratoma); a large peak in young adults (all tumor varieties); and another in older men, in whom seminoma is most common (Mostofi, 1973). The age-specific mortality rates for U.S. whites (Mason *et al.*, 1975) show a small peak at 0–4 years (0.09 per

100 000), a large one at 25–29 years (1.93 per 100 000) and a steady rise above age 60 (reaching 1.90 at 85+ years).

Mortality rates for U.S. black males differ from those for whites in being generally lower and particularly lower in the young adult years (Grumet and MacMahon, 1958) and, therefore, lacking the distinctive young-adult peak.

International comparisons of age-specific rates for testis cancer morbidity show considerable variation, particularly in the incidence at ages 15–44 (Clemmesen, 1968). The age curves are similar in shape for most countries, but in those with very low incidence (e.g. Finland and Israel) the curve shape resembles that for U.S. blacks.

Petersen and Lee (1972) noted that the pattern of mortality among whites in the U.S. and England in the second decade of this century was like that of low-incidence populations today, lacking the young adult peak. From 1911-1915 to 1967-1969 the mortality rate in the 15–44 year age group rose steadily while that in the group over 64 years fell. The maximum rate occurred at decreasing ages in successive cohorts. They suggested that the increasing mortality in younger adults removed susceptible persons from the population, causing the fall in rates in the elderly. A similar reciprocal pattern was seen in Connecticut (Lutes *et al.*, 1980). The mortality from testis cancer in Japan in the period 1951-1955 was low compared to U.S. whites, except in the 0–5 year group, and did not show a peak in the early adult years (Lee *et al.*, 1973). By the 1966-1970 period, however, testis cancer mortality had increased substantially and the young-adult peak had appeared, a pattern of increase much like that seen earlier in the U.S. and England. There were some differences, particularly a considerable increase in mortality in childhood and a slowly rising, instead of falling rate in the elderly. The rise in mortality, marked particularly in the 15–44 year age group, also paralleled the English and U.S. experience in being a gradual yearly change. Increasing incidence has been reported in California (Krain, 1973), Los Angeles (Ross *et al.*, 1979), and Connecticut (Lutes *et al.*, 1980).

A variety of factors have been reported to be associated with the development of testicular cancer, although the relatively low frequency of the disease has made it difficult to study large numbers of cases. The best established correlation is with cryptorchidism (Batata *et al.*, 1980; Morrison, 1976a). There appears to be an association with inguinal hernia or other genitourinary defects (Li and Fraumeni, 1972; Morrison, 1976).

A variety of population characteristics have been reported to be associated with elevated rates of testicular cancer incidence or mortality. In their study of cancer mortality in the U.S., Mason *et al.* (1975) found that testis cancer tended to be elevated in northern rural areas and that it was relatively less common in the South. A significant rural preponderance was noted in England and Wales for seminomas, but not for other testicular neoplasms (Lipworth and Dayan, 1969); in the Netherlands for seminoma, teratoma, and all testicular neoplasms combined (Talerman *et al.*, 1974); and in upstate New York (Graham *et al.*, 1977). In California, however, there was no significant urban-rural difference (Krain, 1973), and Clemmesen (1968) reported a substantially higher rate in Copenhagen than in Danish rural areas. It seems likely that 'rural' and 'urban' may be associated with different characteristics of occupation, environment and life-style in different parts of the world. Graham *et al.* (1977) found rural residence was one of several factors which seemed to be additive in influencing testis cancer risk. Other factors associated with higher risk were marriage (especially earlier marriage), a professional occupation, native birth and native parentage. They provide a good discussion of the possibilities of interactions among the variables and of the values and cautions of this epidemiologic approach. The association with marriage was not found by Grumet and MacMahon (1958) or Morrison (1976b). An increased risk associated with higher socioeconomic status, as measured by various indicators, has been seen in several studies. Morrison (1976b) noted an association of seminoma incidence with more education, and Ross *et al.* (1979) found a positive association of both embryonal carcinoma and seminoma with social class judged by residence tract. A higher risk was seen among men employed in professional and managerial occupations (Graham *et al.*, 1977; Mustacchi and Millmore, 1976; and Ross *et al.*, 1979). Petersen *et al.* (1977) found an elevated testis cancer mortality risk associated with higher social status in England and Wales in 1951 but not in 1961. In both periods, however, the mean age of death was lower for the higher social class (professionals and administrators). An earlier age of incidence for professionals, managers and skilled workers was seen in San Francisco (Mustacchi and Millmore, 1976). In a related observation in Los Angeles, Ross *et al.* (1979) noted that the intermediate social classes showed the usual age peaks in young adults and the elderly, but the highest class lacked the old-age peak while the lowest class had a single broad peak delayed to 45–55 years.

Testis tumors have not been related often to particular occupations. The association with professional and managerial classes was noted above, and the rural preponderance in the Netherlands was in a largely agricultural district (Talerman *et al.*, 1974). Rhomberg and Schmoll (1976) noted a high proportion of metalworkers in their series of 45 patients and suggested that metal dusts and metal-organic complexes might play an important role in testicular cancer.

Studies of testis carcinogenesis in experimental animals have dealt chiefly with interstitial cell tumors. Such tumors can be induced by treatment of mice with estrogens (Andervont *et al.*, 1957; Huseby, 1980). Temporary occlusion of the spermatic vessels in dogs caused interstitial cell atrophy, followed by regeneration and neoplasia if both testes were damaged (Hinman and Smith, 1960). They suggested that an outpouring of pituitary gonadotrophins followed loss of the germinal epithelium and was involved in the neoplasia. Subcutaneous inoculation of cadmium salts in mice and rats also led to testicular atrophy followed by interstitial cell hyperplasia and, in the rat, to neoplasia (Roe *et al.*, 1964). The tumors induced in the rat by ligation or by cadmium were similar (Gunn *et al.*, 1965). Administration of zinc reduced tumor incidence due to cadmium treatment, but not to ligation. Interstitial cell tumors have also been reported after treatment of rats with aflatoxin B1 (Zawirska, 1979).

Hormonal stimulation appears to play a significant role in all of these experimental studies, with the possible exception of the aflatoxin work. In the case of cadmium treatment or seminal vessel ligation, there is also a period of atrophy with neoplasia developing during regeneration of the interstitial cells.

The few cases of experimental induction of germ cell tumors also involve hormonal influence. Intratesticular inoculation of zinc salts induced germ cell tumors in roosters (Michalowsky, 1928) and in hamsters (Guthrie and Guthrie, 1974) if administered during seasonal testicular growth.

Mulvihill (1975) pointed out that the role of genetic factors in human testicular cancer is suggested by the observation that cryptorchidism, which carries a much increased risk, is often associated with other testicular abnormalities, and that in unilateral maldescent, it is often the properly descended testis which develops neoplasia. It is likely that genetic and local factors both play roles in the association with maldescent. Wang *et al.* (1980) have noted that changes in chromosome number one are frequent in human testicular tumors.

An important consideration in examining the potential role of exogenous agents in testicular carcinogenesis was pointed out by Dixon and Lee (1980) in their discussion of the testis-blood barrier, which markedly restricts the access of blood-borne materials to the germ cells. Toxication and detoxication reactions differ in different compartments of the testis, and DNA repair capability appears to be present in spermatogonia and spermatocytes, but not in spermatids.

Taking into account the generally rising testicular cancer incidence and mortality, and the reciprocal relation between rates for young adults and the elderly, Petersen and Lee (1972) and Petersen *et al.* (1977) have suggested that most testicular germ cell tumors arise from clones of cells with a high risk of undergoing malignant change and that these clones are established in childhod. Environmental factor(s), which they call the technology factor, may operate to accelerate tumor development. It appears that men in industrial societies have been increasingly exposed to the factor(s) over the past several decades and that exposure is greatest among the more affluent. This hypothesis is not inconsistent with the possibility of an important role for hormonal influence, particularly in utero (Ross *et al.*, 1979). Our knowledge of carcinogenesis in general suggests that the interaction between a target cell and a potential carcinogen will be influenced critically by the genetic constitution of the cell, the hormonal environment, and a variety of other factors, all of which may be involved in the initial establishment of clones of cells with neoplastic potential.

7. CARCINOMA OF THE PENIS

Most penile malignancies are squamous cell carcinomas, more than 96% in the large Danish series (Jensen, 1977), and this section will be limited to these tumors. Little is known about the etiology of urethral tumors, other than those of the transitional epithelium which resemble the other urothelial tumors discussed earlier.

The incidence of penile cancer varies widely among different populations and it is a serious and common health problem in some parts of the world. The incidence is very low in Israel, only 0.1 per 100 000 males. In the U.S. the incidence rate is about 0.5–1.0 per 100 000 males (Persky, 1977) or about 0.5% of all male cancer (Jensen, 1977). Rates in Canada and Europe are similar to that in the U.S. (Jensen, 1977; Persky, 1977). The disease is far more common in some other parts of the world. In Paraguay penile cancer was the fourth most common malignancy diagnosed at the Institute of Pathology (Riveros and Lebron, 1963). It constituted 15% of all cancer in males in North Vietnam (Shabad, 1964), almost 20% of all cancer in males in Puerto Rico (Persky, 1977), and was the most common epithelial tumor among male Ugandans in the Kampala Tumor Registry (Dodge and Linsell, 1963).

The most important factor affecting incidence in a population is the practice of circumcision. The disease is extremely rare among Jewish males, who are routinely circumcised at 8 days of age. Boczko and Freed (1979) recently reported only the ninth recorded case of penile cancer in a man who had been circumcised in infancy. Somewhat higher, but still very low, rates are seen in Moslem men who are usually circumcised between 3 and 14 years of age (Boczko and Freed, 1979; Kennaway, 1947). Low rates have been reported from other areas where circumcision is practiced, Kazachstan (Shabad, 1964), and parts of Africa (Persky, 1977). Schrek and Lenowitz (1947) observed that circumcison before age 6 provided almost complete protection from carcinoma of the penis, while later operation was less effective.

Riveros and Lebron (1963) concluded that circumcision in infancy was very nearly a guarantee against later penile carcinoma, before age 14 was highly protective, and between 14 and 18 was partially protective. Kennaway (1947) summarized studies suggesting that when penile cancer followed circumcision done at ages 14 to 45, it did so with a long latent period (mean 23 years). Cases in which the latent period was less than 8 years were omitted from the computation on the ground that carcinoma might already have been present. Dagher *et al.* (1973), on the other hand, concluded from their study that circumcision at any age would virtually prevent the onset of squamous cell carcinoma of the penis if the neoplasm was not already present at the time of circumcision, and the prepuce was completely removed. The protective value of circumcision seems clear, and only the degree of protection provided by postpubertal operation is in question.

Incidence of penile cancer is by no means uniform among populations which do not circumcise, depending on the other major factor, viz. adequate penile hygiene. The highest incidence rates of this type of cancer are usually found where poor hygiene facilities and practices are common (Persky, 1977; Riveros and Lebron, 1963; Schrek and Lenowitz, 1947). In Sweden, where circumcision has not been routine, but where personal standards of hygiene are high, penile cancer is relatively rare (Persky, 1977). A history of phimosis is frequently associated with cancer of the penis (Jensen, 1977; Persky, 1977; Shabad, 1964; Thomas and Small, 1968). The effect is probably not due to the phimosis *per se,* but rather to its interference with penile hygiene and, perhaps, a consequent chronic irritation from retained smegma (Persky, 1977; Thomas and Small, 1968). The role of retention of a potentially carcinogenic agent was shown in rabbits treated on the glans and inner surface of the foreskin with the carcinogen 7,12-dimethylbenz(a)anthracene. Those animals given artificial phimosis had a higher incidence of malignant change (Shabad, 1964).

While the accumulation of smegma is widely thought to play a contributing role in penile cancer, the question as to whether it contains actual carcinogens remains undecided. Plaut and Kohn-Speyer (1947) treated 400 mice with horse smegma applied in a skin tunnel, injected subcutaneously, or painted on the skin. Three carcinomas and one sarcoma were induced at the site of treatment, as well as 4 papillary warts, one of which had carcinoma-like areas. Pratt-Thomas *et al.* (1956) inoculated human smegma into the vaginas of mice twice weekly for 19 months and found 4 invasive carcinomas, 1 early carcinoma, and one intraepithelial carcinoma in 12 evaluable mice. Application once a week was less effective. Reddy and Baruah (1963), however, applied human smegma to the vaginas and penises of mice thrice weekly for 16 months without inducing neoplasia. Because of differences in techniques and mouse strains, and problems with animal survival, the studies are not entirely comparable. Reddy and Baruah conclude that if human smegma is carcinogenic it is weakly so.

A possible relation between carcinoma of the uterine cervix and circumcision of the husband led Pratt-Thomas *et al.* (1956) to undertake the mouse studies described above. They noted that cervical carcinoma was rare in Jewish women; and that in the Fiji Islands it was 8 times more frequent among immigrant Indian women, whose husbands were not circumcised, than among native Fiji Islanders who routinely circumcise males. Their experimental studies with mice tended to support a contributing role of smegma in cervical cancer.

The relation between carcinoma of the uterine cervix and carcinoma of the penis has been examined in studies in Puerto Rico (Martinez, 1969), in New York State (Graham *et al.*, 1979), and in England and Wales (Smith *et al.*, 1980). In all three studies women whose husbands had penile cancer were at higher risk of cervical neoplasia, but this was not true of other cancer sites in the women. The mechanism of the association remains to be determined. Smith *et al.* (1980) noted that in general the epidemiologic characteristics of the two diseases were not similar, and there was little international correlation between the two. To put the matter in perspective, they calculated that if their risk estimates were correct, then of the 4000 new cases of cervical cancer seen in England and Wales in a year, 10 or 11 would be associated with cancer of the penis.

Factors other than circumcision and hygienic customs may play roles in the incidence of penile cancer. Schmauz and Jain (1971) noted substantial differences in incidence among Ugandan tribes that did not circumcise. While some differences appeared to be related to hygienic practices, others appeared to be more related to geographic location. Some studies have found an association with lower socioeconomic status. While this is probably true on an international level (Riveros and Lebron, 1963), related in part to bathing facilities and customs, it seems not to be true within a rather homogeneous population. Jensen (1977) reported an excess of patients in the middle class in Denmark, as judged by occupation. There was no higher frequency in the lower social classes. Prior venereal disease has been reported to be associated with penile cancer in some studies (Jensen, 1977), but not in all (Persky, 1977).

It appears a well-established fact that poor penile hygiene, with the accumulation of smegma, is a major etiologic factor in squamous cell carcinoma of the penis, although the mechanism remains uncertain. Either consistently good hygiene or circumcision is a satisfactory preventive. It seems likely that environmental factors may also play a role.

8. EPILOGUE

While a review such as this points out how little we know about the detailed etiology of urogenital cancers, it also indicates that much has been learned, especially in recent years. We have a growing understanding of basic mechanisms and their role in the induction of urogenital tumors (Paulson, 1978). More broadly-based and more precise epidemiologic information is providing better guides for laboratory studies which, in turn, help guide the epidemiologist. By combining the varied research tools available, from organic chemistry through tissue culture and experimental animal work to epidemiology, we can enhance the value of each one. As we understand better the carcinogenic mechanisms, and the complex interactions of the many factors involved, we become better able to identify the critical elements in the induction of each kind of neoplasm. We then become increasingly able to devise rational strategies for avoiding or countering key steps in the initiation and development of the various cancers. Whether genetic or epigenetic mechanisms are crucial in a given tumor (Ashby *et al.*, 1978), whether intervention in the initiation (Campbell, 1980) or promotion (Hicks, 1980) phases offers the better chances for prevention, the more complete knowledge and understanding now being acquired offer real promise of helping to reduce cancer morbidity and mortality.

ACKNOWLEDGEMENTS

The unpublished research was supported by the Medical Research Service of the Veterans Administration and by PHS Grant CA14930 from the National Cancer Institute through the National Bladder Cancer Project.

REFERENCES

1. Ablin RJ, Bhatti RA, Guinan PD, Bush IM: Effect of human seminal plasma on tumour-associated immunity in prostatic cancer. A preliminary report. Experientia 35:1510-1511, 1979.
2. Ablin RJ, Danaher J, Soanes WA, Gonder MJ: Antibodies reactive with autologous prostatic tissue in adenocarcinoma of the prostate. Urology 3:491–493, 1974.
3. Akazaki K, Stemmerman GN: Comparative study of latent carcinoma of the prostate among Japanese in Japan and Hawaii. J Natl Cancer Inst 50:1137–1144, 1973.
4. Anders A, Anders F: Etiology of cancer as studied in the platyfish-swordtail system. Biochim Biophys acta 516:61–95, 1978.
5. Abderson DE: Familial susceptibility. In: Persons at High Risk of Cancer (Fraumeni JF, ed.). New York: Academic Press, pp. 39-54, 1975.
6. Andervont HB, Shimkin MB, Canter HY: Effect of discontinued estrogenic stimulation upon the development and growth of testicular tumors in mice. J Natl Cancer Inst 18:1–39, 1957.

7. Armenian HK, Lilienfeld AB, Diamond EL, Bross IDJ: Relation between benign prostatic hyperplasia and cancer of the prostate. Lancet 2:115–117, 1974.
8. Armenian HK, Lilienfeld AM, Diamond EL, Bross IDJ: Epidemiologic characteristics of patients with prostatic neoplasms. Am J Epidemiol 102:47–54, 1975.
9. Armstrong B, Doll R: Environmental factors and cancer incidence and mortality in different countries, with special reference to dietary practices. Int J Cancer 15:617–631, 1975.
10. Armstrong B, Garrod A, Doll R: A retrospective study of renal cancer with special reference to coffee and animal protein consumption. Br J Cancer 33:127–136, 1976.
11. Ashby J, Styles JA, Anderson D, Paton D: Saccharin: An epigenetic carcinogen/mutagen? Food Cosmet Toxicol 16:95–103, 1978.
12. Bannasch P, Mayer D, Krech R: Neoplastic and preneoplastic lesions in rats after oral administration of a single dose of N-nitrosomorpholine. J Cancer Res Clin Oncol 94:233–248, 1979.
13. Batata MA, Whitmore WF Jr, Chu FCH, Hilaris BS, Loh J, Grabstald H, Golbey R: Cryptorchidism and testicular cancer. J Urol 124:382–387, 1980.
14. Bennington JL: Cancer of the kidney – Etiology, epidemiology, and pathology. Cancer 32:1017–1029, 1973.
15. Bennington JL, Laubscher FA: Epidemiologic studies on carcinoma of the kidney. I. Association of renal adenocarcinoma with smoking. Cancer 21:1069–1071, 1968.
16. Berenblum I, Shubik P: The persistence of latent tumour cells induced in the mouse's skin by a single application of 9,10-dimethyl-1,2-benzanthracene. Br J Cancer 3:384–386, 1949.
17. Berg JW: Can nutrition explain the patterns of international epidemiology of hormone-dependent cancers? Cancer Res 35:3345–3350, 1975
18. Blair A, Fraumeni JF: Geographic patterns of prostate cancer in the United States. J Natl Cancer Inst 61:1379–1384, 1978.
19. Blot WJ, Fraumeni JF: Geographic patterns of renal cancer in the United States. J Natl Cancer Inst 63:363–366, 1979.
20. Boczko S, Freed S: Penile carcinoma in circumcized males. NY State J Med 79:1903–1904, 1979.
21. Bonar RA, Paulson DF: Response of chick-embryo kidney cells in vitro to two avian tumor viruses. J Natl Cancer Inst 53:711–718, 1974.
22. Boyland E: The history and future of chemical carcinogenesis. Br Med Bull 36:5–10, 1980.
23. Breslow N, Chan CW, Dhom G, Drury RAB, Franks LM, Gellei B, Lee YS, Lundberg S, Sparke B, Sternby NH, Tulinius H: Latent carcinoma of prostate at autopsy in seven areas. Int J Cancer 20:680–688, 1977.
24. Brown DE, Warren S, Chute RN, Ryan KJ, Todd RB: Hormonally induced tumors of the reproductive system of parabiosed male rats. Cancer Res. 39:3971–3976, 1979.
25. Bryan GT: The role of urinary tryptophan metabolites in the etiology of bladder cancer. Am J Clin Nutr 24:841–847, 1971.
26. Bryan GT: Bladder cancer – Etiology. Adv Med Oncol Res Educ 11:207–212, 1979.
27. Bulay O, Patil K, Wilson R, Shubik P: Kidney tumors induced in rats by the antischistosomal drug niridazole. Cancer Res 39:4996–5002, 1979.
28. Campbell TC: Chemical carcinogens and human risk assessment. Fed Proc 39:2467–2484, 1980.
29. Case RAM, Hosker ME, McDonald DB, Pearson JT: Tumours of the urinary bladder in workmen engaged in the manufacture and use of certain dyestuff intermediates in the British chemical industry. Part I. The role of aniline, benzidine, alpha-naphthylamine, and beta-naphthylamine. Br J Ind Med 11:75–104, 1954.

30. Catalona WJ: Immunobiology of carcinoma of the prostate. Invest Urol 17:373–377, 1980.
31. Chandler JA, Timms BG: The effect of testosterone and cadmium on the rat lateral prostate in organ culture. Virchows Arch B 25:17–31, 1977.
32. Chapman WH, Kirchheim D, McRoberts JW: Effect of the urine and calculus formation on the incidence of bladder tumors in rats implanted with paraffin wax pellets. Cancer Res 33:1225–1229, 1973.
33. Chevlen EM, Awwad HK, Ziegler JL, Elsebai I: Cancer of the bilharzial bladder. Int J Radiat Oncol Biol Phys 5:921–926, 1979.
34. Chopra DP, Wilkoff LJ: Induction of hyperplasia and anaplasia by carcinogens in organ cultures of mouse prostate. In Vitro 13: 260–267, 1977.
35. Clayson DB, Cooper EH: Cancer of the urinary tract. Adv in Cancer Res 13:271–381, 1970.
36. Clemmesen J: A doubling of morbidity from testis carcinoma in Copenhagen, 1943-1962. Acta Path Microbiol Scand 72:348–349, 1968.
37. Cohen AJ, Li FP, Berg S, Marchetto DJ, Tsai S, Jacobs SC, Brown, RS: Hereditary renal-cell carcinoma associated with a chromosomal translocation. N Engl J Med 301:592-595, 1979.
38. Cohen SM, Arai M, Jacobs JB, Friedell GH: Promoting effect of saccharin and DL-tryptophan in urinary bladder carcinogenesis. Cancer Res 39:1207–1217, 1979.
39. Cole P: Coffee-drinking and cancer of the lower urinary tract. Lancet 1:1335–1337, 1971.
40. Cole P, Cramer D: Diet and cancer of endocrine target organs. Cancer 40:434–437, 1977.
41. Cole P, Hoover R, Friedell GH: Occupation and cancer of the lower urinary tract. Cancer 29:1250–1260, 1972.
42. Cole P, Monson RR, Haning H, Friedell GH: Smoking and cancer of the lower urinary tract. N Engl J Med 284:129–134, 1971.
43. Creagen ET, Fraumeni JF: Cancer mortality among American Indians, 1950-1967. J Natl Cancer Inst 49:959–967, 1972.
44. Dagher R, Selzer ML, Lapides J: Carcinoma of the penis and anticircumcision crusade. J Urol 110:79–80, 1973.
45. Dixon RL, Lee IP: Pharmacokinetic and adaptation factors involved in testicular toxicity. Fed Proc 39:66–72, 1980.Dodge OG, Linsell CA: Carcinoma of the penis in Uganda and Kenya Africans. Cancer 16:1255–1263, 1963.
46. Dodge OG, Linsell CA: Carcinoma of the penis in Uganda and Kenya Africans. Cancer 16:1255–1263, 1963.
47. Doll R: Cancer in five continents. Proc Roy Soc Med 65:49–55, 1972.
48. Dunn JE: Cancer epidemiology in populations of the United States – with emphasis on Hawaii and California – and Japan. Cancer Res 35:3240–3245, 1975.
49. Dunning WF, Curtis MR, Maun ME: The effect of added dietary tryptophan on the occurrence of 2-acetylaminofluorene induced liver and bladder cancer in rats. Cancer Res 10:454–459, 1950.
50. Dunning WF, Curtis MR, Segaloff A: Methylcholanthrene squamous cell carcinoma of the rat prostate with skeletal metastases, and failure of the rat liver to respond to the same carcinogen. Cancer Res 6:256–262, 1946.
51. Enstrom JE: Cancer and total mortality among active Mormons. Cancer 42:1943–1951, 1978.
52. Epstein SM, Bartus B, Farber E: Renal epithelial neoplasms induced in male Wistar rats by oral aflotoxin B. Cancer Res 29:1045–1050, 1969.

53. Ernster VL, Sacks ST, Selvin S, Petrakis NL: Cancer incidence by marital status: U.S. Third National Cancer Survey. J Natl Cancer Inst 63:567–585, 1969.
54. Ernster VL, Selvin S, Brown SM, Sacks ST, Winkelstein W, Austin DF: Occupation and prostatic cancer. A review and retrospective analysis based on death certificates in two California counties. J Occup Med 21:175–183, 1979.
55. Ernster VL, Selvin S, Winkelstein W: Cohort mortality for prostatic cancer among United States nonwhites. Science 200:1165–1166, 1978a.
56. Ernster VL, Selvin S, Sacks ST, Austin DF, Brown SM, Winkelstein W: Prostatic cancer: Mortality and incidence rates by race and social class. Am J Epidemiol 107:311–320, 1978b.
57. Evans IA: The bracken carcinogen. In: Chemical Carcinogens (Searle CE, ed.). ACS Monograph 173. Washington, D.C.: American Chemical Society, 1976, pp. 690–700.
58. Fokkens W: Phenacetin abuse related to bladder cancer. Environ, Res 20:192–198, 1979.
59. Fraley EE, Elliott AY, Castro AE, Cleveland P, Hakala T, Stein N: Ribonucleic acid virus associated with human urothelial tumors: significance for diagnosis and treatment. J Urol 111:378–381, 1974.
60. Franks LM: Etiology, epidemiology, and pathology of prostatic cancer. Cancer 32:1092–1095, 1973.
61. Fraumeni JF, Mason TJ: Cancer mortality among Chinese-Americans, 1950-1969. J Natl Cancer Inst 52:659–665, 1974.
62. Friedell GH, Cohen SM: Experimental models of cancer of the urinary bladder. Adv Med Oncol Res Educ 11:233–240, 1979.
63. Frith CH, Farmer JH, Greenman DL, Shaw GW: Biologic and morphologic characteristics of urinary bladder neoplasms induced in BALB/c female mice with 2-acetylaminofluorene. J Environ Pathol Toxicol 3:103–119, 1979.
64. Geder L, Rapp F: Herpesvirus and prostate carcinogenesis. Arch Androl 4:71–78, 1980.
65. Govan DE, Donaldson SS, Wilbur J: Pediatric oncology. In: Campbell's Urology (Harrison JH, Gittes RF, Perlmutter AD, Stamey TA, Walsh PC, eds.), Vol. 2. Philadelphia: W.B. Saunders, 1979, pp. 1795–1822.
66. Graham S, Gibson R, West D, Swanson M, Burnett W, Dayal H: Epidemiology of cancer of the testis in upstate New York. J Natl Cancer Inst 58:1255–1261, 1977.
67. Graham S, Priore R, Graham M, Browne R, Burnett W, West D: Genital cancer in wives of penile cancer patients. Cancer 44:1870–1874, 1979.
68. Greenwald P, Damon A, Kirmss V, Polan AK: Physical and demographic features of men before developing cancer of the prostate. J Natl Cancer Inst 53:341–346, 1974a.
69. Greenwald P, Kirmss V, Polan AK, Dick VS: Cancer of the prostate among men with benign prostatic hyperplasia. J Natl Cancer Inst 53:335–340, 1974b.
70. Greenwald P, Kirmss V, Burnett WS: Prostate cancer epidemiology: Widowerhood and cancer in spouses. J Natl Cancer Inst 62:1131–1136, 1979.
71. Grumet RF, MacMahon B: Trends in mortality from neoplasms of the testis. Cancer 11:790–797, 1958.
72. Gunn SA, Gould TC, Anderson WAD: Comparative study of interstitial cell tumors of rat testis induced by cadmium injection and vascular ligation. J Natl Cancer Inst 35:329–337, 1965.
73. Guthrie J, Guthrie OA: Embryonal carcinomas in Syrian hamsters after intratesticular inoculation of zinc chloride during seasonal testicular growth. Cancer Res 34:2612–2614, 1974.
74. Habib FK, Hammond GL, Lee IR, Dawson JB, Mason MK, Smith PH, Stitch SR: Metal-androgen interrelationships in carcinoma and hyperplasia of the human prostate. J Endrocrinol 71:133–141, 1976.

75. Haenszel W, Kurihara M: Studies of Japanese migrants. I. Mortality from cancer and other diseases among Japanese in the U.S. J Natl Cancer Inst 40:43–68, 1968.
76. Hakky SI, Chisholm GD, Skeet RG: Social class and carcinoma of the prostate. Br J Urol 51:393–396, 1979.
77. Hamilton JM: Renal carcinogenesis. Adv. Cancer Res 22:1–56, 1975.
78. Hanis NM, Stavraky KM, Fowler JL: Cancer mortality in oil refinery workers. J Occup Med 21:167–174, 1979.
79. Hard GC: Tumours of the kidney, renal pelvis and ureter. IARC Sci Publ 1:73–101, 1977.
80. Hard GC: The nature of experimentally induced renal tumors of the rat, and possible implications for human renal cancer. In: Prevention and Detection of Cancer (Neiburgs HR, ed.), Part 1, Prevention; Vol. 2, Etiology-Prevention Methods. New York: Marcel Dekker, 1978, pp. 1435–1442.
81. Hecht SS, Chen CB, McCoy GD, Hoffman D: Tobacco specific N-nitrosamines: Occurence, carcinogenicity, and metabolism. ACS Symp Ser 101:125–152, 1979.
82. Heine U, de The G, Ishiguro H, Sommer JR, Beard D, Beard JW: Multiplicity of cell response to the BAI Strain A (myeloblastosis) avian tumor virus. II. Nephroblastoma (Wilms' tumor): Ultrastructure. J Natl Cancer Inst 29:41–105, 1962.
83. Heshmat MY, Kovi J, Herson J, Jones GW, Jackson MA: Epidemiologic association between gonorrhea and prostatic carcinoma. Urology 6:457–460, 1975.
84. Hicks RM: Multistage carcinogenesis in the urinary bladder. Br Med Bull 36:39–46, 1980.
85. Higginson J: Present and future developments in environmental carcinogenesis. Adv Med Oncol Res Educ 3:203–213, 1979.
86. Hill MJ: *In vivo* bacterial N-nitrosation and its possible role in human cancer. In: Naturally Occurring Carcinogens-Mutagens and Modulators of Carcinogenesis. (Miller EC, Miller JA, Hirono I, Sugimura T, Takayama S, eds.) Baltimore: University Park Press, 1979, pp. 229–240.
87. Hill PB, Wynder EL: Effect of a vegetarian diet and dexamethasone on plasma prolactin, testosterone and dehydroepiandrosterone in men and women. Cancer Lett 7:273–282, 1979.
88. Hill P, Wynder EL, Garbaczewski L, Garnes H, Walker ARP: Diet and urinary steroids in black and white North American men and black South African men. Cancer Res 39:5101–5105, 1979.
89. Hinman F, Smith GL: Leydig cell neoplasia in experimental testicular Atrophy. J Urol 83:706–712, 1960.
90. Hirayama T: Changing patterns of cancer in Japan with special reference to the decrease in stomach cancer mortality. In: Origins of Human Cancer. (Hiatt HH, Watson JD, Winsten JA, eds.) Cold Spring Harbor Laboratory, Cold Spring, 1977, pp. 55–75.
91. Hirose F, Takizawa S, Watanabe H, Takeichi N: Development of adenocarcinoma of the prostate in ICR mice locally irradiated with X-rays. Gann 67:407–411, 1976.
92. Hoover R: Saccharin – bitter aftertaste? N Engl J Med 302:573–575, 1980.
93. Hoover R, Cole P: Temporal aspects of occupational bladder carcinogenesis. N Engl J Med 288:1040–1043, 1973.
94. Hoover R, Fraumeni JF: Cancer mortality in U.S. counties with chemical industries. Environ Res 9:196–207, 1975.
95. Hoover RN, Strasser PH: Artificial sweeteners and human bladder cancer. Preliminary results. Lancet 1:837–840, 1980.
96. Horning ES: Induction of glandular carcinomas of the prostate in the mouse. Lancet 1:829–830, 1946.

97. Howe GR, Burch JD, Miller AB, Cook GM, Esteve J, Morrison B, Gordon P, Chambers LW, Fodor G, Winsor GM: Tobacco use, occupation, coffee, various nutrients, and bladder cancer. J Natl Cancer Inst 64:701–713, 1980.
98. Hueper WC: Occupational and environmental cancers of the urinary system. New Haven: Yale University Press, 1969.
99. Hueper WC, Wiley FH, Wolfe HD: Experimental production of bladder tumors in dogs by administration of beta-naphthylamine. J Indust Hyg Toxicol 20:46–84, 1938.
100. Huseby RA: Demonstration of a direct carcinogenic effect of estradiol on Leydig cells of the mouse. Cancer Res 40:1006–1013, 1980.
101. Hutchison GB: Epidemiology of prostatic cancer. Sem Oncol 3:151–159, 1976.
102. Ishiguro H, Beard D, Sommer JR, Heine U, de The G, Beard JW: Multiplicity of cell response to the BAI Strain A, (myeloblastosis) avian tumor virus. I. Nephroblastoma (Wilms' tumor): Gross and microscopic pathology. J Natl Cancer Inst 29:1–39, 1962.
103. Ivankovic S: Teratogenic and carcinogenic effects of some chemicals during prenatal life in rats, Syrian golden hamsters, and minipigs. Natl Cancer Inst Monogr 51:103–115, 1979.
104. Jackson MA, Ahluwalia BS, Herson J, Heshmat MY, Jackson AG, Jones GW, Kapoor SK, Kennedy J, Kovi J, Lucas AO, Nkposons EO, Olisa E, Williams AO: Characterization of prostatic carcinoma among blacks. A continuation report. Cancer Treat Rep 61:167–172, 1977.
105. Jacobs JB, Arai, M, Cohen SM, Friedell GH: A long-term study of reversible and progressive urinary bladder cancer lesions in rats fed N-[14-(5-nitro-2-furyl)-2-thiazolyl] formamide. Cancer Res 37:2817–2821, 1977.
106. Jensen MS: Cancer of the penis in Denmark 1942 to 1962 (511 cases). Danish Med Bull 24:66–72, 1977.
107. Jurgelski W, Hudson P, Falk HL: Tissue differentiation and susceptibility to embryonal tumor induction by ethylnitrosourea in the opossum. Natl Cancer Inst Monogr 51:123–158, 1979.
108. Kanarek MS: Asbestos in drinking water and cancer incidence. Diss Abstr Int B 40:147, 1979.
109. Kantor AF: Current concepts in the epidemiology and etiology of primary renal cell carinoma. J Urol 117:415–417, 1977.
110. Kantor ALF, Meigs JW, Heston JF, Flannery JT: Epidemiology of renal cancer in Connecticut, 1935–1973. J Natl Cancer Inst 57:495–500, 1976.
111. Kennaway EL: Cancer of the penis and circumcision in relation to the incubation period of cancer. Br J Cancer 1:335–344, 1947.
112. Kessler II, Clark JP: Saccharin, cyclamate, and human bladder cancer. No evidence of an association. J Am Med Assoc 240:349–355, 1978.
113. Kipling MD, Waterhouse JAH: Cadmium and prostatic carcinoma. Lancet 1:730–731, 1967.
114. Kmet J: The role of migrant population in studies of selected cancer sites: a review. J Chronic Dis 23:305–324, 1970.
115. Knudson AG: Mutagenesis and embryonal carcinogenesis. Natl Cancer Inst Monograph 51:19–24, 1979.
116. Knudson AG, Strong LC: Mutation and cancer: A model for Wilms' tumor of the kidney. J Natl Cancer Inst 48:313–324, 1972.
117. Kolonel LN: Association of cadmium with renal cancer. Cancer 37:1782–1787, 1976.
118. Kolonel L, Winkelstein W: Cadmium and prostatic carcinoma. Lancet 2:566, 1977.
119. Koss LG: Tumors of the urinary bladder. Atlas of Tumor Pathology, second series, fascicle 11. Washington, D.C.: Armed Forces Institute of Pathology 1975.
120. Kovi J, Heshmat MY: Incidence of cancer in Negroes in Washington, D.C. and selected African cities. Am J Epidemiol 96:401–413, 1972.

121. Krain LS: Testicular cancer in California from 1942 to 1969: The California Tumor Registry experience. Oncology 27:45–51, 1973.
122. Lasnitzki I: Growth pattern of the mouse prostate gland in organ culture and its reponse to sex hormones, vitamin A and 3-methylcholanthrene. Natl Cancer Inst Monogr 12:381–403, 1963.
123. Lee JAH, Hitosugi M, Petersen GR: Rise in mortality from tumors of the testis in Japan, 1947–1970. J Natl Cancer Inst 51:1485–1490, 1973.
124. Lemen RA, Lee JS, Wagoner JK, Blejer HP: Cancer mortality among cadmium production workers. Ann NY Acad Sci 271:273–279, 1976.
125. Li FP, Fraumeni JF: Testicular cancers in children: Epidemiologic characteristics. J Natl Cancer Inst 48:1575–1582, 1972.
126. Li JJ, Cuthbertson TL Li SA: Inhibition of estrogen tumorigenesis in the Syrian golden hamster kidney by antiestrogens. J Natl Cancer Inst 64:795–800, 1980.
127. Lipworth L, Dayan AD: Rural preponderance of seminoma of the testis. Cancer 23:1119–1121, 1969.
128. Lower GM, Nilsson T, Nelson CE, Wolf H, Gamsky TE, Bryan GT: N-acetyltransferase phenotype and risk in urinary bladder cancer: approaches in molecular epidemiology. Preliminary results in Sweden and Denmark. Environ Health Perspect 29:71–79, 1979.
129. Lutes R, Meigs JW, Heston JF, Flannery JT: Increasing testicular cancer incidence in Connecticut. Conn Med 44:327–328, 1980.
130. Lynch HT, Walzak MP, Fried R, Domina AH, Lynch JF: Familial factors in bladder carcinoma. J Urol 122:458–461, 1979.
131. Lyon JL, Gardner JW, Klauber MR, Smart CR: Low cancer incidence and mortality in Utah. Cancer 39:2608–2618, 1977.
132. Macklin AW, Welch RM, Cuatrecasas P: Drug safety: Phenacetin. Science 205:144–148, 1979.
133. Martinez I: Relationship of squamous cell carcinoma of the cervix uteri to squamous cell carcinoma of the penis among Puerto Rican women married to men with penile carcinoma. Cancer 24:777–780, 1969.
134. Mason TJ, McKay FW, Hoover R, Blot WJ, Fraumeni JF: Atlas of cancer mortality for U.S. counties: 1950–1969. Washington, D.C.: U.S. Dept of Health, Educ and Welfare. DHEW Publication No. (NIH) 75–780, 1975.
135. Matsumoto H: Carcinogenicity of cycasin, its aglycone methylazoxymethanol, and methylazoxymethyl-glucosiduronic acid. In: Naturally Occurring Carcinogens-Mutagens and Modulators of Carcinogenesis. (Miller EC, Miller JA, Hirono I, Sugimura T, Takayama S, eds.) Baltimore: University Park Press, 1979, pp. 67–77.
136. Maugh TH: Chemicals: how many are there? Science 199:162, 1978.
137. Menck HR, Henderson BE, Pike MC, Mack T, Martin SP, SooHoo J: Cancer Incidence in the Mexican-American. J Natl Cancer Inst 55:531–536, 1975.
138. Meneely GR: Saccharin and cancer. J Am Med Assoc 242:2178–2179, 1979.
139. Mettlin C, Graham S: Dietary risk factors in human bladder cancer. Am J Epidemiol 110:255–263, 1979.
140. Michalowsky I: Eine experimentelle Erzeugung teratoider Geschwulste der Hoden beim Hahn. Zweite Mitteilung. Virchow's Arch Path Anat 267:27–62, 1928.
141. Mihatsch MJ, Manz T, Knusli C, Hofer HO, Rist M, Guetg R, Rutishauser G, Zollinger HU: Phenacetin abuse III. Malignant urinary tract tumor from phenacetin abuse in Basel 1963–1977. Schweiz Med Wochenschr 110:255–264, 1980.
142. Miller EC: Some current perspectives on chemical carcinogenesis in humans and experimental animals: Presidential address. Cancer Res 38:1479–1496, 1978.
143. Mladenov Z, Heine U, Beard D, Beard JW: Strain MC29 avian leukosis virus. Myelocy-

toma, endothelioma, and renal growths: Pathomorphological and ultrastructural aspects. J Natl Cancer Inst 38:251–285, 1967.
144. Moore MR, Meredith PA: The carcinogenicity of lead. Arch Toxicol 42:87–94, 1979.
145. Morgan RW, Jain MG: Bladder cancer: Smoking, beverages and artificial sweeteners. Can Med Assoc J 111:1067–1070, 1974.
146. Morrison AS: Some social and medical characteristics of Army men with testicular cancer. Am J Epidemiol 104:511–516, 1976.
147. Morrison AS: Cryptorchidism, hernia, and cancer of the testis. J Natl Cancer Inst 56:731–733, 1976.
148. Morrison AS: Geographic and time trends of coffee imports and bladder cancer. Eur J Cancer 14:51–54, 1978.
149. Morrison AS, Buring JE: Artificial sweeteners and cancer of the lower urinary tract. N Engl J Med 302:537–541, 1980.
150. Morrision AS, Cole P: Epidemiology of bladder cancer. Urol Clin North Am 3:13–29, 1976.
151. Mostofi FK: Testicular tumors. Epidemiologic, etiologic, and pathologic features. Cancer 32:1186–1201, 1973.
152. Mulvihill JJ: Congenital and genetic diseases. In: Persons at High Risk of Cancer. An approach to cancer etiology and control. Fraumeni JF Jr, ed.), New York: Academic Press, 1975, pp. 3–37.
153. Mustacchi P, Millmore D: Racial and occupational variations in cancer of the testis: San Francisco, 1956–1965. J Natl Cancer Inst 56:717–720, 1976.
154. Noble RL: The development of prostatic adenocarcinoma in Nb rats following prolonged sex hormone administration. Cancer Res 37:1929–1933, 1977.
155. Noronha RFX, Goodall CM: Enhancement of liver and kidney carcinogenesis by dimethylnitrosamine in thyroidectomized NZR/GD rats. In: Prevention and Detection of Cancer. Part 1, Prevention, Vol. 2, Etiology-Prevention Methods (Nieburgs HR, ed.), New York: Marcel Dekker, 1978, pp. 1273–1282.
156. Orell SR, Nanra RS, Ferguson NW: Renal pelvic cancer in the Hunter valley. Med J Aust 2:524–557, 1979.
157. Oyasu R, Hirao Y, Izumi K: Promotion by urine of urinary bladder carcinogenesis. Proc Am Assoc Cancer Res 21:70, 1980.
158. Pamukcu AM, Bryan GT: Bracken fern, a natural urinary bladder and intestinal carcinogen. In: Naturally Occurring Carcinogens-Mutagens and Modulators of Carcinogenesis (Miller EC, Miller JA, Hirono I, Sugimura T, Takayama S, eds.), Baltimore: University Park Press, 1979, pp. 89–99.
159. Parkes HG: The epidemiology of the aromatic amine cancers. Am Chem Soc Monogr 173:462–480, 1976.
160. Paulson DF: Carcinogenesis in urogenital sites. Invest Urol 16:77–86, 1978.
161. Paulson DF, Rabson AS, Fraley EE: Viral neoplastic transformation of hamster prostate tissue *in vitro*. Science 159:200–201, 1968.
162. Persky L: Epidemiology of cancer of the penis. Recent Results Cancer Res 60:97–109, 1977.
163. Petersen GR, Lee JAH: Secular trends of malignant tumors of the testis in white men. J Natl Cancer Inst 49:339–354, 1972.
164. Peterson GR, Lee JAH, Weathersby ME: Malignant tumors of the testis. J Natl Cancer Inst 58:173, 1977.
165. Petkovic SD: Epidemiology and treatment of renal pelvic and ureteral tumors. J Urol 114:858–865, 1975.
166. Phillips RL: Role of life-style and dietary habits in risk of cancer among Seventh-Day Adventists. Cancer Res 35:3513–3522, 1975.

167. Plaut A, Kohn-Speyer AC: The carcinogenic action of smegma. Science 105:391–392, 1947.
168. Pliss GB, Volfson NI: Carcinogenic properties of dicarboxydine (Gamma, gamma'-3,3'-benzidine dioxydibutyric acid). Arch Geschwulstforsch 49:229–239, 1979.
169. Pollard M: Spontaneous prostate adenocarcinomas in aged germ-free Wistar rats. J Natl Cancer Inst 51:1235–1241, 1973.
170. Potts CL: Cadmium proteinuria – The health of battery workers exposed to cadmium oxide dust. Ann Occup Hyg 8:55–61, 1965.
171. Pratt-Thomas HR, Heins HC, Latham E, Dennis EJ, McIver FA: The carcinogenic effect of human smegma: an experimental study I. Preliminary report. Cancer 9:671–680, 1956.
172. Purtilo DT, McCarthy B, Yang JPS, Friedell GH: Familial urinary bladder cancer. Semin Oncol 6:254–256, 1979.
173. Radomski JL, Radomski T, MacDonald WE: Co-carcinogenic interaction between D,L-tryptophan and 4-amino-biphenyl or 2-naphthylamine in dogs. J Natl Cancer Inst 58:1831–1834, 1977.
174. Radovanovic Z, Krajinovic S: The Balkan endemic nephropathy and urinary tract tumors. Arch Geschwulstforsch 49:444–447, 1979.
175. Rapp F: Virology and cancer. Prev Med 9:244–251, 1980.
176. Rapp F, Geder L, Murasko D, Lausch R, Ladda R, Huang E-S, Webber M: Long-term persistence of cytomegalovirus genome in cultured human cells of prostatic origin. J Virol 16:982–990, 1975.
177. Reddy BS, Cohen LA, McCoy GD, Hill P, Weisburger JH, Wynder EL: Nutrition and its relationship to cancer. Adv Cancer Res 32:237–345, 1980.
178. Reddy DG, Baruah IKSM: Carcinogenic action of human smegma. Arch Path 75:414–420, 1963.
179. Redmond CK, Ciocco A, Lloyd JW, Rush HW: Long-term mortality study of steel workers. VI. Mortality from malignant neoplasms among coke oven workers. J Occup Med 14:621–629, 1972.
180. Rehn L: Blasengenschwülste bei Fuchsin-Arbeitern. Arch klin Chir 50:588–600, 1895.
181. Reuber MD: Carcinogenicity of chloroform. Environ Health Perspect 31:171–182, 1979.
182. Reznik G, Ward JM, Hardisty JF, Russfield A: Renal carcinogenic and nephrotoxic effects of the flame retardant tris(2,3-dibromopropyl) phosphate in F344 rats and (C57BL/6N X C3H/HeN)F_1 mice. J Natl Cancer Inst 63:205–212, 1979.
183. Rhomberg W, Schmoll HJ: High incidence of metalworkers among patients with testicular cancer. In: Prevention and Detection of Cancer. Part 1, Prevention; vol. 2, Etiology-Prevention Methods (Nieburgs HE, ed.), New York: Marcel Dekker, 1976, pp. 1737–1743.
184. Riveros M, Lebrón RF: Geographical pathology of cancer of the penis. Cancer 16:798–811, 1963.
185. Roberts JJ: Cellular responses to carcinogen-induced DNA damage and the role of DNA repair. Br Med Bull 36:25–31, 1980.
186. Roe FJ: Food and cancer. J Hum Nutr 33:405–415, 1979.
187. Roe FJC, Dukes CE, Cameron KM, Pugh RCB, Mitchley BCV: Cadmium neoplasia: Testicular atrophy and Leydig cell hyperplasia in rats and mice following the subcutaneous injection of cadmium salts. Br J Cancer 18:674–681, 1964.
188. Ross RK, McCurtis JW, Henderson BE, Menck HR, Mack TM, Martin SP: Descriptive epidemiology of testicular and prostatic cancer in Los Angeles. Br J Cancer 39:284–292, 1979.
189. Rotkin ID: Studies in the epidemiology of prostatic cancer: expanded sampling. Cancer Treat Rep 61:173–180, 1977.

190. Sadeghi A, Behmard S, Vesselinovitch SD: Opium: a potential urinary bladder carcinogen in man. Cancer 43:2315–2321, 1979.
191. Sanefuji H, Heatfield BM, Trump BF: Studies on carcinogenesis of human prostate. V. Effects of the carcinogen, N-methyl-N'-nitro-N-nitrosoguanidine (MNNG), on normal prostate during long-term explant culture. Scan Electron Microsc 1979:657–663, 1979.
192. Sanford EJ, Geder L, Laychock A, Rohner TJ, Rapp F: Evidence for the association of cytomegalovirus with carcinoma of the prostate. J Urol 118:789–792, 1977.
193. Schmauz R, Jain DK: Geographical variation of carcinoma of the penis in Uganda. Br J cancer 25:25–32, 1971.
194. Schrek R, Lenowitz H: Etiologic factors in carcinoma of the penis. Cancer Res 7:180–187, 1947.
195. Selikoff IJ, Hammond EC: Asbestos and smoking. J Am Med Assoc 242:458–459, 1979.
196. Selikoff IJ, Hammond EC, Seidman H: Mortality experience of insulation workers in the United States and Canada, 1943–1976. Ann NY Acad Sci 330:91–116, 1979.
197. Shabad AL: Some aspects of etiology and prevention of penile cancer. J Urol 92:696–702, 1964.
198. Shain SA, McCullough B, Segaloff A: Spontaneous adenocarcinomas of the ventral prostate of aged AXC rats. J Natl Cancer Inst 55:177–180, 1975.
199. Shank RC, Wogan GN, Gibson JB, Nondasuta A: Dietary aflatoxins and human liver cancer. II. Aflatoxins in market foods and foodstuffs of Thailand and Hong Kong. Food Cosmet Toxicol 10:61–69, 1972.
200. Sharief Y, Reich CF, Bonar RA: Polyploidy in mammalian urothelial cells. Urol Res 8:153–161, 1980.
201. Sieber SM, Correa P, Dalgard DW, McIntire R, Adamson RH: Carcinogenicity and hepatotoxicity of cycasin and its aglycone methylazoxymethanol acetate in nonhuman primates. J Natl Cancer Inst 65:177–189, 1980.
202. Silverberg E: Cancer statistics 1980. CA 30:23–28, 1980.
203. Sivak A: Cocarcinogenesis. Biochim Biophys Acta 560:67–89, 1979.
204. Smith PG, Kinlen LJ, White GC, Adelstein AM, Fox AJ: Mortality of wives of men dying with cancer of the penis. Br J Cancer 41:422–428, 1980.
205. Somerville SM, Davies JM, Hendry WF, Williams G: Bladder cancer as a prescribed industrial disease: a guide for clinicians. Br Med J 280:540–542, 1980.
206. Sporn MB, Squire RA, Brown CC, Smith JM, Wenk ML, Springer S: 13-cis-Retinoic acid: inhibition of bladder carcinogenesis in the rat. Science 195:487–489, 1977.
207. Stark AA, Demain AL: Genetic activity and hazards of mycotoxins. ASM News 46:80-83, 1980.
208. Staszewski J: Cancer of the urinary bladder: International mortality patterns and trends. World Health Stat 33:27–41, 1980.
209. Staszewski J, Haenszel W: Cancer mortality among the Polish-born in the United States. J Natl Cancer Inst 35:291–297, 1965.
210. Stein-Werblowsky R: On the etiology of cancer of the prostate. Eur Urol 4:370–373, 1978.
211. Stevens RG, Moolgavkar SH: Estimation of relative risk from vital data: smoking and cancers of the lung and bladder. J Natl Cancer Inst 63:1351–1357, 1979.
212. Svoboda DJ, Azarnoff DL: Tumors in male rats fed ethyl chlorophenoxyisobutyrate, a hypolipidemic drug. Cancer Res 39:3419–3428, 1979.
213. Swann PF, Kaufman DG, Magee PN, Mace R: Induction of kidney tumors by a single dose of dimethylnitrosamine: Dose response and influence of diet and benzo(a)pyrene pretreatment. Br J Cancer 41:285–294, 1980.

214. Takizawa S, Hirose F: Modification of renal tumorigenesis by gonadal ablation in rats treated with N-butylnitrosourea or dimethylnitrosamine. Hiroshima J Med Sci 27:247–252, 1978.
215. Talerman A, Kaalen JGAH, Fokkens W: Rural preponderance of testicular neoplasms. Br J Cancer 29:176–178, 1974.
216. Taylor JM, Weinberger JA, Friedman L: Chronic toxicity and carcinogenicity to the urinary bladder of sodium saccharin in the in utero-exposed rat. Toxicol Appl Pharmacol 54:57–75, 1980.
217. Teulings FAG, Peters HA, Hop WCJ, Fokkens W, Haije WG, Portengen H, Van Der Werf-Messing B: A new aspect of the urinary excretion of tryptophan metabolites in patients with cancer of the bladder. Int J Cancer 21:140–146, 1978.
218. Thomas JA, Small CS: Carcinoma of the penis in Southern India. J Urol 100:520–526, 1968.
219. Tomatis L: Evaluation of the carcinogenic risk of chemicals to humans. Adv Med Oncol Res Educ 1:191–198, 1979.
220. Van Duuren BL: Tumor-promoting and co-carcinogenic agents in chemical carcinogenesis. Am Chem Soc Monogr 173:24–51, 1976.
221. Vaught JB, King CM: Phenacetin studies. Science 206:637, 639, 1979.
222. Wang N, Trend B, Bronson DL, Fraley EE: Nonrandom abnormalities in chromosome 1 in human testicular tumors. Cancer Res 40:796–802, 1980.
223. Waterhouse JAH: Current status of cancer risk in the rubber industry. Adv Med Oncol Res Educ 3:97–105, 1979.
224. Watt BK, Merrill AL: Composition of foods – raw, processed, prepared. Agriculture handbook No. 8, Washington, D.C.: US Dept of Agriculture, 1963.
225. Watts SL, Smith RE: Pathology of chickens infected with avian nephroblastoma virus MAV-2(N). Infect Immun 27:501–522, 1980.
226. Weinstein RS: Origin and dissemination of human urinary bladder carcinoma. Sem Oncol 6:149–156, 1979.
227. Winklestein W, Kantor S: Prostatic cancer – relationship to suspended particulate air pollution. Am J Public Health 59:1134–1138, 1969.
228. Wogan GN: Aflatoxin carcinogenesis. In: Methods in Cancer Research (Harris Busch, ed.), Vol. 7. New York: Academic Press, 1973, pp. 309–344.
229. Wynder EL, Goldsmith R: The epidemiology of bladder cancer: A second look. Cancer 40:1246–1268, 1977.
230. Wynder EL, Gori GB: Contribution of the environment to cancer incidence: An epidemiologic exercise. J Natl Cancer Inst 58:825–832, 1977.
231. Wynder EL, Mabuchi K, Whitmore WF: Epidemiology of cancer of the prostate. Cancer 28:344–360, 1971.
232. Wynder EL, Mabuchi K, Whitmore WF: Epidemiology of adenocarcinoma of the kidney. J Natl Cancer Inst 53:1619–1634, 1974.
233. Wynder EL, Stellman SD: Artificial sweetener use and bladder cancer: A case-control study. Science 207:1214–1216, 1980.
234. Yoshida O, Miyakawa M: Etiology of bladder cancer: 'Metabolic' aspects. In: Analytic and Experimental Epidemiology of Cancer (Nakahara W, Hirayama T, Nishioka K, Sugano H, eds.) Tokyo: University of Tokyo Press, 1973, pp. 31–39.
235. Zawirska B: The particular traits of carcinogenesis induced in Wistar rats by aflatoxin B1. 1. Morphological changes and gamma-glutamyltranspeptidase activity. Patol Pol 30:439–456, 1979.

2. Marker Proteins as a Guide in Clinical Management of Genitourinary Cancer

PAUL H. LANGE

1. INTRODUCTION

Most of the noninvasive methods heretofore used to detect cancer entail identification of the images or anatomic effects of masses of tumor cells. Although this anatomical approach has been improved by such methods as computed tomography (CAT), it probably still is not able to detect masses of tumor cells smaller than 10^9 cells [1, 2]. Thus, there is a pressing need for better methods of detecting cancer, not only for earlier diagnosis of tumors or recurrences but also for staging and judging the response to treatment. This necessarily has stimulated a search for molecular probes; that is, tumor markers.

Strictly speaking, a tumor marker is any molecule whose presence may herald a malignancy. At first, however, tumor markers were usually considered to be substances produced only by the tumor itself and secreted into body fluids. As more became known about many of the putative tumor markers, however, it became apparent that most are also found in the normal state and that their utility as markers depends on quantitative rather than on qualitative differences. For example, for many years hCG was considered to be unique to tumors except in pregnant women. Recent evidence shows that hCG or a similar substance is produced normally by the testes, although it is usually detectable only by exquisitely sensitive assays [3].

The substances now classified as tumor markers comprise a heterogenous group. They may be derived from the tumor, in which case they may or may not be appropriate for the tissue of origin, or they may merely be associated with the tumor and originate in some other tissue (e.g., alkaline phosphatase in liver metastasis). Moreover, a marker may be specific to one or a group of tumors or be associated nonspecifically with any malignancy. The marker may have a recognized function, as with tumor-associated hormones, or, as is usually the case, its function may be unknown. Finally,

D.F. Paulson (ed.), Genitourinary Cancer 1, 45-72. All rights reserved.

tumor markers may be detectable primarily in body fluids such as urine or blood (the classical view), or they may be noncirculating substances confined to the malignant cell itself.

Most of the putative tumor markers, including most of those of interest in genitourinary oncology, are proteins. (Exceptions include shed cells, as in cytological studies for urothelial cancer, chromosome abnormalities, certain lipids, and some nucleic acids or their degradation products.) Because proteins usually are immunogenic, particularly in another species, and because antibody-based methods of detection often are far more sensitive and specific than are the strictly biochemical methods, detection of tumor markers has come to depend greatly on the production of xenogeneic antibodies. Tests for tumor markers, especially those assays used clinically, usually entail radioimmunoassay (RIA) or some other immunoassay or immunohistochemical staining. In a sense, immunodetection of markers is a branch of tumor immunology, although, in contrast to the classical field in which the emphasis is on the host's immunological response to putative tumor antigens, the science of tumor markers usually considers antigens that are poorly, if at all, immunogenic in the tumor host [4].

2. NECESSARY CHARACTERISTICS OF TUMOR MARKERS

In addition to a knowledge of immunological methods, an understanding of tumor markers requires familiarity with the terms used to assess their clinical utility, viz. sensitivity, specificity, false-positive and false-negative rates, and predictive value.

The sensitivity of a marker is the proportion of subjects known to have the disease who have the marker. The false-negative rate is the complement of this, the percentage of patients known to have the disease in whom the marker is not detected. The specificity of a marker, a measure of its uniqueness, is the proportion of patients known to be free of the disease who do not have the marker. Again, the false-positive rate is the complement: the proportion of this same population in whom the marker is detected. (In practice, specificity is determined in relation to the frequency of the marker in a population of age-matched controls, patients with nonmalignant diseases, and, most important, patients known to be cured of the disease rather than in an unselected population of normal people.) Obviously, the ideal marker would be 100% sensitive (all patients with the disease have the marker) and 100% specific (no patients without the disease have the marker). Unfortunately, no such marker has been found, although in a clinical context other causes of false-positive marker results often can be ruled out easily, as will be explained.

Finally, the predictive value (shown in the formula as the positive predictive value) is calculated as follows:

$$+\ PV = \frac{(Sen \times P)}{(Sen \times P) + (1 - Spec) \times (1 - P)}$$

in which Sen is the sensitivity and Spec the specificity of the marker and P is the prevalence of the disease in the population being studied. In other words, the positive predictive value of a marker assay is the probability that a person with a positive test for that marker actually has the disease [5].

Because the predictive value of a marker obviously depends not only on its sensitivity and specificity but also on the prevalence of the disease, marker assays have not been practical as screening tests for genitourinary cancers because the prevalences are usually low. However, when the prevalence is high, as in a population suspected of having a particular cancer or being monitored for disease recurrence, prevalence becomes less of a factor; and the predictive value of a marker often becomes great enough to make it useful clinically.

In addition to sensitivity and specificity, a tumor marker should have the following additional characteristics to be useful clinically. First, it should be readily detectable in body fluids or easily accessible tissues or cells. Second, it should appear early, preferably before the disease is detectable by the anatomical methods (i.e., fewer than 10^9 cells). Third, levels should reflect the size of the tumor burden yet be able to reveal micrometastases. Fourth, the half-life should be short enough so that the marker does not accumulate in the body and thus obscure changes in the rate of its production. And fifth, the levels should correlate with the response (or lack thereof) to treatment. These additional criteria are not all met by any one of the available markers, but genitourinary oncologists are fortunate in having some of the markers that come closest: prostatic acid phosphatase and alpha-fetoprotein (AFP) plus human chorionic gonadotropin (hCG).

3. CATEGORIES OF TUMOR MARKERS

3.1. Tumor-specific Transplantation Antigens (TSTA)

The TSTA have been defined primarily by the immunological responses they elicit in syngeneic animals and are usually considered to be those antigens that never appear on normal cells. As such, they have been the traditional focus of tumor immunology. However, as knowledge of TSTA grew, many were found to be present on normal cells also under some conditions and so were renamed 'tumor-associated antigens,' or TAA. In my opinion, this term should be avoided, because it overlaps with many other, more specific, categories to be mentioned subsequently and thus is confusing.

As recently as five years ago, there appeared to be much evidence that TSTA are present on human tumors. This conclusion derived primarily from *in vitro* studies such as the cell-mediated microcytotoxicity assay. Transitional cell carcinoma (TCC) had been studied with particular fervor, and detailed theories had been offered about the patterns and meanings of apparently tumor-specific immunological reactions in TCC patients. However, recent re-evaluation of *in vitro* tests such as the cell-mediated cytotoxicity assay caused a drastic revision in the interpretation of the earlier results, and today the very existence of TSTA in human tumors is in doubt. To date, true TSTA have been proved to exist only in animals, and then mostly in tumors that have been induced by viruses or chemicals rather than in those that arise spontaneously. The status of our knowledge of human and animal TSTA has been reviewed extensively [6–8].

3.2. Oncodevelopmental Antigens

These antigens, formerly called oncofetal antigens, are secreted by, or present on, tumor cells but are also associated with normal cells at some time during development and occasionally at maturity. Because these antigens normally are expressed primarily during development, their presence on tumor cells is not considered to result from mutation (as is assumed for many TSTA) but rather from re-expression of genes that were repressed during later stages of development. (This is referred to variously as derepression, dedifferentiation, retrodifferentiation, and antigenic reversion.) Oncodevelopmental antigens are rarely immunogenic in the species of origin and so must be identified through the production of xenogeneic antibodies.

Most of the oncodevelopmental antigens relevant to genitourinary oncology pertain primarily to testicular cancer (as will be discussed below), but a few words must be said about a well-known member of the class, carcinoembryonic antigen (CEA), because it has been said to be associated with many genitourinary tumors and there is much confusion about its measurement and clinical value. It is a cell-surface glycoprotein isolated initially from human colonic carcinoma [9] and found soon thereafter by immunological techniques to be associated with human embryonic and fetal organs and adult colonic carcinomas, although not with normal adult colon. The advent of sensitive RIAs generated immense initial enthusiasm for CEA as a marker for human gastrointestinal malignancies, but subsequent experience revealed that serum CEA levels were raised, not only in other, nonendodermally derived, malignancies, but also in various inflammatory diseases; and the enthusiasm faded. However, the reputation of CEA now is probably lower than it should be [10]. What is commonly designated 'CEA' is in fact several substances including not only CEA but more than ten compounds that cross-react to some extent with purified CEA in immunoassays. Some of these CEA-like substances strikingly resemble CEA in both amino-acid sequence and type and number of carbohydrate side chains, but there are some significant differences. It is postulated that an ancestral CEA gene underwent reduplication and mutation, so that several closely related CEA-like compounds are now produced in varying amounts at different stages from the early embryo to the adult. Malignant transformation thus could cause increased production of one of these cross-reacting substances, through either dedifferentiation or increased production of those compounds normally present at that stage of life. Because the CEA antibodies in the assays often do not distinguish clearly among these various compounds, it is not surprising that widespread clinical use of assays from various sources has produced such confusing data. However, as more is learned about the individual CEA-like compounds, more accurate methods of distinguishing them probably will be found so that they become more useful markers [10, 11]. The reasons for hope that this is true in prostatic cancer are discussed later in this chapter.

Although most oncodevelopmental antigens are not immunogenic, there may be some fetal antigens that are; i.e., ones that can elicit tumor-associated transplantation immunity [12]. These antigens are documented by *in vitro* techniques, as it is difficult to confirm their presence entirely by *in vivo* methods. At best, they are much weaker than are the TSTA of either chemically or virally induced tumors or the normal histocompatibility antigens, and not all investigators agree that they exist. Accordingly, such immunogenic fetal antigens have not been explored as markers for any human tumor.

3.3. Enzymes and Isoenzymes

These substances may be normal for the tissue in which the cancer originates (and thus be markers because an abnormal amount is produced) or be re-expressed from an earlier development period (and thus be a kind of oncodevelopmental antigen) or be expressed inappropriately either by the tumor or by normal tissue that has been altered by the tumor. Formerly, these substances were detected by methods that measured their enzymatic activity, but immunological methods are now available for several, increasing both sensitivity and specificity. Prostatic acid phosphatase is an example of this category and will be discussed further later in this chapter.

3.4. Major Histocompatibility Complex (MHC) Antigens

These antigens usually are thought of only in connection with transplantation, but they are becoming important to the study of tumor immunology also [6, 13–15]. Certain MHC types are associated with certain diseases (as in ankylosing spondylitis), and associations between an MHC type and cancer would thus implicate genetic factors in the pathogenesis of cancer. Second, the MHC in mice, and probably also in man, contains an Ir region, which influences the ability of the organism to respond immunologically to certain antigens. Because immune potential may be important in the human response to neoplasia, the Ir region could contain markers of susceptibility to cancer. Third, the MHC locus in mice (and, again, probably also in man) is linked to other genetic loci that are important in neoplasia. Finally, in virally induced animal tumors, recognition of TSTA by the immune system is 'MHC-restricted,' in that cytotoxic T lymphocytes will destroy only those tumor cells that both have been transformed by a virus to which the lymphocytes are sensitized and bear histocompatibility antigens identical to those on the T lymphocytes. It is not known whether this occurs in man also.

Mention should be made here of two recent observations about the MHC and cancer in man. First, among men with testicular tumors, more patients with teratocarcinoma have the MHC D-locus antigen HLA-Dw7 than would be expected by chance. This is reminiscent of the linkage between the murine MHC locus and the T region, which controls several features of development, including expression of the F9 antigen, which also is associated with murine teratocarcinoma [16]. Second, a study of MHC types in patients with renal cell carcinoma (RCC) suggested an association between this tumor and another locus, HLA-Dw5 [17]. These HLA types are too common to permit their use as markers for these tumors, but the findings have stimulated speculation about the pathogenesis of the tumors. To my knowledge, no HLA typing studies of patients with TCC or prostate cancer have been reported.

3.5. Serum Proteins

Some normally occurring serum proteins are altered by malignancy. Foremost among them are the acute-phase proteins, including a variety of alpha-1, alpha-2, and beta globulins such as haptoglobin, $alpha_1$-antitrypsin, $alpha_1$-acid glycoprotein, fibrinogen, seromucoid, ceruloplasmin, C-reactive protein, transferrin, and the C_2, C_3, and C_4 components of complement. As a rule, they have been of little use as cancer markers, because changes of similar type and magnitude often occur in inflammatory or degenerative disorders and benign tumors, but several have been or are claimed to be of some use in some genitourinary cancers (Table 1) [13].

Table 1. Possible markers of genitourinary cancer

Tumor	Marker	Mode *	Prevalence	Clinical utility
RCC	Renin	B	low	poor
	Erythropoietin	B	low	poor
	Polyamines	U	unknown	poor
	Cholesterol	B, T	high	undetermined
	hCG	B	low	poor
	GGT	U, T	low	undetermined
	Prostaglandins	T	low	poor
	Calcitonin	T	low	poor
	Parathormone	B, T	low	poor
	Glucagon	B	low	poor
	ACTH	B	low	poor
	Prolactin	B	low	poor
	Acute-phase proteins	B	high	poor
	CEA	B, U	high	poor
	LDH	U	low	poor
TCC	Blood-group antigens	T	high	good
	CEA	B, U	high	poor
	Polyamines	U	unknown	undetermined
	Beta-glucuronidase	U	unknown	poor
	Beta-aminoisobutyrate	U	unknown	poor
	Rheumatoid factor	B	high	poor
	Fibrin degradation products	U	high	undetermined
	hCG	B	low	poor
	Acute-phase proteins	U	high	poor
CAP	Prostatic acid phosphate	T, B	high	good
	Prostatic tissue-specific antigen	T, B	high	undetermined
	Hydroxyproline	U	high	undetermined
	CK-BB	B	high	poor (?)
	Cholesterol	U	high	poor
	LDH, C_3 + transferrin	T	high	undetermined
	CEA	B, U	high	poor
	Acute-phase proteins	B	unknown	poor
	Polyamines	U	unknown	undetermined
	Fibronectin	U	unknown	undetermined
TT	AFP	B, T	high	good
	hCG	B, T, U	high	good
	SP-1	B, T, U	high	good

Table 1. (cont.)

Tumor	Marker	Mode *	Prevalence	Clinical utility
	CEA	B, T	high	poor
	PlAP	B, T	high	undetermined
	Placental lactogen	T, B	low	poor
	SSEA-1	T	low	undetermined
	LDH	B	high	good
	Alpha-1-antitrypsin	B, T	high	poor
	Histocompatibility antigens	T, B	high	undetermined

* B : Blood
T : Tissue
U : Urine

3.6. *Markers of Rapid Growth or Membrane Leakage*

Increases in the amounts of the substances associated with rapid growth or membrane leakage would be expected to accompany cancer, because increased cell growth and destruction are hallmarks of the disease. Accordingly, some of these substances have been offered as cancer markers. For example, because the bases of tRNA are methylated only after the macromolecule has been assembled, increased levels of methylated nucleosides could be a measure of tRNA turnover. Indeed, increased levels of N,N-dimethylguanosine and 1-methylinosine have been found in the tumors, blood, and urine of patients with cancer. Also, pseudouridine (Ψ), another component of tRNA, which is not reutilized after tRNA breakdown, has been detected in patients with cancer. Finally, beta-aminoisobutyrate, a degradation product from the thymine of DNA, has been studied as a measure of the rate of cell turnover. However, the excretion varies among normal persons, presumably as a result of genetic factors, thereby compromising its usefulness as a marker. At present, none of the products of nucleic acid turnover has been established as a tumor marker in man, in part because of difficulties in measuring the amounts and defining the limits of normal [18–20]. The work done on them in genitourinary cancer is discussed further later in this chapter.

The polyamines, especially spermidine, spermine, and putrescine, are another example of something that appeared to be a promising tumor marker that so far has not been helpful. Polyamines are thought to be important in regulating the biosynthesis and functioning of the nucleic acids. Increased production is associated with increased protein synthesis, and because polyamines are not metabolized extensively, they can be detected in the urine, blood, and some tissues. Increased levels are present in tumors and in body fluids from cancer patients, but the levels also are increased during inflammation and tissue regeneration. Therefore, although polyamines have been helpful in the laboratory (rising levels may be the earliest sign of malignant transformation in carcinogen-treated tissues), they do not appear to be promising human tumor markers [18, 20].

Hydroxyproline, an amino acid found primarily in collagen, is concentrated in the skeleton (two-thirds of the body stores), and the amount excreted in the urine (especially when expressed as the hydroxyproline/creatinine ratio) can be a sensitive indicator of bony metastases. In some cases, this measure of bone matrix turnover can reveal metastases better than any other method, irrespective of the histologic type of the primary tumor [18].

3.7. Fibrin Degradation Products

These substances have received little attention as markers of human tumors except in bladder cancer. Their possible value arises from the frequent presence around a tumor of a rich extravascular fibrin network and from the tendency of tumor cells to leak cytoplasmic enzymes, among them plasminogen activator, thus increasing the level of fibrinolytic activity.

3.8. Fibronectin

This is a high-molecular-weight glycoprotein, found primarily on cell surfaces and in the blood, that is produced by many differentiated cells. It appears to assist in adhesion of cells to the extracellular matrix; in the circulation, it may serve as an opsonin, binding stray particles of fibrin or collagen for phagocytosis by the reticuloendothelial system. Transformed cells *in vitro* tend to lack surface fibronectin, and there are suggestions that the more malignant the cell, the less fibronectin it has. However, results of other studies do not support these conclusions. Preliminary results of studies of fibronectin as a tumor marker have not been encouraging, but they have suggested that there are different kinds of fibronectin that need to be explored [21, 22].

3.9. Surface Glycolipid and Glycoprotein Antigens

Many cell-surface components are glycosphingolipids or glycoproteins, and often the carbohydrate side chains are the antigenic determinants used to detect the entire molecule. Some of these components change in structure or amount during malignant transformation, making them potential tumor markers.

It is apparent that this category of tumor-related substances overlaps extensively with other categories. For example, most of the oncodevelopmental antigens, including CEA and AFP, are glycoproteins (although some are secretion products rather than cell-surface antigens). However, there are reasons to preserve it as a separate category. Implicit in it is the assumption that one is characterizing, not antigens that are unique to or which reappear on tumor cells, but rather those that arise from changes in the structure of normal cell-surface molecules. For example, there have been many studies of the alterations in the oligosaccharides of animal tumor-cell surfaces, although these have not yet provided information that can be exploited clinically [22].

An important group of 'normal' antigens that have been studied clinically is the blood-group (such as the ABO[H]) substances. These are genetically determined, carbohydrate-containing, polymorphic determinants associated with the glycoproteins and glycosphingolipids in body fluids and secretions and on cellular membranes. Like the MHC antigens, the blood-group antigens are alloantigens, and much of what is known about them has been learned with alloantisera and immunologic techniques. Several studies of blood-group antigens in human carcinomas showed an absence of host blood-group – especially ABH – reactivity on some tumor cells; accumulation of precursor substances such as the Lewis antigen, blood-group core structures, and T antigens of the MN blood group; and, in some tumors, the appearance of inappropriate blood-group substances. The extensive work on ABO antigens in TCC is reviewed in the section on that tumor.

3.10. Immune Complexes

After the failure to measure specific cell-mediated or humoral antitumor immunity reliably and consistently in man, several laboratories shifted their attention to the detection of circulating immune complexes. It is assumed (without much evidence) that these complexes consist of circulating immunogenic tumor-cell antigens combined with antibody. The assays most commonly used are the complement-binding assay (I^{125} CIq assay) and the Raji-cell-binding assay, both of which measure circulating immune complexes nonspecifically. Elevated levels have been reported in 40–70% of patients with tumors of the breast, lung, or colon or with gynecologic tumors, osteogenic sarcoma, melanoma, or neuroblastoma. Most of these studies included only patients with advanced disease, and, although there is some evidence that elevated immune complex levels are an adverse prognostic sign, the value of this measurement in clinical follow-up is not known. The evaluation is complicated by the fact that elevated levels of immune complexes are also found in patients with infections, inflammation, and autoimmune diseases [23]. To my knowledge, no one has studied the levels of circulating immune complexes in patients with genitourinary tumors.

4. MARKERS OF SPECIFIC GENITOURINARY TUMORS

The remaining discussion reviews the markers that have been evaluated most thoroughly in the common types of genitourinary cancer (Table 1). Nonetheless, in most instances, the information available is less than definitive. A reader of the literature can conclude either that further work needs to be done or, more likely, that later investigations revealed the marker to be of little value but that these results, like so many negative results, were never published. Indeed, the usual history of a 'tumor marker' is a burst of enthusiasm accompanied by many favorable data, followed by disillusionment. The explanation is that often too few patients are studied, the collection of sera is not sufficiently representative of the clinical spectrum of the disease, and, perhaps most important, the marker results are not placed in the proper clinical context. For example, a marker, no matter how well its levels reflect disease status and prognosis, is no good if it tells us only what we already know.

4.1. Renal Cell Carcinoma (RCC)

The kidney produces many things besides urine: polypeptides such as renin and erythropoietin, lipids such as prostaglandins, and steroids such as 1,25-dihydroxycholecalciferol. Predictably, these secretory products have been explored as tumor markers for RCC. For example, after several studies had shown elevated erythropoietin levels in only 5% of patients, a study with a bioassay found elevated levels in 63% of 57 patients [24]. They occurred most often in patients without erythrocytosis and did not appear to result from severe anemia. However, although the levels usually declined after the primary tumor was removed, the levels did not correlate well with the grade or stage of the disease. No sequential studies were included in this report, and the lack of further reports suggests that erythropoietin does not have great potential as a marker in RCC, although the more sensitive RIA now available perhaps should be applied more extensively before the substance is abandoned as a marker for this tumor.

Serum renin levels, as measured by RIA, were also elevated in 37% of the patients in this series, including many of those with elevated erythropoietin levels, and appeared to correlate with the stage of the disease and with the presence, although not the site, of metastases [24]. Surprisingly, elevated renin levels usually were seen in patients with normal blood pressure even though as a group they had low serum potassium levels (suggesting that the substance detected was an active form of renin and not a cross-reacting prohormone or other inactive form). The patients with elevated renin levels tended to do poorly. Again, no serial studies were reported, and the lack of other publications since this article was published in 1977 makes it difficult to conclude that renin is a clinically valuable marker for RCC.

In some cases, RCC is associated with hypercalcemia. This may result from the bony metastases that often occur in this disease, in which case alkaline phosphatase and other usual markers of bony metastasis are useful tumor markers. However, as in certain other cancers, RCC can be associated with hypercalcemia in the absence of bony metastases. Usually, these tumors are found to produce any of a variety of substances that influence calcium metabolism, such as parathormone, prostaglandins, osteoclast-activating factor, or calcitonin. Parathormone and prostaglandins E and F have been found in the serum of patients with RCC and in the tumors and cells cultured from them. Although these substances have not been evaluated thoroughly as markers, in most cases the serum calcium level probably is a sufficient marker [25–27].

Several years ago, studies were made of CEA in the serum and urine of patients with RCC. Elevated levels were found in 40–60%, with the higher prevalences in patients with metastatic disease [28, 29]. However, some patients who were free of disease also had elevated levels, and the few serial studies did not indicate much usefulness. Again, the absence of further reports makes one suspect that this oncodevelopmental antigen is not of great value in RCC with the methods now available.

The enzyme gamma-glutamyltranspeptidase (GGT) is present in considerable amounts in normal kidney tissue and can be detected in the urine. In a preliminary study, the urine and renal tissue levels were found to be decreased in patients with RCC in comparison with those who had other renal diseases [30]. More recent work has revealed apparent tumor-associated isoenzymes of GGT in liver cancer and RCC [31, 32]. Attempts are being made to purify and characterize these isoenzymes; the work is aided by the fact that a human RCC cell line produces the renal form. This work is still too basic for clinical studies to be made.

One histological hallmark of many RCCs is their clear-cell appearance, which reflects their accumulation of lipids, particularly cholesterol, apparently as the result of improperly regulated synthesis and transport [33–35]. Efforts are being made to translate this knowledge into markers or other staging methods, so far without success. For example, arterial-venous cholesterol gradients have not been useful in locating metastases, nor have attempts at radioimmunodetection with radiolabelled cholesterol (Ralph V. Clayman, personal communication). The primary difficulty with the latter is that RCCs take up very little cholesterol from their surroundings. However, other possibilities remain to be explored, and the cholesterol metabolism of RCC may yet be exploitable either in diagnosis or in treatment.

Several other substances have been discovered in patients with RCC, usually as the result of an unusual clinical presentation. For example, prolactin was found in cultured RCC cells from a patient with galactorrhea, ACTH in several patients with Cushing's syndrome, glucagon in a patient suffering from enteropathy, and hCG in patients with gynecomastia. In our experience and that of others [25] hCG is not prevalent in patients with RCC, nor is it useful in serial studies. Urinary polyamines were found to be elevated in nine of eleven patients and of clinical value in two of these [36], and other investigators also have said they are a useful marker [37]. However, as I mentioned earlier, many people have studied polyamines as tumor markers with disappointing results, and the difficulty of measuring them makes it even less likely that they will become useful markers of RCC.

For the sake of completeness, mention should be made of some other substances reported to be markers for RCC. First, the acute-phase proteins haptoglobin and alpha-2-globulin have been reported in patients with RCC and, in the case of the latter particularly, have been claimed to be useful prognostically. In my opinion, the record of these substances in other cancers suggests that they are of doubtful value. Also, fibrin degradation products have been found in the serum and urine of patients with RCC, but nothing further has been reported for several years. Finally, lactate dehydrogenase (LDH) and alkaline phosphatase, as measured in specially processed urine specimens, appear to be elevated in some RCC patients, but this probably is an epiphenomenon and does not indicate their value as markers [38–40].

4.2. Transitional Cell Carcinoma (TCC)

Transitional cell carcinoma is an unusual cancer in that its clinical spectrum encompasses several stages, each of which can contain tumors in various grades, with most of the low-stage low-grade tumors recurring, often in more invasive form. The difficulty this causes urologists is well known and has encouraged a search for ways to predict the behavior of low-stage tumors.

Normal urothelium is rich in ABH blood-group antigens, and some time ago it was suggested that the presence or absence of these substances on TCC might have prognostic value [41–43]. Specifically, it was postulated that patients whose low-stage TCC retain their blood-group antigens have a good prognosis, whereas those whose tumors lose their reactivity are likely to have recurrences in a higher stage. Testing of this hypothesis has been facilitated by the fact that there are easily applicable immunological methods, such as the red-cell adherence (RCA) assay, that can detect ABH antigens even on tissue that was formalin-fixed and paraffin-embedded many years ago. Such retrospective studies have lent support to the hypothesis (Table 2) [44–48]. Of particular significance is the finding that when ABH

Table 2. Prediction of invasiveness of TCC by blood-group antigen

Reference	(BGAg) status		
	Invasion		% Predicted correctly
	BGAg +	BGAg −	
42	0/13	8/9	95
44	1/8	8/20	54
45	0/9	5/7	88
46	0/15	9/15	80
47	9/223	71/99	89
48	4/34	30/47	74
Total	14/302 (5%)	131/197 (66%)	84

reactivity is analyzed in tandem with the histologic grade, the ABH study provides additional information. (In other words, ABH reactivity is a function of something other than histologic grade.) In our experience, this is especially true for grade II and grade III tumors. For example, in our series, among the (rare) low-stage, grade III lesions, the ABH-negative tumors almost always became invasive later, whereas if the tumor was ABH-positive the risk of invasion was only 20%. (Of course, analysis of many more cases is required to establish the validity of these numbers.) Another important point is that sequential ABH analysis of recurring bladder tumors appears to provide additional prognostic information.

Unfortunately, several problems make widespread clinical application of ABH analysis inappropriate at present [49]. First, the RCA assay is cumbersome and subjective, and, although the results are reproducible, this requires considerable expertise. Thus, it is difficult to standardize, especially among laboratories in different institutions. Second, some apparently normal urothelium does not react well for ABH antigens; the frequency of these 'false negatives' differs greatly among laboratories. In our experience, it is most common among patients with blood group O (i.e., the H antigen). If these problems are to be solved – and this brings us to the third difficulty – the mechanism of ABH loss must be determined; at present, it is but poorly understood.

Our laboratories have been trying to unravel the mechanism of ABH loss, with results that will only be summarized here [50, 51]. First, fresh-frozen tissue, both normal urothelium and, especially, TCC, sometimes reacts positively for ABH antigens before fixation and negatively afterward. Thus, the method of tissue fixation, especially exposure to alcohol, appears to affect the results. Second, the loss of ABH reactivity apparently does not result from masking of the antigens by sialic acids, as has been proposed for some tumor-associated antigens. Third, ABH loss is quantitative, so that there is a range of detectability among normal tissues and TCC, with the latter, as a group, having less reactivity. Factors other than malignant transformation undoubtedly influence the extent of reactivity. For example, our preliminary evidence shows that the patient's secretor status (whether he or she is genetically disposed to release blood-group substances into the internal secretions) affects the results [51]. Fourth, the loss of antigen backtracks along the biosynthetic pathway for blood-groups substances, with the A and B substances being lost first, then H, and finally the precursor substances. Thus, patients with blood-groups A, B, or AB whose tumors have 'lost' their blood-group antigen often paradoxically show increased reactivity for the H antigen. These results suggest a biosynthetic defect such as aberrant transferase or glycosidase enzymes.

Clearly, then, much remains to be learned about blood-group reactivity in TCC. In particular, the enormous amount of work done on blood-group-related glycolipids and glycosphingolipids on cancer-cell surfaces is only now being applied to TCC. Also, there is promise of new techniques for measuring tissue ABH reactivity that may solve some of the problems of the RCA assay [52]. We are confident that ABH analysis will be applied routinely in the near future to assist in the management of patients with low-stage TCC.

Other putative tumor markers for TCC are listed in Table 1. Most have not fulfilled their early promise. For example, CEA (or CEA-like substances) have been found in bladder tumors but not in normal urothelium, and it was suggested that CEA was a useful marker, especially for high-stage disease [53]. In later studies, measurements of CEA in urine and serum did not prove helpful in screening for TCC, in evaluating patients with hematuria, or in follow-up of most patients with known TCC [54, 55]. However, in some patients, particularly those with initially high-stage TCC who may have persistent tumor after potentially curative treatment, serial CEA measurements may be helpful [53, 56]. Exploration of the value of CEA in such patients is complicated by the fact that levels are elevated in infected urine and in urine from bowel conduits [53]. As mentioned earlier, better CEA assays and greater understanding of the forms of this marker are needed before the place, if any, of CEA can be determined.

Urinary polyamines have received little attention in TCC, in part because of the difficulties in measuring them and of the large numbers of false-positive results found in other cancers. However, they may be of value, especially as a predictor of recurrence [20, 37]. Urinary fibrin degradation products appear to correlate with disease activity, although there is a false-negative rate of 23%. Significantly, when the data are combined with the results of urinary cytology, further information is obtained. In 30 patients with negative cytology and normal levels of fibrin degradation products, 93% were free of tumor, whereas in the 14 patients in whom both studies were positive 86% had TCC [57]. Both of these possible markers require further work before they can be recommended for clinical use.

Another substance that may help predict recurrence is beta-aminoisobutyrate (BAIB), a breakdown product of thymine. Levels have been found to be significantly elevated, independent of genetic factors, in the urine of patients with invasive bladder tumors in comparison with levels in persons free of disease or with noninvasive tumors. The size of the elevation appears to be related to the histologic grade. Recurrences often are preceded by a fall in BAIB excretion; if the BAIB level is low and the pseudouridine (ψ) level is high, recurrences can be expected in 70% of cases [20]. However, BAIB does not appear to be useful in screening for bladder cancer.

Several investigators have reported finding beta-glucuronidase in urine from patients with TCC or bilharzial disease and in TCC tissue. However, as it also is found in the urine of patients with urinary tract infections, its value as a tumor marker is doubtful [58].

Rheumatoid factor was detected in 29 of 47 patients with either squamous cell carcinoma or TCC of the bladder but in none of 44 patients with nonmalignant bladder diseases [59, 60]. However, the titers were low, and rheumatoid factor is found in many normal persons, especially among the elderly, and in some patients with other malignancies. Because rheumatoid factor is essentially an IgM antibody against immunoglobulin, it is probably a response to the circulating immune complexes that appear to be common among cancer patients, as previously indicated. To my knowledge, the circulating immune complexes themselves have not been measured directly in bladder cancer patients with the better, recent methods such as CIq or Raji-cell-binding assays.

Several groups of investigators, particularly Monaco and his associates, have attempted to discover bladder-cancer-associated antigens with xenogeneic antisera against partially purified bladder-tumor tissue or urine from TCC patients [61–63]. To date, the antibodies produced react with materials from a majority of patients with TCC, thereby advancing the hope that such antibodies might be useful in diagnosis. However, these antibodies also react with materials from almost half the patients with urinary tract infections. The same lack of specificity has plagued studies by this same group on acute-phase proteins, including transferrin, alpha-2-macroglobulin, orosomucoid, plasminogen, haptoglobin, and immunoglobulin. Although these proteins are not common in urine from normal persons, they are very often found in those with urinary tract infections, suggesting that they are not useful markers.

Finally, a word should be said about the role of oncodevelopmental proteins in bladder cancer. There are reports that the hCG level is elevated in patients with TCC [64], but our experience is that this is rare and of no clinical significance. There are no reports of elevated AFP levels. These data, together with the studies on CEA mentioned previously, suggest that oncodevelopmental proteins will not be useful clinically in TCC.

4.3. Carcinoma of the Prostate (CAP)

More than 40 years ago, acid phosphatase was established as a valuable marker for metastatic CAP. Assays that measured its enzymatic activity showed elevated levels in 60–70% of patients with bony metastases but in only 10–20% of patients with apparently localized (stages A-B and C) disease. (It is believed that these few patients probably have unrecognized spread through the prostatic capsule or into regional pelvic lymph nodes.) No fully satisfactory explanation has been given of the association of elevated acid phosphatase levels with metastatic disease only. Presumably, the arrangement of the enzyme-rich prostatic tissue normally permits leakage of such small amounts that blood levels remain below the limit of sensitivity of the enzymatic assays. Thus, elevated levels occur only when malignant tissue appears in well-perfused (but abnormal) sites such as bony metastases or destroys the normal anatomic barriers around the prostate, such as in extensive stage C disease. The normal serum acid phosphatase levels that are sometimes seen in patients with extensive metastatic disease result because the cancer has largely lost its ability to synthesize acid phosphatase. Thus, false-negative results are usually associated with anaplastic tumors.

There have been many efforts to refine the acid phosphatase marker. The enzyme exists in several isoenzymatic forms throughout the body, and investigators tried to create an assay that would measure only the activity of the prostatic isoenzyme(s). The first attempts made use of 'specific' inhibitors such as L-tartrate. Unfortunately, these methodological variations on the enzymatic assay were neither sufficiently specific nor significantly valuable [65–68].

More successful are the assays that take advantage of the structural differences between prostatic acid phosphatase (PAP) and other acid phosphatases and of PAP's antigenicity in other species. These immunologic assays are more specific for PAP, detect smaller amounts of it (are more sensitive), and allow more latitude in specimen collection, because there is no need to be concerned about loss of enzymatic activity. Today, energized in part by clinical overoptimism and by the commercial potential of a CAP assay, there is a plethora of data on many different RIAs for PAP, causing much confusion and uncertainty. Because there are several recent discussions of the state-of-the-art of RIA for PAP [65–69], and because the field is changing so rapidly, only a summary is warranted here.

First, the RIAs have made sample collection easier and more reliable. Second, they are indeed more sensitive than are enzymatic ones. In patients with obvious bony metastases, the sensitivity has increased from 60–80% with enzymatic assays to 95% with RIAs. However, the initial belief of Foti and coworkers that the RIAs would make it possible to detect localized disease (stages A and B) has been tempered by later findings. The RIAs identify only 8–44% of the cases of localized CAP. (The wide range results from differences in the assays – widely differing sources of antigens and purification methods – in the population of patients studied, and, especially, in the criteria used in staging, particularly whether pelvic lymphadenectomy was used and, if so, how extensive the operation was.) Nevertheless, even with the most thorough and precise staging methods, some patients with apparently localized disease do indeed have elevated PAP levels by RIA. Whether they truly have localized disease or, as is suspected with the older enzymatic assays, there are still-undiscovered metastases cannot be determined without studies on the patients' fates. Third, the increased sensitivity of the RIA unfortunately has also brought decreased specificity. The false-positive rate is at least 8% in patients with benign prostatic hyperplasia. Fourth, despite the large numbers of men with CAP, it is such an uncommon disease that the positive predictive value of RIA for PAP will be approximately 7% only, even in men older than 50. This calculation militates against the use of this assay in screening, even in such selected populations as patients with prostatic induration on rectal examination. Fifth, enzymatic determinations of PAP in bone-marrow aspirates failed as a useful method of detecting early bony metastases because there were too many false-positive results. However, RIAs have increased the specificity and promise to make this approach a significant prognostic, and possibly staging, tool, despite the rare false-positive results [65, 66].

In summary, then, newer methods of measuring PAP, especially RIA, have been a significant methodological, if not yet clinical, advance. Further refinements, such as enzyme-linked immunosorbent assays (ELISA), will undoubtedly simplify PAP analysis and probably increase the sensitivity and specificity as well. For a time, this increased specificity will confound clinicians, especially in the management of apparently localized CAP, but eventually these new assays will improve clinical management as the data accumulate showing us how to use them.

Some other possible markers of CAP deserve comment. Recently, a prostatic tissue-specific antigen, called PA, was isolated that is distinct from PAP. Sensitive assays indicate that it is indeed specific to normal and tumorous prostate and is found only in men with benign prostatic hyperplasia or CAP. In the latter, the amount and the frequency of elevated levels increase with advancing stage. The place of this marker in clinical management is being studied [70].

The BB isoenzyme of creatine kinase (CK-BB) also has been proposed as a CAP marker. Several studies show that it is elevated in at least half of patients with advanced disease but only rarely in those with localized disease, that levels correlate with PAP levels (by RIA) and with the clinical course, that combining CK-BB and PAP (RIA) data reduces the number of false-positive PAP results, and that CK-BB levels are elevated occasionally in other malignant diseases. Experience to date has not demonstrated that knowledge of CK-BB serum levels contributes any unique clinical information, but more study appears appropriate [71–73].

Urinary levels of hydroxyproline, a collagen constituent, are a sensitive index of bone matrix turnover and of bony metastases from lung and breast cancers. In CAP, elevated levels occur primarily in untreated patients with bony metastases; changes in the levels are said to reflect the clinical course [74, 75]. However, measurement is cumbersome, and evidence that hydroxyproline excretion levels add anything to data from bone scintigraphy and serum PAP assays is still anecdotal.

Urinary levels of total cholesterol and nonesterified cholesterol have been suggested as a marker for CAP. Levels are elevated in 45–50% of patients in all stages, regardless of the histologic grade of the tumor, and in most patients with elevated PAP levels (by enzymatic assay). However, elevated levels are also found in many patients with benign prostatic hyperplasia who have large residual urine volumes and in some patients with germ-cell tumors or RCC [76, 77]. Although the value of cholesterol levels in screening for CAP has not been assessed, it is not likely to be great.

Doctor Grayhack and his associates have evidence suggesting that substances in prostatic fluid (obtained by massage) may be useful markers for CAP. These workers discovered that the ratio of LDH isoenzymes 5 and 1 (LDH 5/LDH 1) is greater than 2 in 80% of patients with CAP, although many men with prostatitis also have high ratios. Fluid from cancer patients also has high levels of C_3, C_4, and transferrin. In these men, 90% have both abnormal LDH ratios and elevated C_3 and transferrin levels, whereas this is true in only 17% of men with prostatitis. Such data suggest that prostatic fluid markers may be useful in the diagnosis of CAP.

Two oncodevelopmental proteins have been mentioned in connection with CAP. Elevated serum CEA levels are present in 25–60% of patients [79], and a cross-reacting CEA-like substance is produced by cultured cells from normal, hyperplastic, and cancerous prostates that may be tissue-specific [80, 81]. Nevertheless, the reports of the clinical utility of CEA are conflicting, although Kane *et al.* indicate that it is superior to PAP in monitoring patients with advanced disease [79]. There is one report of elevated serum hCG levels [82], but in our experience this is too rare to be useful. Urinary fibronectin levels may be elevated, especially in repeated determinations, and wide fluctuations in the levels have been observed in serial studies. The cause, presumably, is fibrinolytic release of material from the fibrin network that supports tumor growth and vascularization [83]. Finally, elevations in several acute-phase proteins, including haptoglobin, alpha-acid glycoprotein, and immunoglobulin, and in urinary polyamines have been reported [40, 84]. To date, none of these findings has produced a useful marker.

4.4. Testicular Cancer

Tumor markers have achieved clinical fruition in testicular cancer as in no other genitourinary (or indeed any other) cancer, primarily as the result of the introduction of sensitive RIAs for the two substances, AFP and hCG. This subject has been reviewed extensively [85–88]; I will mention only the most salient points.

1. In patients with nonseminomatous testicular cancer (NSTC), AFP levels are elevated in approximately 60% and hCG levels in approximately 50% when RIAs are used. However, these figures vary considerably with the stage of the tumor and the clinical situation. For example, various other diseases, benign and malignant, can raise the level of one or the other of the markers and would have to be ruled out. However, in practice this is not a problem, and AFP and hCG prove very specific in patients who have or who might have a testicular cancer.

2. Markers can be helpful in diagnosis and staging, but they cannot substitute for radiographic and operative evaluation. For example, in a man with an intrascrotal mass, markers are useful in differential diagnosis only if the levels are abnormal, because normal levels are found in most patients with seminoma and in at least 40% of those with Stage I nonseminomatous tumors. Also, at least 40% of men with only microscopic retroperitoneal metastases from NSTC have normal marker levels before lymphadenectomy.

3. Both markers must be measured throughout the clinical course. They are produced by different types of tumor cells, and discordance is often seen at some point.

4. There are no false-positive results (elevated marker levels in a patient free of tumor), providing other diseases have been ruled out and two caveats are remembered. First, the metabolic half-life must be considered. An elevated AFP level obtained two days after orchiectomy could represent either residual marker produced by the primary tumor that has not been metabolically cleared or marker synthesized by metastases. Second, even the best

beta-hCG assays have some cross-reactivity with high levels of luteinizing hormone. Slight elevations of the hCG level in testicular cancer patients thus must be regarded with suspicion, as these men are prone to high luteinizing-hormone levels because of hypogonadism.

5. The most valuable use of the markers undoubtedly is in the follow-up of initial treatments and the monitoring of chemotherapy. Often, changes in marker levels presage clinical events. Because there have been no true false-positive results, many oncologists now begin or continue chemotherapy for NSTC solely on the basis of elevated marker levels, especially if pathologic confirmation would require a major operation. Also, when persistently normal marker levels occur in the presence of stable or growing masses in Stage III disease, the diagnosis may be benign disease, mature teratoma, or seminoma, especially in previously treated patients. False-negative marker levels do occur in Stage III disease, however, so a biopsy is necessary. (In our series, the frequency of normal marker levels in patients with untreated Stage III NSTC is approximately 10%).

During chemotherapy, marker levels often become normal quickly (*vide infra*), but of course this does not mean that chemotherapy should be stopped. Even when the initial chemotherapy courses are completed, patients who have cytoreductive operations to remove residual masses that are found to contain viable NSTC have normal marker levels approximately half the time.

Newer methods of using AFP and hCG data are being introduced into the management of testicular cancer. For example, the rate of decline of a marker level during treatment, particularly with chemotherapy, appears to have prognostic significance. Our preliminary data suggest that patients with long actual marker half-lives (AHL), that is, slower-than-normal rates of marker decay, usually do not respond completely to chemotherapy, even if the marker levels become normal temporarily, whereas patients with shorter AHLs usually do respond completely [89]. Significantly, this determination can be made within the first month [89, 90]. Another new application is a more sensitive hCG assay. Because this marker is excreted primarily in the urine, concentrating techniques and a specialized assay can be used to achieve a level of sensitivity at least 20 times greater than heretofore possible with RIAs for serum levels. Preliminary evidence suggests that this increased sensitivity can be helpful in defining complete responses to chemotherapy and in the early detection of relapses [91].

Another promising new use of markers is in radioimmunodetection. The method involves injection of radiolabelled antimarker antibody, which concentrates in the tumor, and the detection of these areas of label with sophisticated imaging and subtraction techniques. Goldenberg and his associates have detected metastatic testicular tumor, including, in some instances, deposits not detectable by other noninvasive techniques, with both anti-AFP and anti-hCG, even in few patients with normal marker levels [92–94].

Tumor markers have been traced to their cells of origin with histochemical techniques such as immunofluorescence and immunoperoxidase staining. hCG is found in the syncytiotrophoblastic cells of NSTC and (occasionally) seminoma and AFP in the yolk sac elements and a few embryonal carcinoma cells not identifiable as yolk sac cells [95]. This has been of considerable interest to those studying the pathogenesis of testicular tumors, and it has been claimed that new classifications will result from this work, although to date the discussions have not produced clinically relevant changes.

Elevated marker levels occur also in patients considered to have pure seminoma. All available data indicate that if the level of AFP is elevated, the patient in fact has NSTC, either in the primary tumor or in metastases. The meaning of elevated hCG levels is less clear. They may signal the presence of NSTC, either at the time or soon thereafter, but abundant clinical and pathologic evidence shows that they may accompany pure seminoma also and that the levels can be greater than 100 ng/ml. The clinical significance of hCG is seminoma is the subject of fierce debate. Our data suggest that low-stage seminomas that produce hCG respond well to conventional therapy whereas high-stage ones do not but will respond to present chemotherapy for NSTC [96]. Whether the production of hCG by a seminoma is an independent sign of a radiation-resistant seminoma is unclear, as failures with radiation have been seen primarily in high-stage tumors, which may be unresponsive even if they do not produce hCG.

Other markers for testicular cancer are becoming important: SP-1, placental alkaline phosphatase (PlAP), and lactate dehydrogenase (LDH). SP-1 is a placental protein, unrelated to the other markers, which is present in high concentrations in the human placenta, the serum of pregnant women, and the serum of 80–100% of women with gestational choriocarcinoma. Elevations have been reported in the serum of men with testicular cancer [97, 98], and histochemical staining shows that SP-1 is produced by cells similar to those that produce hCG [99]. We showed that approximately 40% of men with active testicular cancer have elevated SP-1 levels, that these are not found in men whose cancers are believed to be cured, and that, although SP-1 levels usually parallel hCG levels, sometimes they provide clinically useful information not available from AFP and hCG determinations [100]. More study is needed before SP-1 is recommended for routine use, however, particularly on the definition of the upper limit of normal.

Placental alkaline phosphatase is an oncodevelopmental enzyme found in the placenta and serum and associated occasionally with various cancers, including those of the testicle. It is sometimes called the Regan isoenzyme. Elevated levels have been found in many patients with testicular cancer, especially those with seminoma, but false-positive results were common [101], and until recently there was no evidence that PlAP was clinically useful. However, our recent study with a new ELISA [102] suggests that PlAP may become a valuable marker for seminoma [103].

Lactate dehydrogenase is, of course, not specific for testicular cancer. However, we have found it useful in some circumstances, particularly in patients with advanced disease. Occasionally, the LDH levels are elevated in patients with active NSTC who have normal levels of both AFP and hCG [104]. We do not have as much faith in LDH as we do in AFP and hCG and would not begin chemotherapy solely on the basis of a rising LDH level, but LDH can be an effective early-warning system.

5. THE FUTURE

The promise of tumor markers has been talked about for many years, but the next decade does indeed appear especially bright. The reason is the new hybridoma technology for producing monoclonal antibodies. Fusion of immunized lymphocytes and immunoglobulin-producing cells can yield a host of hybrid 'cells' capable of producing only one antibody each. Subsequent cloning results in cell lines (hybridomas) that produce truly monoclonal antibodies [105]. Hybridomas can be developed against individual components of complex immunogens such as cell membranes, permitting their identification, and monoclonal antibodies against some apparent human TAA have been reported already. Several monoclonal antibodies against the proteins unique to genitourinary tumors can be expected soon for clinical testing as serum and tissue markers and in radioimmunodetection. Tumor markers will then truly come of age.

REFERENCES

1. Hill BT: Cancer chemotherapy: the relevance of certain concepts of cell cycle kinetics. Biochim Biophys Acta 516:389–417, 1978.
2. Husband J: Diagnostic techniques: their strengths and weaknesses. Br J Cancer 41 (Suppl 4):21–9, 1980.
3. Yoshimoto Y, Wolfsen AR, Odell WD: Glycosylation, a variable in the production of hCG by cancers. Am J Med 67:414–20, 1979.
4. Lange PH: Immunologic testing of patients with genitourinary malignancies. Urol Clin North Am 6:587–97, 1979.
5. Watson RA, Tang DB: The predictive value of prostatic acid phosphatase as a screening test for prostatic cancer. N Engl J Med 303:497–9, 1980.

6. Lange PH: Tumor immunology: a review of basic concepts with special reference to bladder cancer. American Urological Association Monogr 1:119–32, 1982.
7. Benacerraf B, Unanue ER. Tumor immunology. In: Textbook of Immunology. (Benacerraf B, ed.) Baltimore: Williams & Wilkins, 1979, pp. 196–213.
8. Old LJ: Cancer immunology: the search for specificity. Cancer Res 41:361–75, 1981.
9. Gold P, Freedman SO: Specific carcinoembryonic antigens of the human digestive system. J Exp Med 122:467–81, 1965.
10. Fuks A, Shuster J, Gold P: Theoretical and practical consideration of the utility of the radioimmunoassay for carcinoembryonic antigen (CEA) in clinical medicine. In: Cancer Markers: Developmental and Diagnostic Significance. (Sell S, ed) Clifton, NJ: Humana Press, 1980, pp. 315–27.
11. Shively JE, Todd CW. Carcinoembryonic antigen A: chemistry and biology. In: Cancer Markers: Developmental and Diagnostic Significance. (Sell S, ed.) Clifton, NJ: Humana Press, 1980, pp. 295–314.
12. Chism SE: Oncofetal transplantation antigens. In: Cancer Markers: Developmental and Diagnostic Significance. (Sell S, ed.) Clifton, NJ: Humana Press, pp. 115–32.
13. Benacerraf B, Unanue ER. Transplantation in Biology. In: Textbook of Immunology. (Benacerraf B, ed.) Baltimore: Williams & Wilkins, 1979, pp. 125–54.
14. Forman J: Antigens and the major histocompatibility complex. In: Cancer Markers: Developmental and Diagnostic Significance (Sell S, ed.) Clifton, NJ: Humana Press, 1980, pp. 133–68.
15. McDevitt HO: Regulation of the immune response by the major histocompatibility system. N Engl J Med 303:1514–7, 1980.
16. DeWolf WC, Lange PH, Einarson ME, Yunis EJ: HLA and testicular cancer. Nature 277:216–7, 1979.
17. DeWolf WC, Lange PH, Shepherd R, Martin-Alosco S, Yunis EJ: Association of HLA and renal cell carcinoma. Hum Immunol 2:41–4, 1981.
18. Neville AM, Cooper EH: Biochemical monitoring of cancer: a review. Ann Clin Biochem 13:283–305, 1976.
19. Borek E: Transfer RNA and its by-products as tumor markers. In: Cancer Markers: Developmental and Diagnostic Significance (Sell S, ed.) Clifton, NJ: Humana Press, 1980, pp. 445–62.
20. Irving CC: Biochemically detectable tumor markers in the urine of bladder cancer patients. Cancer Res 37:2872–4, 1977.
21. Ruoslahti E, Hayman EG, Engvall E: Fibronectin. In: Cancer Markers: Developmental and Diagnostic Significance (Sell S, ed.) Clifton, NJ: Humana Press, 1980, pp. 485–506.
22. Yogeeswaran G: Surface glycolipid and glycoprotein antigens. In: Cancer Markers: Developmental and Diagnostic Significance (Sell S, ed.) Clifton, NJ: Humana Press, 1980, pp. 371–402.
23. Baldwin EW, Robins RA: Circulating immune complexes in cancer. In: Cancer Markers: Developmental and Diagnostic Significance (Sell S, ed.) Clifton, NJ: Humana Press, 1980, pp. 507–31.
24. Sufrin G, Mirand EA, Moore RH, Chu TM, Murphy GP: Hormones in renal cancer. J Urol 117:433–8, 1977.
25. Marshall FF, Walsh PC: Extrarenal manifestations of renal cell carcinoma. J Urol 117:439–40, 1977.
26. Lubensky JD, Gangai MP: The hypercalcemia of genitourinary malignancy. J Urol 121:259–61, 1979.
27. Cummings KB, Robertson RP: Prostaglandin: increased production by renal cell carcinoma. J Urol 118:720–3, 1977.

28. Chu TM, Skulka SK, Mittleman AO, Murphy GP: Plasma carcinoembryonic antigen in renal cell carcinoma patients. J Urol 111:742–4, 1974.
29. Guinan PD, Ablin RJ, Dubin A, Nourkayham S, Bush IM: Carcinoembryonic antigen test in renal cell carcinoma. Urology 5:185–7, 1975.
30. Hautmann R, Kisters R, Lutzeyer W: Diagnosis of renal tumor by gamma-glutamyltranspeptidase (EC 2.3.2.2). Urology 7:12–6, 1976.
31. Hada T, Hagashino K, Yamamoto H *et al.*: The presence of novel gamma-glutamyltranspeptidase in newly established cell line from human renal cell carcinoma OUR-10. Surrey, UK: Int Soc Oncodev Biol Med, 7th Annual Meeting, 1979.
32. Veith F, Page M, Marceau N: Gamma-glutamyltranspeptidase isoenzyme in human hypernephromas. Surrey, UK: Int Soc Oncodev Biol Med, 7th Annual Meeting, 1979.
33. Clayman RV, Gonzalez R, Elliott AY, Dempsey ME: Differences in cholesterol transport by normal and malignant human kidney cells. Biochem Biophys Res Comm 92:1355–61, 1980.
34. Gonzalez R, Goldberg ME: Origins of intracellular cholesterol in renal-cell carcinoma. Lancet 1:912, 1977.
35. Clayman RV, Gonzalez R, Elliott AY, Gleason DE, Dempsey ME: Cholesterol uptake in heterotransplanted human renal cell cancer. (submitted).
36. Sanford EJ, Drago JR, Rohner TJ, Kessler GF, Sheehan L, Lipton A: Preliminary evaluation of urinary polyamines in the diagnosis of genitourinary tract malignancy. J Urol 113:218–21, 1975.
37. Milano G, Schneider M, Cassuto J-P *et al.*: Polyamines: comments on clinical utility in cancer: a review. Tumordiagnostik 3:121–5, 1980.
38. de Iriarte EG, Lopez Garcia JA, Hidalgo L, Mendoza M, Martinez-Pineiro JA: L'alpha-2 globuline: un marqueur biologique potentiel dans le cancer du rein? Ann Urol (Paris) 13:102–5, 1979.
39. Grubb W, Drylie DM, Cade R, Fuller TJ: Reversible systemic abnormalities associated with renal cell carcinoma. Urology 9:269–72, 1977.
40. Wahren B: Tumour markers in urology: aids in cancer diagnosis and management. Urol Res 7:57–67, 1979.
41. Kovarik S, Davidsohn I, Strjskal R: ABO antigens in cancer: detection with the mixed cell agglutination reaction. Arch Pathol 86:12–21, 1968
42. DeCenzo JM, Howard P, Irish CE: Antigenic deletion and prognosis of patients with stage A transitional cell bladder carcinoma. J Urol 114:874–8, 1975.
43. Lange PH, Limas C, Fraley EE: Tissue blood-group antigens and prognosis in low stage transitional cell carcinoma of the bladder. J Urol 119:52–5, 1978.
44. Emmott RC, Javadpour N, Bergman SM, Soares T: Correlation of the cell surface antigens with stage and grade in cancer of the bladder. J Urol 121:37–9, 1979.
45. Richie JP, Blute RD Jr, Waisman J: Immunologic indicators of prognosis in bladder cancer: the importance of cell surface antigens. J Urol 123:22–4, 1980.
46. Johnson JD, Lamm DL: Prediction of bladder tumor invasion with the mixed cell agglutination test. J Urol 123:25–8, 1980.
47. Newman AJ Jr, Carlton CE Jr, Johnson S: Cell surface A, B or (O)H blood group antigens as an indicator of malignant potential in stage A bladder carcinoma. J Urol 124:27–9, 1980.
48. Limas C, Lange PH: Reactivity of transitional cell carcinoma of the urinary bladder for A, B, H isoantigens: its prognostic significance. In: Tumor Progression, (Crispen RG, ed.) Amsterdam: Elsevier/North-Holland Biomedical Press, 1980, pp. 101–23.
49. Lange PH, Limas C: Tissue blood-group antigen testing in transitional cell carcinoma of the bladder. J Urol 124:304, 1980.

50. Limas C, Lange PH: Altered reactivity for A, B, H antigens in transitional cell carcinomas of the urinary bladder: a study of the mechanisms involved. Cancer 46:1366–73, 1980.
51. Limas C, Lange PH: A, B, H antigen detectability in normal and neoplastic urothelium: influence of methodological factors. Cancer (in press).
52. Weinstein RS, Coon J, Alroy J, Davidsohn I: Detection and significance of tissue-associated blood group antigens (ABH(O)) in human carcinomas. In: Diagnostic Immunology. (DeLellis RA, Stenberg SS, eds). New York: Masson Publishing (in press).
53. Zimmerman R, Wahren B, Edsmyr F: Assessment of serial CEA determinations in urine of patients with bladder carcinoma. Cancer 46:1802–9, 1980.
54. Turner AG, Carter S, Higgins E, Glashan RW, Neville AM: The clinical diagnostic value of carcinoembryonic antigen (CEA) in haematuria. Br J Urol 49:61–6, 1977.
55. Murphy WM, Vandevoorde JP, Rao MK, Soloway MS: The clinical value of urinary carcinoembryonic antigen-like substances in urothelial cancer. J Urol 118:806–8, 1977.
56. Ørjasaeter H, Fossa SD, Schjølseth SA, Fjaestad K. Carcinoembryonic antigen (CEA) in plasma of patients with carcinoma of the bladder/urethra. Cancer 42:287–95, 1978.
57. Wajsman Z, Merrin CE, Chu TM, Moore RH, Murphy GP. Evaluation of biological markers in bladder cancer. J Urol 114:879–83, 1975.
58. Javadpour N: Tumor markers in urologic cancer. Urology 16:127–36, 1980.
59. Pyrhönen S, Timonen T, Heikkinen A, Penttinen K, Alftan O, Saksela E, Wager O: Rheumatoid factor as an indicator of serum blocking activity and tumour recurrences in bladder tumours. Eur J Cancer 12:87–94, 1976.
60. Gupta N, Malavija N, Singh SM: Rheumatoid factor in bladder tumors. J Urol 120:296–7, 1978.
61. Gozzo JJ, Gottschalk R, O'Brien P, Cronin W, Monaco AP: Use of heterogenous and monospecific antisera for the diagnosis of bladder cancer. J Urol 118:748–51, 1977.
62. Gozzo JJ, Cronin WJ, O'Brien P, Monaco AP: Detection of tumor-associated antigens in urine from patients with bladder cancer. J Urol 124:804–7, 1980.
63. O'Brien P, Gozzo JJ, Monaco AP: Urinary proteins as biological markers: bladder cancer diagnosis versus urinary tract infection. J Urol 124:802–3, 1980.
64. Civantos F, Rywlin AM: Carcinomas with trophoblastic differentiation and secretion of chorionic gonadotrophins. Cancer 29:789–98, 1972.
65. Bruce AW, Mahan DE, Belville WD. The role of radioimmunoassay for prostatic acid phosphatase in prostatic carcinoma. Urol Clin North Am 7:645–52, 1980.
66. Belville WD, Sepulveda RA, Bruce AW *et al.*: Bone marrow acid phosphatase by radioimmunoassay – three years' experience. San Francisco: American Urological Association Annual Meeting, 1980.
67. Cooper JF: The radioimmunochemical measurement of prostatic acid phosphatase: current state of the art. Urol Clin North Am 7:653–5, 1980.
68. Pontes JE: State of the art in immune diagnosis of early adenocarcinoma of the prostate. Urol Clin North Am 7:667–73, 1980.
69. Vihko P, Lukkarinen O, Kontturi M, Vihko R: Effectiveness of radioimmunoassay of human prostate-specific acid phosphatase in the diagnosis and follow-up of therapy in prostatic carcinoma. Cancer Res 41:1180–3, 1981.
70. Kuriyama M, Wang MC, Papsidero LD *et al.*: Immunologic detection of a prostate specific antigen in human prostate cancer (abstract 826). Proc Amer Soc Clin Oncol 1980.
71. Fair WR, Catalona WC, Ratliff TR, Heston WDW: Tumor markers for prostatic carcinoma: prostatic acid phosphatase (PAP) and creatine kinase (CK-BB). San Francisco: American Urological Association Annual Meeting, 1980.
72. Narayana AS, Feld R, Loening SA, Culp DA: A new serum marker for carcinoma of the prostate. San Francisco: American Urological Association Annual Meeting, 1980.

73. Hindsley JP Jr, Fried FA, Zweig MH *et al.*: Creatine kinase BB in prostatic carcinoma. San Francisco: American Urological Association Annual Meeting, 1980.
74. Bishop MC, Fellows GJ: Urine hydroxyproline excretion – a marker of bone metastases in prostatic carcinoma. Br J Urol 49:711–6, 1977.
75. Mooppan MMU, Wax SH, Kim H, Wang JC, Tobin MS: Urinary hydroxyproline excretion as a marker of osseous metastasis in carcinoma of the prostate. J Urol 123:694–6, 1980.
76. Juengst D, Pickel A, Elsaesser E, Marx FJ, Karl HJ: Urinary cholesterol excretion in men with benign prostatic hyperplasia and carcinoma of the prostate. Cancer 43:353–9, 1979.
77. Belis JA, Cenedella J: Urinary nonesterified cholesterol excretion in adenocarcinoma of the prostate. Cancer 43:1840–6, 1979.
78. Grayhack JT, Wendel EF, Oliver L, Lee C: Analysis of specific proteins in prostatic fluid for detecting prostatic malignancy. J Urol 121:295–9, 1979.
79. Kane RD, Mickey DD, Paulson DF: Serial carcinoembryonic antigen assays in patients with metastatic carcinoma of prostate being treated with chemotherapy. Urology 8:559–62, 1976.
80. Williams RD, Bronson DL, Elliott AY, Fraley EE: Production of carcinoembryonic antigen by human prostate epithelial cells *in vitro*. J Natl Cancer Inst 58:1115–6, 1977.
81. Williams RD, Bronson DL, Myl AD, Vandevoorde JP, Elliott AY: Carcinoembryonic antigen-like substance derived from human prostate. Cancer Res 39:2447–50, 1979.
82. Broder LE, Weintraub BD, Rosen SW, Cohen MH, Tejada F: Placental proteins and their subunits as tumor markers in prostatic carcinoma. Cancer 40:211–6, 1977.
83. Webb K, Lin GH: Urinary fibronectin: potential as a biomarker in prostatic cancer. Invest Urol 17:401–4, 1980.
84. Ablin RJ, Gonder MH, Soanes WA: Levels of immunoglobulins in the serum of patients with carcinoma of the prostate. Neoplasma 19:61–5, 1972.
85. Lange PH: Cancer markers in germ-cell testicular tumors. In: Cancer Markers: Developmental and Diagnostic Significance. (Sell S, Wahren B, eds.) vol 2. Clifton, NJ: Humana Press (in press).
86. Lange PH, McIntire KR, Waldmann TA: Tumor markers in testicular tumor: current status and future prospects. In: Testicular Tumors: Management and Treatment (Einhorn LE, ed.) New York: Masson, 1980, pp. 69–81.
87. Nørgaard-Pedersen B, Raghavan D: Germ-cell tumours: collaborative review. Oncodev Biol Med 1:327–58, 1980.
88. Javadpour N: Applications of biological markers in testicular cancer. Cancer Treat Rep 63:1643–7, 1979.
89. Lange PH, Vogelzang NJ, Goldman A, Kennedy BJ, Fraley EE: Marker half-life analysis in testicular tumor: a prognostic tumor. J Urol (in press).
90. Kohn J: The value of apparent half-life assay of alpha-1 fetoprotein in the management of testicular teratoma. In: Carcino-Embryonic Proteins. (Lehmann FG, ed.) vol 2. Amsterdam: Elsevier/North-Holland Biomedical Press, 1979, pp. 383–6.
91. Javadpour N, Chen HC: Radioimmunoassay of urinary chorionic gonadotropin: a sensitive marker in testicular cancer. J Urol 126:176–81, 1981.
92. Goldenberg DM, Kim EE, Deland FH, van Nagell JR Jr, Javadpour N: Radioimmunodetection of cancer with radioactive antibodies to human chorionic gonadotropin. Science 207:1284–6, 1980.
93. Goldenberg DM, Kim EE, Deland F *et al.*: Clinical studies on the radioimmunodetection of tumors containing alpha-fetoprotein. Cancer 45:2500–5, 1980.
94. Goldenberg DM, Deland FH, Kim EE, Primus FJ: Xenogeneic antitumor antibodies in cancer radioimmunodetection. Transplant Proc 12:188–91, 1980.

95. Kurman RJ, Scardino PT, McIntire KR, Waldmann TA, Javadpour N: Cellular localization of alpha-fetoprotein and human chorionic gonadotropin in germ cell tumors of the testis using an indirect immunoperoxidase technique: a new approach to classification utilizing tumor markers. Cancer 40:2136–51, 1977.
96. Lange PH, Nochomovitz LE, Rosai J *et al.*: Serum alpha-fetoprotein and human chorionic gonadotropin in patients with seminoma. J Urol 124:472–8, 1980.
97. Johnson SAN, Grudzinskas JG, Gordon YB *et al.*: Pregnancy-specific $beta_1$-glycoprotein in plasma and tissue extract in malignant teratoma of the testis. Br Med J 1:951–2, 1977.
98. Rosen SW, Javadpour N, Calvert I, Kaminska J: Increased 'pregnancy-specific' $beta_1$-glycoprotein in certain nonseminomatous germ cell tumors. JNCI (J Natl Cancer Inst) 62:1439–41, 1979.
99. Javadpour N Utz M, Soares T: Immunocytochemical discordance in localization of pregnancy specific beta-1 glycoprotein, alpha-fetoprotein and human chorionic gonadotropin in testicular cancers. J Urol 124:615–6, 1980.
100. Lange PH, Bremner RD, Horne CHW, Vessella RL, Fraley EE: Is SP-1 a marker for testicular cancer? Urology 15:251–5, 1980.
101. Wahren B, Holmgren PA, Stigbrand T: Placental alkaline phosphatase, alphafetoprotein and carcinoembryonic antigen in testicular tumors: tissue typing by means of cytologic smears. Int J Cancer 24:749–53, 1979.
102. Millan JL, Stigbrand T: 'Sandwich' enzyme immunoassay for placental alkaline phosphatase. Clin Chem 27:2014–8, 1981.
103. Lange PH, Millan JL, Stigbrand T, Vessella RL, Ruoslahti E, Fishman WH: Placental alkaline phosphatase as a tumor marker for seminoma. Cancer Res (in press).
104. Bosl, GJ, Lange PH, Nochomovitz LE *et al.*: Tumor markers in advanced nonseminomatous testicular cancer. Cancer 47:572–6, 1981.
105. Milstein C: Monoclonal antibodies. Sci Am 243(4):66–74, 1980.

3. Assessment of Biologic Hazard of Urologic Tumors

DAVID F. PAULSON and MATTHEW S. SMITH

1. RENAL CELL CARCINOMA

Rational assay of the impact of any specific disease control method can be established only after it has been determined that the patients in each of the treatment groups are equal with respect to disease risk. Five broad categories: (1) the tumor pathology, (2) the stage of the disease, (3) biologic markers, (4) the type of treatment, and (5) the pattern of metastatic disease have been shown to have prognostic significance.

1.1. Tumor Pathology

Size, cell type, growth pattern, and pathology grade are four characteristics with prognostic importance.

1.2. Size

Tumor size is an indirect prognostic indicator of disease hazard being correlated closely with stage. Although primary renal tumors of tubular origin less than 2.5 cm in diameter are considered benign adenomas and tumors greater than 2.5 cm in diameter are classified as adenocarcinomas, Mostofi has demonstrated renal tumors less than 2 cm which have histologic criteria for malignancy and other large renal tumors greater than 3 cm which were clearly benign [1]. Size alone does not seem to be an appropriate criterion for definition of malignancy, although there does appear to be a direct relationship between tumor size and prognosis [2–4]. Katz demonstrated a five-year survival rate of 89.8% for patients with tumors less than 8 cm in diameter with only 10% surviving 5 years if the tumor diameter was greater than 8 cm. Arner noted five-year survivals of 69.4% for tumors less than 7 cm, 39.6% for tumors 7–15 cm, and 20.4% for tumors greater than 15 cm in diameter [5]. Bell identified the relationship of size and metastatic disease [6]. Only one of 45 patients with tumors less than 3 cm had

D.F. Paulson (ed.), Genitourinary Cancer 1, 73-100.

demonstrable metastases, while 5 of 69 patients with tumors 3–5 cm in diameter showed metastatic lesions, but 70 of 84 patients with tumors greater than 10 cm showed metastatic disease. Size itself is not sufficient to determine the benign or malignant nature of a specific tumor but size does correlate loosely with patient survival, probably relecting the relationship between size and metastases.

1.3. Cell Type

Renal cell carcinomas usually display one of three distinct cell types, clear, granular or spindle cell with a five-year survival of 58% for pure clear cell carcinoma, 46% for granular cell tumors and 23% for tumors of the carcinomatoid spindle cell type [1, 7–9]. The difference between 58% and 46% for clear cell and granular cell tumors is not felt to be statistically significant. However, the presence of fusiform or spindle cells in even small quantity within the tumor decreases the survival statistics dramatically (Table 1).

Table 1. Five-year survival by cell type

	Skinner [7] 1971	Boxer [10] 1979	Patel [9] 1978
Clear	58%	53%	23%
Granular	46%	58%	28%
Spindle	23%	28%	

1.4. Growth Pattern

The histologic growth pattern of the tumor appears related to survival. Tubular, acinar, papillary, or cystic patterns are signs of tumor differentiation and as such provide a survival advantage over those tumors which display a sheet-like pattern of solid cells without organization [3]. Mancilla-Jinenez demonstrated an improved survival in 34 of 224 patients whose tumors displayed a papillary pattern [11]. Pathologic stage I tumors were noted in 85.3% of the papillary group and in only 42.6% of the non-papillary group. The five-year survival of 84% and 52% for papillary and non-papillary tumors, respectively, appears to correlate with the pathologic stage suggesting that the tumors with a papillary pattern are less aggressive. The majority of angiographically avascular renal cell carcinomas are papillary or tubular [12]. The incidence of capsular invasion is less among papillary tumors (18%) as compared to non-papillary tumors (50%). Only 18% of the papillary tumors demonstrated renal vein invasion as compared to 43% of the non-papillary tumors. Although these studies showed a relationship between tumor vascularity and clinical stage, a subsequent report failed to demonstrate any relationship between tumor vascularity and prognosis [12].

However, it is felt generally that hypovascular tumors have a better prognosis than hypervascular tumors.

1.5. Histologic Grade

The histologic grade of renal carcinoma, examined independantly, is related to survival. Increased nuclear atypia with nuclear enlargement, irregularity, and hyperchromatism is associated with an adverse prognosis [4, 5, 7, 10, 13]. Although different grading systems are used, a decreased survivorship with increasing pathologic grade is evident (Table 2). This adverse survival with increased tumor grade is constant both with and across clinical stage [7].

Table 2. Five-year survival by histologic grade

Grade	Skinner [7]	Grade	Böttiger [13]	Arner [5]	Grade	Robson [15]	Boxer [10]	
							General	Nuclear
I	75%	I	100%	93%	I	57%	61%	50%
II	65%	IIA	59%	63%	II	47%	36%	32%
		IIB	36%	41%				
III	56%	III	0%	7%	III	40%	14%	25%
IV	26%							

1.6. Stage of Disease

Clinical and pathologic staging is an accepted method of categorizing the biologic hazard of renal cell carcinoma. The Robson modification of the Flocks and Kadesky staging system is widely used (Figure 1). Stage I tumors are confined to the kidney and do not extend through the renal capsule. Stage II lesions extend to the perinephric fat but are contained within Gerota's fascia and show no evidence of metastases. Stage III disease involves regional lymph node metastases and/or renal vein or inferior vena cava extension of tumor. Stage IV disease is defined as tumor extension into adjacent organs other than the adrenal gland and/or evidence of distant metastases [15–17]. Skinner, demonstrating that the presence of tumor in the lumen of the renal vein or inferior vena cava without actual invasion into the substance of the vessel did not alter the prognosis for those patients with stage II tumors, urged that the patients be classified as stage II [7]. Skinner's observations were in contrast to other reports which associated decreased survival opportunity in patients with tumor extension into the renal vein [5, 6, 19–22]. Waters and Richie reported an overall five-year survival rate of 58.5% for stage II tumors but a 64% five-year survival for

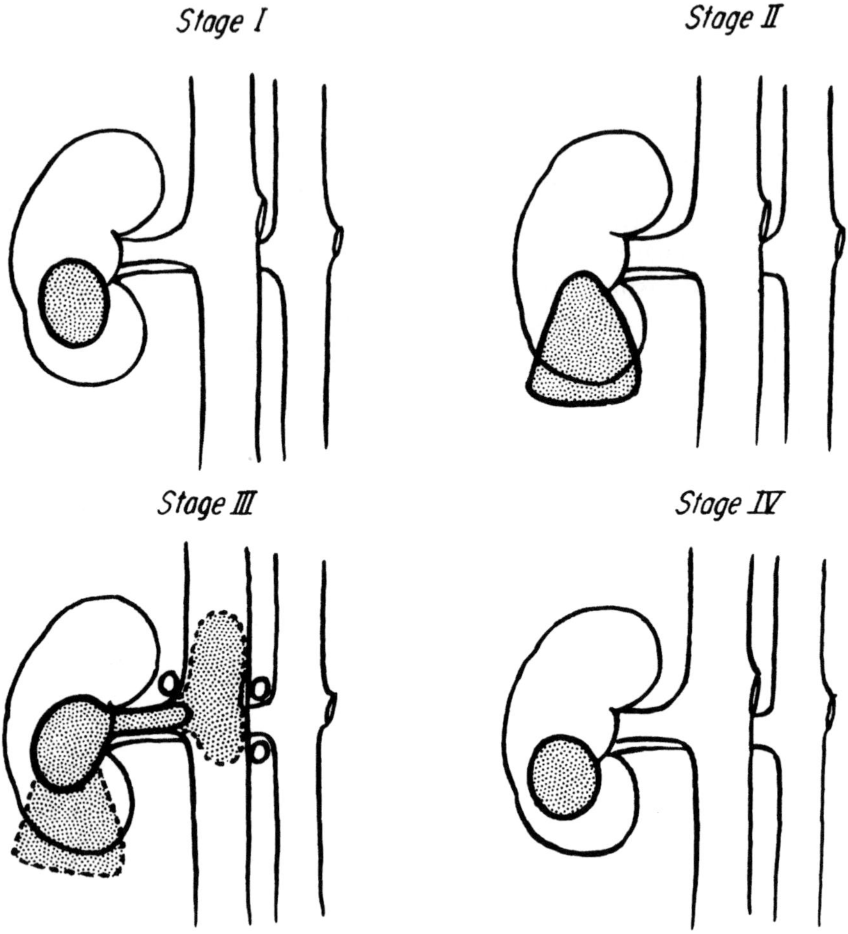

Figure 1. Staging of renal adenocarcinoma.

stage II tumors with inferior vena cava involvement [22]. This must be contrasted to a 12.3% five-year survival for stage III disease with or without vein involvement. Schefft reports a 50% five-year survival in 12 patients who presented with tumor extension into the inferior vena cava without evidence of distant metastases who received radical nephrectomy and either venacavotomy or tumor thrombectomy [23]. Although a recent report by Patel reports survival decreased from 66% to 32% at five years in patients with renal vein involvement, no effort was made to segregate these patients by other staging criteria [9].

Tumor stage as a prognostic index for cure and survival is well established [4, 7, 14, 24, 25] (Table 3). The involvement of regional lymph nodes, distant metastases, or the involvement of contiguous viscera are adverse

Table 3. Five-year survival by tumor stage

	Flochs & Kadesky * [179	Robson [14]	Skinner [17]	Katz [4]	Böttiger [13]	Boxer [10]	Waters [22]
No. of Pts.	353	88	309	164	100	96	130
Stage 1	55%	66%	65%	64	76	56	51
Stage 2	40.5%	64%	47%	56	65	100	58.5
Stage 3	14%	42%	51%	27	35	50	12.3
Stage 4	3.5%	11%	8%	0	5	8	0

* Treated cases.

prognostic indicators. Although improvement in survival has occurred since the introduction of radical nephrectomy, extension of tumor into the perinephric fat decreases survival (Figure 2). Invasion through the renal capsule alone decreases survival at five-years to 45% with regional nodal extension further depressing the five-year survival to 33% [25].

1.7. Biologic Markers

One of the most exciting areas of development in tumor biology has been

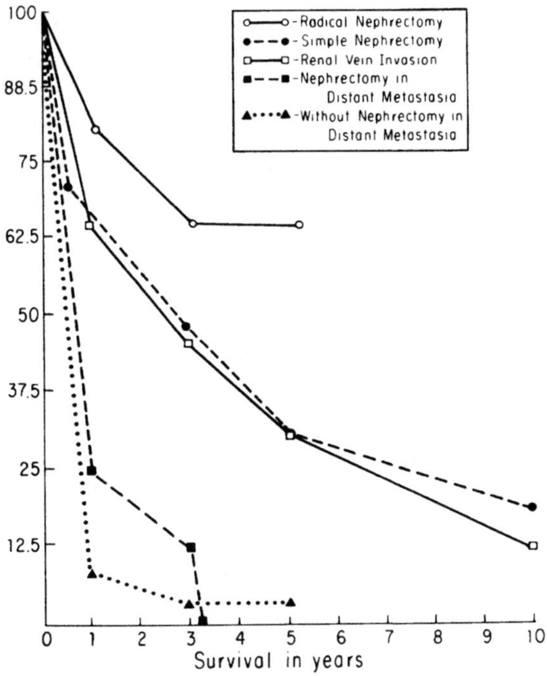

Figure 2. Modified from reference 9.

the identification of marker proteins. In several malignant diseases, markers are useful in diagnosis, prognosis, and as adjuncts in following and treating patients. However, there is no evidence to date that renal cell carcinoma either produces or contains any tumor-specific or tumor-associated antigens. Unlike prostatic and testicular malignancy, renal cell carcinoma does not produce any specific abnormal serum biochemical marker.

There are, however, other biologic characteristics which accompany the disease and which have survival significance. Hypertension occurs in about 15% of all patients with renal cell carcinoma. Most probably this elevation in blood pressure is due to an elevation in serum renin levels either produced by the tumor itself or from adjacent ischemic renal tissue. Prospective studies have demonstrated elevated plasma renin levels in 37% of 57 patients with renal adenocarcinoma [26]. Peripheral serum renin elevation was associated with a high grade and a high stage renal cancer. Patients with elevated renin levels experience a decreased survival even if the cancer levels decreased after nephrectomy. Erythrocytosis may be an early manifestation of occult renal cell carcinoma. Sixty-three percent of patients examined by Sufrin showed serum elevation of this hormone, however, no correlation could be demonstrated between erythropoietin levels and tumor grade or stage, or to prognosis [26]. Elevated levels of serum chorionic gonadotropin have been reported in 2 patients with renal cell carcinoma, however none of the 57 patients studied by Sufrin showed elevations of this hormone [26, 28]. Elevation in the erythrocyte sedimentation rate seems associated with decreased survival; however, ESR seems more likely to reflect the stage of disease [13, 28]. The ESR can be expected to be elevated in about 42% of patients with stage I and II disease, and in about 81% of patients with stage III and IV disease. A syndrome of hepatosplenomegaly with hepatic dysfunction as demonstrated by elevated liver function tests in the absence of obvious metastatic disease has been described [8, 29, 30]. The etiology of this syndrome is unknown but in those who manifest it, there is a decrease in survival. At least three of the following enzyme abnormalities are seen: increased alkaline phosphatase, retention of sulfobromophthalein, an albumin/globulin ratio of less than one, elevated serum haptoglobin level, or an increased serum prothrombin time. Most patients with this syndrome are dead within five years of diagnosis, unless the liver function tests return to normal after nephrectomy [8]. Renal adenocarcinomas have been known to secrete a parathormone-like substance producing hypercalcemia. While elevated serum calcium levels most frequently are due to widespread metastatic disease and not to hormone elevation, elevated calcium levels in the absence of stage D disease causes no adverse prognosis. Lymphocyte counts, measured pre and postnephrectomy, are not of prognostic value [31]. Elevated levels of plasma fibrinogin correlate with more

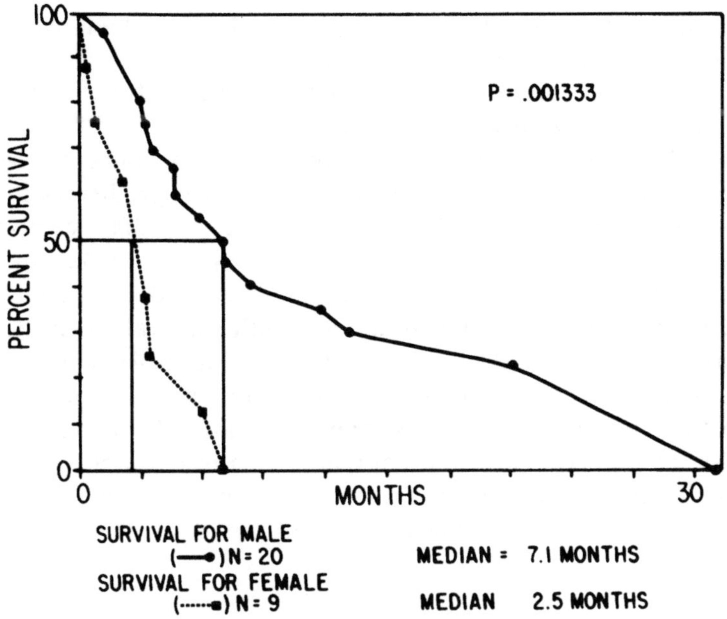

Figure 3. Survival by sex. Modified from reference 32.

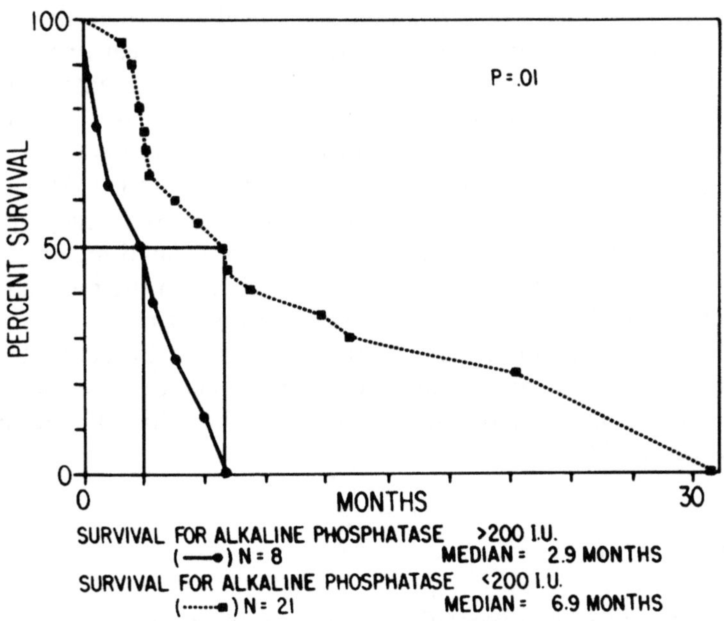

Figure 4. Survival of alkaline phosphatase levels. Modified from reference 32.

advanced stages of disease as do fibrin degradation products when platelet counts and prothrombin times are normal [31].

In patients with metastatic disease, there are well-defined characteristics which are associated with enhanced survival. Paulson and co-workers demonstrated that sex, the level of the initial alkaline phosphatase, initial hematocrit, and the site of metastases were survival predictors in patients receiving chemotherapy [32]. Men demonstrated a median survival of 7.1 months as compared to 2.5 months for women (Figure 3). An elevated alkaline phosphatase prior to treatment was associated with a median survival of 2.5 months as compared to a 6.9 month survival when the alkaline phosphatase was below 200 international units (Figure 4). The elevation of this enzyme did not correlate with either liver or bony metastases. The presence of anemia (hematocrit less than 36) produced survival statistics of 2.9 months on the average when compared to those patients with normal hematocrits who survived for an average of 7.1 months. Poor survival was also associated with bone metastases as opposed to other parenchymal sites.

1.8. Metastatic Disease

The available data would indicate that cell type, growth pattern, pathologic grade, tumor size, clinical stage, specific biochemical, physiologic and anatomic characteristics can be used to predict survival in patients presenting with renal cell carcinoma and should be considered when different treatments are compared. While there is much discussion regarding the significance of early versus delayed single metastatic sites, the data is based on small numbers of patients observations. Middleton reports a 34% fiveŒear survival rate in patients with isolated metastatic disease undergoing simultaneous nephrectomy and resection of the metastatic site [33]. Tolia and Whitmore report a 35.3% five-year survival in similar patients [34]. Thus it would seem that the patient who presents with an isolated metastatic lesion and is treated with radical nephrectomy and excision of the metastasis has a survival similar to that of the patient with positive regional nodes. While it has been reported that the aggressive treatment of an isolated site is associated with prolonged survival, this occurs only when survival is calculated from the date of the original nephrectomy rather than the date of the delayed procedure [7, 35].

2. BLADDER CANCER

Many factors have been identified which are of prognostic value in transitional cell carcinoma of the bladder. These can be used to identify patients with non-invasive tumors who are at greatest risk for recurrence with or without invasion, and to identify patients with invasive disease who are at greatest risk for death.

2.1. Tumor Pathology

Growth pattern, tumor size and number, pathologic grade, and clinical stage of the disease are customary predictors of the biologic course of the disease.

2.2. Growth Pattern

Urothelial malignancies can be divided into either exophytic or endophytic lesions with the former group predominating. Approximately 70% of exophytic tumors are papillary in nature and usually are non-infiltrating lesions carrying a favorable prognosis. Twenty percent are papillary, but infiltrate the bladder wall and have an intermediate prognosis. A poor outcome is seen in the remaining 10% of tumors which display a sessile and infiltrating pattern. Endophytic tumors in general show decreased survival rates and are often non-transitional in cell type. Invasive bladder tumors which grow in a solid cohesive pattern have a better prognosis than those tumors which grow in an infiltrating manner. The latter tend to show tongues of tumor cells advancing into normal body tissues. This type of growth is associated with earlier metastatic disease and decreased survival.

2.3. Tumor Size and Number

A single papillary lesion regardless of size, carries a 50–85% chance of recurrence [36, 37]. Four percent of patients with a single tumor at first presentation subsequently will develop tumors showing bladder muscle invasion. If multiple superficial tumors are observed at first presentation 40% of patients subsequently will develop invasive bladder disease [38]. Initial tumors with a diameter of less than 1 cm have a 35% recurrence rate. The frequency of tumor recurrence increases to 80% for lesions greater than 3 cm in diameter [38]. A recurrence rate of 100% is noted when the initial lesion is greater then 4 cm [38, 39]. Approximately 10% of these recurrences will show invasion of the bladder musculature.

2.3. Grade

Pathologic grade, based on the degree of anaplasia correlates well with prognosis [40–44]. As with most malignancies, patients with low grade bladder carcinomas experience a better survival then do those with high grade tumors, ranging from a 71% five-year survival for patients with low grade transitional cell tumors to a 37% five-year survival for patients with high grade lesions [45]. The presence of nuclear pleomorphism, increased

Table 4. Staging of bladder cancer

		Jewettt & Strong (1946)	Jewett (1952)	Marshall (1952)	TNM (1974) Clinical (T)	Pathologic (P)
O	Confined to mucosa			O	ToN × Mo+	PoNoMo
Ps	Carcinoma *in situ*				TIS	PIS
A	Infiltration of submucosa	A	A	O	$T_1N \times Mo$	P_1NoMo
B	Infiltration of:					
	Superficial muscle		B_1	B_1	$T_2N \times Mo$	P_2NoMo
	Deep muscle		B_2	B_2	$T_{3a}N \times Mo$	$P_{3a}NoMo$
	Both	B				
	Perivesical infiltration	C	C	C	$T_{3b}N \times Mo$	$P_{3b}NoMo$
	Prostate				$T_{4a}N \times Mo$	$P_{4a}NoMo$
	Uterus/vagina				$T_{4b}N \times Mo$	$P_{4b}NoMo$
	Adjacent organ			D_1	Pelvic abdominal wall	
	Nodes + (pelvic only)			D_1	T(any)N × Mo	$P(any)N_{1-3}$
	Distant metastases, or Nodes + (above aoetic bifurcation)			D_2	$T(any)N \times M_{1a-d}$	$T(any)N_{(4)}$
	Pelvic, abdominal wall fixation					

T, primary tumor; N, nodal involvement; M, distant metastases; + ×, cannot be assessed.

nuclear to cytoplasmic ratio, prominence of nuclear chromatin, prominent nucleoli, increased mitotic activity, and disturbance in the maturation process from the basement membrane to the epithelial surface are factors which contribute to a more advanced tumor grade.

Grade and stage parallel each other closely in bladder cancer, thus it is difficult to separate these two parameters in a statistically meaningful way. Approximately 10% of grade I tumors demonstrate muscle invasion. The incidence of muscle invasion increases to 50% for grade II tumors and 80% for grade III tumors. Benign papillomas, tumors with thin fibrovascular stalks lined by normal transitional cell epithelium, have a 47% recurrence rate and approximately 10% recurring as transitional cell carcinoma [46, 47]. Only 5% of patients with non-invasive grade I tumors subsequently died of their disease, as compared with 16% of patients with non-invasive grade II tumors and 35% of patients with non-invasive grade III tumors [46].

2.4. Stage of Disease

The best indicator of disease risk is the clinical stage. Although clinical staging of bladder cancer may be inaccurate in 50% of all cases, it does provide assessment of hazard. The currently accepted clinical staging of the disease is based on the depth of invasion and the presence or absence of distant metastases (Table 4). While the depth of muscle invasion classically has been related to prognosis, recent study has shown little advantage of superficial over deep muscle invasion [40, 48]. Any muscle invasion predicts decreased survival. If the initial tumor is stage O, there is a 20% chance of recurrent disease. If the tumor is either stage O or A, there is a 70% recurrence rate. Stage A tumors show a 40% incidence of invasive recurrence with approximately one third of these patients subsequently dying of metastatic disease. Disease risk as a function of clinical stage is identified in Table 5.

2.5. Carcinoma In Situ

The adverse prognostic impact of carcinoma *in situ* is recognized but poorly quantitated [49, 50]. Carcinoma *in situ* is, by definition, a non-papillary, non-invasive (located above the basement membrane), grade III lesion. This disease often is multifocal. Carcinoma *in situ* is found adjacent to invasive disease in over two thirds of patients [51]. Carcinoma *in situ* adjacent to a low grade, low stage tumor predicts invasive recurrence in 80% of patients at some future date. Carcinoma *in situ* in a patient with no visual evidence of tumor but a previous history of tumor predicts invasive recurrence in 40% of patients. Carcinoma *in situ* alone with no previous history of visible tumor predicts future invasion in 13% of patients [37, 49, 51, 52]. The time sequence for subsequent invasion recurrence is unknown; consequently aggressive surgical intervention based only on the identification of carcinoma *in situ* may be ill advised.

2.6. Chromosomal Pattern

The chromosomal pattern can be a useful indicator of the biologic potential of the tumor [53–58]. Tumor cells with a diploid number of chromosomes tend to be non-invasive, while euploid nuclear chromatin patterns are characteristic of invasive tumors. Several marker chromosomes have been identified. Ring and A-1 chromosomes when present in the initial non-invasive tumor predict invasive recurrence rate of approximately 90%. When no chromosomal abnormalities exist, the rate drops to 10% [55]. Chromosome number crudely parallels tumor grade; the greater the chromosome number the worse the prognosis [54–56]. The appearance of marker chromosomes in patients with well-differentiated non-invasive tumors

Table 5. Five-year survival by stage and treatment [a]

Treatment	Series	O and A	(%)	B_1	(%)	B_2	(%)	B	(%)	C	(%)
TUR	Flocks (1951)	130/168	(77)					68/142	(47)		
TUR	Barnes (1967)	146/233	(63)					46/114	(40)	3/57	(5)
S.R.	Utz *et al.* (1973)	17/25	(68)	18/38	(47)	14/35	(40)	32/72	(44)	11/38	(29)
S.R.	Riches (1960)	7/12	(58)					16/44	(36)	0/6	(0)
S.R.	Norvick and Stewart (1976)	10/15	(67)					8/15	(53)	1/6	(17)
RAD	Miller (1971)			10/39	(36)	12/40	(30)	22/79	(28)	5/32	(16)
CYST	Cordonnier (1974)	31/67	(46)	24/46	(52)	12/30	(40)	36/76	(47)	11/36	(31)
CYST	Richie *et al.* (1975)	43/54	(79)	14/36	(40)	9/22	(40)	23/58	(40)	4/24	(20)
CYST	Pearse *et al.* (1975)			7/14	(50)	5/12	(42)	12/26	(42)	2/15	(13)
CYST	Prout *et al.* (1976)			16/51	(31)	19/61	(31)	35/112	(31)	5/24	(21)
	Total	348/574	(67)	89/224	(40)	71/200	(36)	298/738	(40)	42/235	(18)

Note the similarity in survival rates between stages B_1 and B_2 both of which are substantially different from stages O and A, and C.

[a] From Skinner DG: Current state of classification and stagin of bladder cancer. Cancer Research 37 : 2838, 1977.

subsequently will identify those to develop recurrent tumors, while patients without marker chromosomes will not develop recurrence [57, 58].

2.7. Cell Surface Antigens

Glycoprotein cell surface antigens are dictated by each patient's particular genetic code and may be specific to a particular tissue or shared in common with several others. Normal bladder epithelium expresses the blood group cell surface isoantigens A, B, or H. These cell surface antigens can be demonstrated by the specific red cell adherence test [59–64]. As tumor cells dedifferentiate, they are less likely to express normal cell surface proteins. Loss of the blood group antigens from the tumor cells correlates with increasing tumor grade [65]. Patients with low grade, low stage bladder tumors subsequently will develop recurrent disease, 10–20% of the patients demonstrating invasion. The presence or absence of blood group antigens identifies those patients who are at increased risk for future invasion. Seventy-five percent of stage A tumors will demonstrate the A, B, H blood group antigens while few invasive tumors are antigen positive [64, 65]. Only 8% of patients with non-invasive pathologic grade I and II tumors which express the blood group antigens can be expected to develop invasive disease while 62% of tumors with a negative red cell adherence test will develop an invasive bladder tumor [65]. Other investigators have confirmed that the presence of blood group antigens on non-invasive low grade tumors predicts the absence of future invasion in 95% of patients while the absence of the blood group antigens is associated with future tumor invasion in 80%

Table 6. Clinical correlation (SRCA) in bladder carcinoma: selected studies *

	No. of patients isoantigen (–)	Comments	Investigator
Disease stage			
Mucosal atypia	Variable	(–) when associated with high grade tumors	Weinstein *et al.* (1979)
Ca *in situ* (CIS)	8/9 (89%)	Material from cystectomy specimen performed for diffuse CIS	Weinstein *et al.* (1979)
Stage O	21/31 (68%)	2/21 died of recurrent invasive bladder tumors	Altoy *et al.* (1978)
Stage A	9/22 (41%)	8/9 isoantigen (–) recurred a higher stage	DeCenzo *et al.* (1975)
Stage B (+)	6/25 (25%)	↑75% with invasive bladder cancer were antigen (+)	Kay and Wallace (1961)
Stage D	47/49 (96%)	Material studied obtained from metastases	Davidsohn (1973)

* Modified from Cummings K: Cancer 45, 1980.

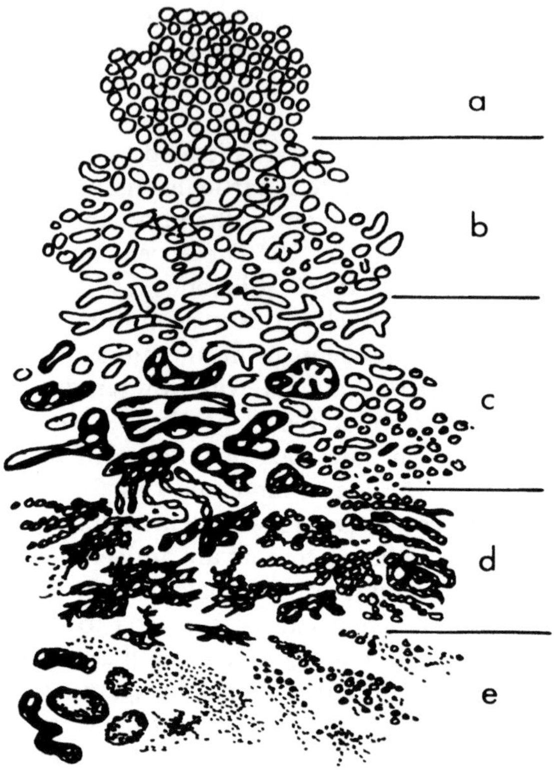

Figure 5. The Gleason pathologic grading scheme. A simplified drawing of histologic grades of prostatic adenocarcinoma, emphasizing the degree of glandular differentiation and relation to stroma. Fundamental criteria: a) single, separate, uniform glands, closely packed; b) single, separate, uniform glands, loosely packed; c) single, separate, varying glands, in varying distribution and/or smoothly-sharply circumscribed, papillary/cribriform masses; d) raggedly infiltrating masses of fused glands (papillary, cribriform or quite solid, dark cells or clear cells); e) raggedly infiltrating anaplastic tumor and/or comedocarcinoma.

of patients [62–65]. Even though a high percentage of patients with a negative specific red cell adherence test go on to develop invasive disease, one is not able to determine the time at which this invasion will occur (Table 6). Consequently, the point at which these high risk patients should be managed with aggressive surgical therapy is not known.

Patients with transitional cell carcinoma of the bladder can be stratified for disease risk based on the presence or chance of invasion. Many factors have been demonstrated to be associated with invasion or invasive recurrence, and these factors are those associated with loss of cellular differentiation as increasing pathologic grade, presence of abnormal chromosomes, loss of the cell surface blood group antigens and carcinoma *in situ*. Therefore, depending on the question being asked of the treatment evaluation, it may be necessary to study patients not only by clinical stage but also by those indicators which are associated with loss of cellular control.

3. CARCINOMA OF THE PROSTATE

The probability of death from prostatic carcinoma can best be assessed as a function of the pathologic grade of the tumor. Although clinical staging of the disease has long been the basis for determining disease risk, recent data would indicate that the pathologic grade of the primary tumor is important in determining the clinical stage of the disease.

3.1. Histologic Grade

Although multiple pathologic grading systems have been developed, the grading system developed by Gleason seems to provide the most accurate assessment of disease risk [66]. The Gleason histologic grading system considers only the degree of glandular differentiation and the growth pattern of the tumor in relation to the prostatic tumors (Figure 5). The grade most extensive in area is defined as the 'primary' grade and the less extensive grade or the 'secondary' grade. The two grades are recorded as two digits for each tumor and summed to provide a final pathologic index. The cancer mortality rates by histologic index, respective of the treatment chosen, demonstrate increasing risk of death with increasing pathologic index (Figure 6).

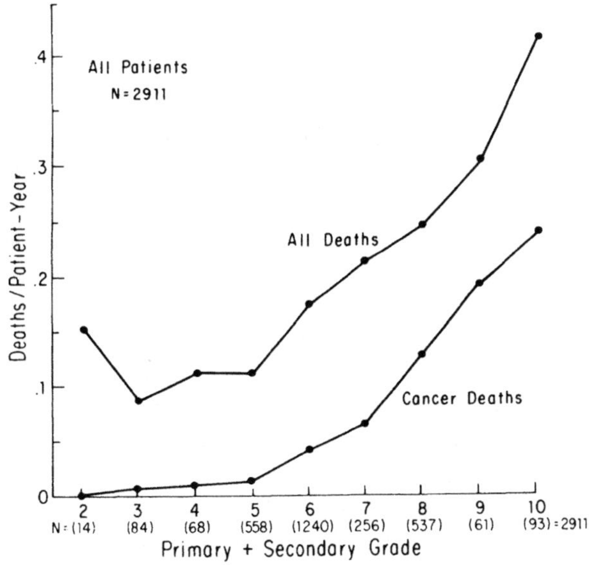

Figure 6. Total and cancer mortality rates by histologic score (sum of primary and secondary grades).

Table 7. Comparison of Gleason sum of the prostatic primary with node biopsy *

	Node biopsy		
Gleason sum	Positive	Negative	N/Group
2–5	13.9%	86.1%	36
6	32.4%	67.6%	34
7	49.9%	50.1%	21
8	75.0%	25.0%	12
9–10	100.0%	0%	7
Diagnosis of cancer only	33.3%	66.7%	12

* Modified from reference 67.
$X^2 = 28.2$; $p < .0005$.

Table 8. Comparison of Gleason patterns as a predictor of nodal metastatic disease *

Pelvic lymphadenectomy	No. Pts.	Gleason patterns		
		(2, 3, 4)	(5, 6, 7)	(8, 9, 10)
Positive	53	0/31 (0%)	26/84 (31%)	27/29 (93%)
Negative	91	31/31 (100%)	58/84 (69%)	2/29 (7%)

* Modified from reference 68.

3.2. Relationship of Histologic Grade and Clinical Stage of Disease

Multiple staging systems for prostatic carcinoma have been devised. They each assess the presence or absence of local spread, of regional node involvement or of distant metastases. Paulson and co-workers examined the relationship of regional node metastases and the Gleason pathologic index of the primary tumor [67, 68]. They were able to demonstrate that the incidence of positive nodes increased as the Gleason pathologic grade increased (Tables 7 and 8). These observations would explain the relationship of decreasing survival with increasing tumor grade after treatment of seemingly localized disease by either radiation therapy or radical perineal prostatectomy because of the increased number of patients with regionally disseminated and hence untreated disease.

Certain biochemical, hematologic and physiologic factors have been identified which can be used to identify disease risk in patients with hormonally unresponsive prostatic carcinoma who are undergoing chemotherapy. Paulson and co-workers examined the survival of a population of patients with

Table 9. Prognostic value of initial patient characteristics [a]

Variable	Group A (number)	Median survival (weeks)	Group B (number)	Median survival	p
Race	White (64)	39.2	Black (22)	44.2	.789
Age	>65 (43)	28.8	<65 (45)	57.0	.014
Stage at diagnosis	I, II or III (31)	28.9	IV (57)	46.0	.432
Duration of disease	>1 year (67)	35.4	⩽1 year (21)	77.1	.071
Prior radiation	No (39)	39.0	Yes (49)	39.6	.653
Prior orchiectomy	Yes (74)	38.5	No (14)	N.R. [b]	.068
Bone pain [c]	Level 4 or 5 (27)	25.0	Level 1, 2, 3 (61)	47.4	.013
Performance status [c]	Level 3, 4, 5 (42)	30.4	Level 1 or 2 (46)	48.6	.020
Sites of metastases	Bone + other organ (22)	28.9	Bone only (63)	45.6	.012
Malignant pleural effusion	Yes (9)	24.5	No (79)	41.9	.041
Liver scan	Abnormal (13)	27.0	Normal (75)	40.3	.058
IVP	Any ureteral obstruction (12)	33.5	Normal (75)	42.3	.376
Hemoglobin	<10 gm/dl (15)	22.5	>10 mg/dl (73)	44.9	.120
LDH	>200 U(53)	29.1	⩽200 U (35)	62.7	.003
SCOT	>50 U(21)	27.2	⩽50 U (67)	48.5	.006
Alkaline phosphatase	>110 U (71)	35.4	⩽110 U (17)	75.9	.013
Acid phosphatase	>5 U (32)	26.5	⩽5 U (56)	51.7	.010
Albumin	<3.5 gm/dl (35)	27.0	≥3.5 gm/dl (53)	48.3	.007
CEA	>2.5 mg/dl (58)	36.5	⩽2.5 mg/dl (30)	48.3	.246
BUN	>23 mg/dl (7)	28.2	⩽23 mg/dl (81)	40.7	.587
Creatinine	>1.2 mg/dl (12)	33.5	⩽1.2 mg/dl (76)	41.5	.846
Prolactin	>10 mg/dl (51)	36.6	⩽10 mg/dl (28)	73.9	.034
LH	⩽10 mIU (32)	38.1	>10 mIU (42)	45.8	.413
FSH	>25 mIU (22)	37.0	⩽25 mIU (59)	47.7	.130
Bone marrow biopsy	Positive (7)	30.1	Negative (14)	N.R. [b]	.207

[a] Modified from reference 70.
[b] N.R.: Median survival not yet reached.
[c] Levels defined in text.

prostatic carcinoma who were undergoing multiagent chemotherapy [69]. Survival was examined as a function of specific serum biochemical, hematologic or physiologic characteristics defined at entry.

Curves representing non-parametric estimates of survival were generated using the Kaplan-Meier method [70]: Survival curves begin at the time of entry into the study, at which time all patients had stage IV disease. On the survival graphs, the median survival is the point at which the time curve intersects the line representing 50% survival. Censored survival values representing patients still alive at the time of last follow-up are represented

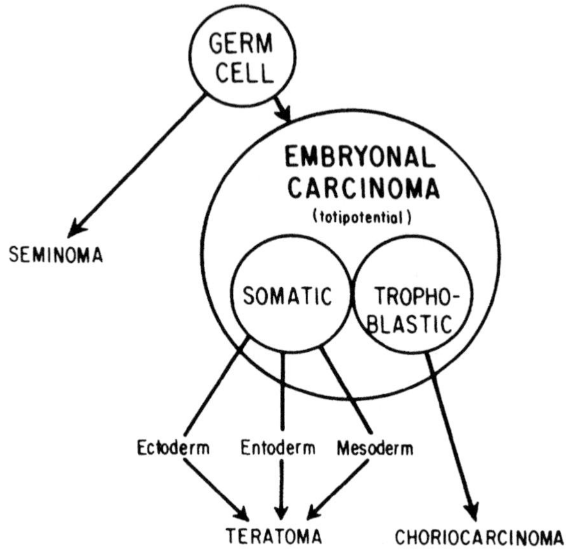

Figure 7. Proposed scheme for differentiation of germ cell tumors.

by single vertical bars on the graphs. When the longest survival value is a censored one, the curve is divided into two parts, representing upper and lower boundaries of survival estimates beyond the last death. Survivals of pairs of subgroups were tested for difference by the Cox-Mantel test [71].

Age, degree of bone pain, performance status, sites of metastases, elevated LDH or SGOT, elevated alkaline or acid phosphatase, hypoalbuminemia, and hyperprolactinemia were factors found to be of prognostic significance in assessing the health risk of the disease (Table 9).

4. GERM CELL TUMORS OF THE TESTICLE

Cell type is the primary prognostic factor in testicular cancer. Although most investigators feel that all primary testicular carcinomas derived from a primitive toti-potential cell, historically it has been the practice to separate testicular carcinomas into seminomatous and non-seminomatous germ cell tumors (Figure 7). Each of these categories has further subdivisions based on cell type and histologic pattern and many tumors will display a mixture of these pure forms. The segregation into seminomatous and non-seminomatous germinal cell tumors is based largely on the differential radiosensitivity of the two tumor types, seminoma being a very radiosensitive tumor.

Disease risk in both seminomatous and non-seminomatous tumors is related to the local and distant extent of disease, to the bulk of local and

Table 10.

Clinical stage	History, physical chest X-ray	Lymphan-giogram IVP	Serum markers	Laparo-tomy	Surg. path. stage
I	Negative	Negative	Negative	Negative	I negative nodes
	Negative	Negative	Negative	Microscopic nodes positive	IIa microscopic nodes positive
II	Negative	Negative	Elevated	Microscopic nodes positive	
	Negative	Positive	Negative or elevated	Macroscopic nodes positive	IIb macroscopic nodes clearly resected
					IIc macroscopic nodes not clearly resected
					IId macroscopic nodes not resected
IIIa IIIb	Positive	Positive/ Negative	Positive/ Negative	Positive/ Negative	Any of the above possibilities

Table 11. Staging definitions

T_1 = Tumor limited to testis and testicular end of spermatic cord.
T_2 = Spermatic cord histologically positive at inguinal ring.
T_3 = Normal tissue barriers broken as by scrotal orchiectomy or invasion through testicular capsule by tumor.
N_1 = Lymph nodes not visibly enlarged at surgery but microscopic disease found on pathologic exam.
- N_{1A} = Five or fewer nodes are positive
- N_{1B} = More than five nodes positive.

N_2 = Lymph nodes enlarged and microscopically contain tumor but no extension beyond the lymph nodes into the areolar tissue.
- N_{2A} = Largest node is 2cm and five or fewer nodes are involved (both criteria).
- N_{2B} = Largest nodes are 2 cm and/or more than five nodes are involved.

N_3 = Extension from lymph nodes into adjacent areolar tissue (microscopic as well as gross). No gross residual tumor remaining after surgery.
N_4 = Tumor present in rectroperitoneal lymph nodes, retroperitoneal areolar tissue with gross residual tumor remaining after surgery.

distal disease and to the cell type. Multiple staging systems have been generated to express these prognostic cancers (Tables 10 and 11). The discussion below will focus on seminomatous and non-seminomatous tumors and the survival by clinical stage.

4.1. Histologic Type

Three histologic patterns are recognized in seminoma: classic, anaplastic, and spermatocytic [72–75]. Although a 93–96% overall survival rate for classic seminoma has been reported as compared to a 70–86% survival rate with anaplastic seminoma, this pooled survival experience fails to acknowledge the greater incidence of high stage disease seen with anaplastic seminoma. The survival of classic and anaplastic seminomas, compared by stage, is similar [76]. Anaplastic seminomas are defined by the presence of an increased mitotic activity (3 mitoses or greater per hpf in 10 microscopic fields). Spermatocytic seminomas experience the best survival statistics, reflecting the relative absence of metastatic tumor seen with this disease.

4.2. Disease Risk or Function of Stage

Seventy-five percent of seminomas present at stage A lesions, 20% present as stage B, and 5% as stage C [72]. The customary treatment for seminoma is surgical removal of the primary and radiation of the distant sites.

The five-year survivals for patients with stage A disease is 93%, for stage B, 69% (including B3), and for stage C, 22% (Table 12).

Elevated levels of human chorionic gonadotrophin have been identified in 13% of patients with histologically pure seminoma, the mortality rate within this subgroup being 20% at 5 years compared to 4% of patients who show no elevation [73, 74, 77–79]. Whether this reflects the presence of

Table 12. Results of treatment by stage of 190 previously untreated patients with seminoma testis (The Royal Marsden Hospital 1963-1975)

Stage	Total patients	Lost to follow-up	Relapsed	Died of inter-current disease	Died seminoma	Died teratoma	Developed second tumor
I	121	13	4	4	1 (second) tumor	0	7
IIA	38	1 (42 months)	6	4	6	0	0
IIB	16	0	4	1	3		0
III	8	1 (67 months)	1/1 *	0	2	2	2 (both died teratoma)
IV	7	1 (9 months)	0/4 *	0	1	1	1 (died teratoma)

* Never controlled by therapy.

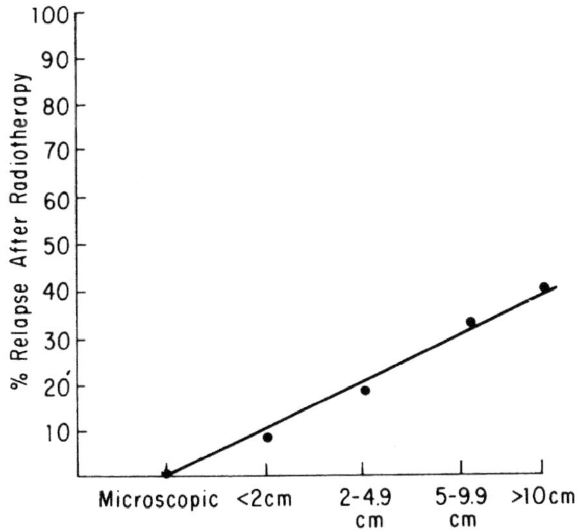

Figure 8. Influence of size of metastases on radiotherapeutic result in seminoma testis. (The Royal Marsden Hospital, 1962–1979).

non-seminomatous disease or a variant of seminoma is unknown. Thirty-five percent of patients with histologically pure seminoma who die of their disease demonstrate non-seminomatous elements at autopsy [75]. Recent studies have shown that the presence of syncytiotrophoblasts with the seminoma predict a mortality rate of almost 30% as compared with 8% for patients with no evidence of these cells [80].

4.3. Non-seminomatous Germ Cell Tumors

Cell Type. Nonseminomatous germ cell tumors can be divided into embryonal carcinoma, teratocarcinoma, teratoma, choriocarcinoma, and yolk sac tumors. Yolk sac tumors also are referred to as juvenile embryonal cell carcinomas and endodermal sinus tumors. Teratocarcinoma is a mixture of teratoma and embryonal cell carcinoma and behaves as embryonal cell carcinoma.

Classically, a decrease in survival was projected as one progressed from teratocarcinoma to embryonal cell carcinoma to choriocarcinoma. This was felt due to the increased propensity for vascular invasion noted at the choriocarcinoma end of the spectrum. However, if choriocarcinoma is excluded, the crude three-year survival rates by tumor type are not significantly different [81]. Pure embryonal tumors carry a 78% three-year crude survival rate, mixed embryonal tumors carry a 69% three-year survival rate, teratocarcinoma an 81% three-year survival rate and mixed teratocarcinoma a 75% three-year survival rate. The mode of treatment and not the tumor type seems the major consideration.

Table 13. Stage II seminoma testis: sites of initial relapse after radiotherapy (The Royal Marsden Hospital, 1962–1979)

Stage	Size of retro-peritoneal node metastases (cm)	Total patients	Lung ± media-stinum	Sites of first relapse				
				Cervi-cal	Scrotum or groin nodes *	Liver	Extra-dural	Multiple sites
IIA	2	31	1	0	2	0	0	0
IIB	2–4.9	11	0	0	1	0	1	0
IIC	5–9.9	9	2	0	0	1	0	0
IID	10	12	1	2	0	0	0	2
Total		63	4	2	3	1	1	2

* Two of three patients who had scrotal interference prior to orchidectomy and who did not receive scrotal and groin node irradiation suffered local relapses.

4.4. Clinical Stage

The bulk of tumor in metastatic sites seems the dominant prognostic factor irregardless of the treatment chosen. The seminoma experience supports this observation (Figure 8, Table 13).

The five-year survival rates after surgery alone for non-seminomatous germ cell tumors are 86–96% for stage I disease, and 56–81% for stage II disease [81–87] (Table 14).

The addition of adjunctive chemotherapy programs has altered the survival rates at three years as follows: Stage A, 91–100%; Stage B, 69–86%, and Stage C, 47–61% [81, 85, 88–91]. As anticipated from the radiotherapeutic data, bulk of disease seems the primary predictor of health risk.

The success of radiation therapy in the treatment of small subclinical deposits of non-seminomatous germ cell tumors within the retroperitoneal nodes seems dependent on tumor volume (Figure 9). The overall survival for stage B disease after radiation therapy alone is 50% at five years. In

Table 14.

Series	Histologicstage I		Histological stage II	
	Number of patients	% Disease free (3 years)	% Disease free (3 years)	% Disease free (e years)
Staubitz *et al.* [85]	17	88	8	87
Skinner [80]	40	92	16	81

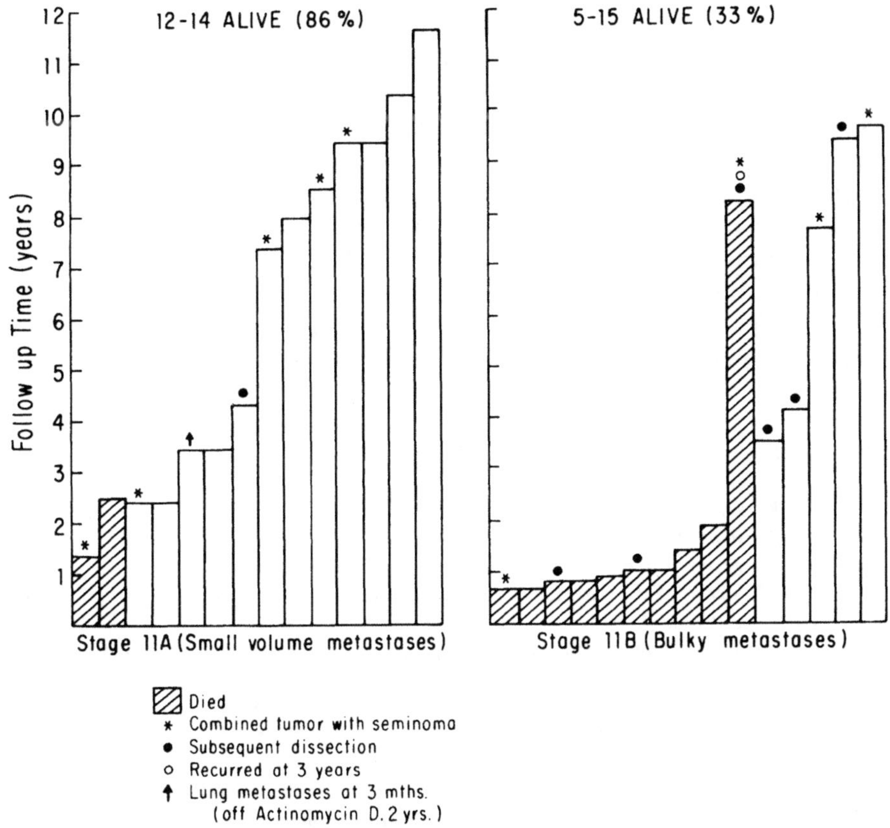

Figure 9. Survival of patients with small volume (2 cm or less in diameter) retroperitoneal node metastases from testicular teratoma treated with post-orchidectomy irradiation.
Survival of patients with bulky (>2 cm in diameter) retroperitoneal node metastases from testicular teratoma treated with post-orchidectomy irradiation.

those patients with abdominal nodes less than 2 cm in diameter the success rate is 85% but this rate drops precipitously to 35% in patients with bulky stage B3 disease. Vanderwerf-Messing reported a 90% cure rate of stage I disease but only a 45% cure rate in patients with positive nodes [91]. Hussey reported a three-year disease cure rate of 78.2% for stage I tumors, 46.7% for stage IIA tumors, and 17.6% for stage IIB tumors [92].

4.5. Tumor Markers

The testicular tumor marker proteins, alpha fetoprotein (AFP) and beta subunit Human Chorionic Gonadotrophin (HCG), are either singly or both elevated in 90% of patients with non-seminomatous germ cell tumors [93, 94]. These marker proteins not only provide a biochemical indicator of treatment effectiveness, but also have prognostic importance.

Patients with elevated tumor markers prior to orchiectomy have a worse prognosis than those who do not show elevated levels [94]. Patients with marker elevation after orchiectomy and lymphectomy are presumed to have failed regional surgical control and are considered at risk from systemic disease.

In conclusion, there are identified factors in renal, bladder, prostate and testicular cancer which permit the clinician to assess the probability of death with reasonable accuracy. An awareness of these predictor variables is important if one is to evaluate the disease control impact of two different treatments or to design a study which seeks to examine the efficacy of two distinct treatments.

REFERENCES

1. Mostofi FK: Pathology and spread of renal cell carcinoma. In: Renal Neoplasia (King JS Jr, ed.). Little, Brown & Co, Boston, 1967, pp. 41–85.
2. Cass AS: Large renal adenoma. J Urol 124:281, 1980.
3. Murphy GP, Mostofi FK: Histological assessment and Clinical prognosis of renal adenoma. J Urol 103:31, 1970.
4. Katz SA, Davis JE: Renal adenocarcinoma: prognostics and treatment reflected by survival. Urology 10:10, 1977.
5. Arner O, Blanck C, Schreeb T von: Renal adenocarcinoma; morphologygrading of malignancy-prognosis. A study of 197 cases. Acta Chir Scand (Suppl) 346:1, 1965.
6. Bell ET: Renal disease. 2nd edn Philadelphia: Lea & Febiger, 1950, p. 435.
7. Skinner DG, Colvin RB, Vermillion CD, Pfister RC, Leadbetter WF: Diagnosis and management of renal cell carcinoma. A clinical and pathologic study of 309 cases. Cancer 28:1165, 1971.
8. Boxer RJ, Waisman J, Lieber MM, Mampaso FM, Skinner DG: Non-metastatic hepatic dysfunction associated with renal carcinoma. J Urol 119:468, 1978.
9. Patel NP, Lavengood RW: Renal cell carcinoma: natural history and results of treatment. J Urol 118:722, 1978.
10. Boxer RJ, Waisman J, Lieber MM, Mampaso FM, Skinner DG: Renal carcinoma: computer analysis of 96 patients treated by nephrectomy. J Urol 122:598, 1979.
11. Mancilla-jimenzez R, Stanley RJ, Blath RA: Papillary renal cell carcinoma: a clinical,radiologic and pathologic study of 34 cases. Cancer 38:2469, 1976.
12. Blath RA, Mancilla-Jimenez R, Stanley RJ: Clinical comparison between vascular and avascular renal carcinoma. J Urol 115:514, 1976.
13. Bottiger LE: Prognosis in renal carcinoma. Cancer 26:780, 1970.
14. Robson CJ, Churchill BM, Anderson W: The results of radical nephrectomy for renal cell carcinoma. J Urol 101:297, 1969.
15. Robson CJ, Churchill BM, Anderson W: The results of radical nephrectomy for renal cell carcinoma. Trans Am Assoc Genitourin Surg 60:122, 1968.
16. Robson CJ: Radical nephrectomy for renal cell carcinoma. J Urol 89:37, 1963.
17. Flocks RH, Kadesky MC: Malignant neoplasms of the kidney: an analysis of 353 patients followed 5 years or more. J Urol 79:196, 1958.
18. Myers GM, Fehrenbaker LG, Kelalis PP: Prognostic significance of renal vein invasion by hypernephroma. J Urol 100:420, 1968.

19. Petkovic S: Significance of venous invasion in renal parenchymal tumor for prognosis. Urol Nephrol 69:707, 1976.
20. Hand JR, Broders AC: Carcinoma of the kidney: the degree of malignancy in relation to factors bearing on prognosis. J Urol 28:199, 1932.
21. McDonald JR, Priestly JT: Malignant tumors of kidney: Surgical and prognostic significance of tumor thrombis of renal vein. Surg, Gynec and Obst 77:295, 1943.
22. Waters WB, Richie JP: Aggressive surgical approach to renal cell carcinoma: Review of 130 cases. J Urol 122:306, 1979.
23. Schefft P, Novick AC, Straffon RA, Stewart BH: Surgery for renal cell carcinoma extending into the inferior vena cava. J Urol 120:28, 1978.
24. Holland JM: Cancer of the kidney-natural history and staging. Cancer 32:1030, 1973.
25. Abdelsayed MA, Bissada NK, Finkbeiner AE, Redman JF: Renal tumors involving the inferior vena cava: plan for management. J Urol 120:153, 1978.
26. Sufrin G, Mirand EA, Moore RH *et al.*: Hormones in renal cancer. J Urol 117:433, 1977.
27. Chisholm GD: Nephrogenic ridge tumors and their syndromes. Ann NY Acad Sci 230:403, 1974.
28. Kaufman JJ, Mims MM: Tumors of the kidney. In: Current Problems in Surgery. (Ravitch MM, Ellison EH, Julian OC, Thal AP, Wangensteen OH, eds.) Chicago: Year Book Medical, 1966, p. 44.
29. Hanash KA, Utz DC, Ludwig J *et al.*: Syndrome of reversible hepatic dysfunction associated with hypernephroma: an experimental study. Invest Urol 8:399, 1971.
30. Utz DC, Warren MM, Gregg JA *et al.*: Reversible hepatic dysfunction associated with hypernephroma. Mayo Clin Proc 45:161, 1970.
31. Sufrin G, Mink I, Fitzpatrick J, Moore R, Murphy JP: Coagulation factors in renal adenocarcinoma. J Urol 119:727, 1978.
32. Paulson DF, Lastinger LB, Cox EB, Hinshaw W, Walker RA: Metastatic renal adenocarcinoma: predictors of treatment response. J Urol (In Press.)
33. Middleton RG: Surgery for metastatic renal cell carcinoma. J Urol)»:)»:, 1)«o».
34. Tolia BM, Whitmore WF Jr: Solitary metastasis from renal cell carcinoma. J Urol 114:836, 1975.
35. Middleton RG, Presto AJ III: Radical thoracoabdominal nephrectomy for renal cell carcinoma. J Urol 110:36, 1973.
36. Farrow GM, Utz DC, Rife CC: Morphological and clinical observations of patients with early bladder cancer treated with total cystectomy. Cancer Res 36:2495, 1976.
37. Althausen AF, Prout GR Jr, Daly JJ: Noninvasive papillary carcinoma of the bladder associated with carcinoma in situ. J Urol 116:575, 1976.
38. Barnes EW, Bergman RT, Hadley HL, Love D: Control of bladder tumors by endoscopic surgery. J Urol 97:864, 1967.
39. Greene LF, Hanash KA, Farrow GM: Benign papilloma or papillary carcinoma of the bladder? J Urol 110:205, 1973.
40. Jewett HJ, Strong GH: Infiltrating carcinoma of the bladder: relation of depth of penetration of the bladder wall to incidence of local extension znd metastases. J Urol 55:366, 1946.
41. Marshall VF: The relation of the preoperative estimate to the pathologic demonstration of the extent of vesicle neoplasms. J Urol 68:714, 1952.
42. Mostofi FK: A study of 2678 patients with initial carcinoma of the bladder. I survival rates. J Urol 75:480, 1956.
43. Mostofi FK: Pathology of malignant tumors of urinary bladder. In: The Biology of Clinical Management of Bladder Cancer. (Cooper EH, Williams RE, eds.) London: Blackwell Scientific, 1975, p. 87.

44. Broders AC: Epithelioma of the genitourinary organs. Ann Surg 75:574, 1922.
45. Marshall VF: Current clinical problems regarding bladder tumors. Cancer 9:543, 1956.
46. Gilbert HA, Logan JL, Kagan AR *et al.*: The natural history of papillary transitional cell carcinoma of the bladder and its treatment in an unselected population on the basis of histologic grading. J Urol 119:488, 1978.
47. Loening S, Narayana A, Yoder L, Slymen D, Weinstein S, Penick G, Gulp D: Factors influencing the recurrence rate of bladder cancer. J Urol 123:29, 1980.
48. Wallace D: Clinicopathological behavior of bladder tumors. In: Wallace D, (Editor) Tumors of Bladder. E & S Livingstone, Edinburgh, 1957.
49. Farrow GM, Utz DC, Rife CC, Greene LF: Clinical observations on 69 cases of in situ carcinoma of the urinary bladder. Cancer Res 37:2794, 1977.
50. Utz DC, Hanash KA, Farrow GM: The plight of the patient with carcinoma in situ of the bladder. J Urol 103:160, 1970.
51. Farrow GM, Utz DC, Rife CC, Greene LF: Clinical observations on 69 cases of in situ carcinoma of the urinary bladder. Cancer Res 37:2791, 1977.
52. Soto EA, Friedell GH, Tiltman AJ: Bladder cancer as seen in giant histologic sections. Cancer 39:447, 1977.
53. Falor WH, Ward Rm: Cytogenetic analysis: a potential index for recurrence of early carcinoma of the bladder. J Urol 115:49, 1976.
54. Tavares AS, Costa J, DeCarvalho A, Reis M: Tumour ploidy and prognosis in carcinoma of the bladder and prostate. Br J Cancer 20:438, 1966.
55. Levi PE, Cooper EH, Anderson CK, Path MC, Williams RE: Analyses of DNA content, nuclear size and cell proliferation of transitional cell carcinoma in man. Cancer 23:1074, 1969.
56. Shigematsu S: Significance of the chromosome in vesicle cancer. In: Proceedings of XIII Congres de la Societe Internationale d'Urologie. Baltimore: Williams & Wilkins, 1965, p. 111.
57. Falor WH, Ward RM: Prognosis in well differentiated, non-invasive carcinoma of the bladder based on chromosomal analysis. Surg Gynec Obst 144:515, 1977.
58. Falor WH, Ward RM: Prognosis in early carcinoma of the bladder based on chromosomal analysis. J Urol 119:44, 1978.
59. Bergman S, Javadpour N: The cell surface antigen A, B, or O (H) as an indicator of malignant potential in stage A bladder carcinomas: preliminary report. J Urol 119:49, 1978.
60. Lange PH, Limas C, Fraley EE: Issue blood group antigens and prognosis in low stage transitional cell carcinoma of the bladder. J Urol 119:52, 1978.
61. Young AK, Hammond E, Middleton AW: The prognostic value of cell surface antigens in low grade, non-invasive, transitional cell carcinoma of the bladder. J Urol 122:462, 1979.
62. Newman AJ Jr, Carlton CE Jr, Johnson S: Cell surface A, B or O (H) blood group antigens as an indicator of malignant potential in stage A bladder carcinoma. J Urol 124:27, 1980.
63. Johnson JD, Lamm DL: Prediction of bladder tumor invasion with the mixed cell agglutination test. J Urol 123:25, 1980.
64. Richie JD, Blute RD Jr, Waisman J: Immunologic indicators of prognosis in bladder cancer: the importance of cell surface antigens. J Urol 123:22, 1980.
65. Emmott RC, Javadpour N, Bergman SM, Soares T: Correlation of the cell surface antigens with stage and grade in cancer of the bladder. J Urol 121:37, 1979.
66. Gleason DF, Mellinger GT, Veterans Administration Cooperative Urological Research Group: Prediction of prognosis for prostatic adenocarcinoma by combined histological grading and clinical staging. J Urol 111:58, 1974.

67. Paulson DF, Uro-Oncology Research Group: Predictors of lymphatic spread in prostatic adenocarcinoma. J Urol 123:697–699, 1980.
68. Kramer SA, Spahr J, Brendler CB, Glenn JF, Paulson DF: Experience with Gleason Histopathologic grading in prostatic cancer. J Urol 124: 223–225, 1980.
69. Paulson DF, Berry WR, Cox EB, Walker A, Laszlo J: Multi-agent chemotherapy in estrogen-Unresponsive prostatic adenocarcinoma. Accept J Urol, 1979.
70. Paulson DF, Berry WR, Cox EB, Laszlo J: Chemotherapy of prostatic cancer. In: Cancer of the Genitourinary Tract. (Johnson, Samuels, eds.) New York: Raven Press, 1979, pp. 261–272.
71. Smith RB: Management of testicular seminoma. In: Genitourinary Cancer. (Skinner DG, DeKernion JB, eds.) Philadelphia: WB Saunders, 1978, p. 470.
72. Dixon FJ, Moore RA: Tumors of the male sex organs. Fasc. 31b and 32, Atlas of Tumor Pathology, 1952. Washington DC: Armed Forces Institute of Pathology.
73. Maier JG, Sulak MH: Radiation therapy in malignant testis tumors. Cancer 32:1217, 1973.
74. Mostofi FK, Price EB Jr: Tumors of the male genital system (Fasc 8) Atlas of Tumor Pathology, 2nd series, Washington, DC Armed Forces Institute of pathology, 1973.
75. Johnson DE, Gomez JJ, Ayala AG: Anaplastic seminoma. J Urol 114:80, 1975.
76. Heyderman E, Neville AM: Syncytiotrophoblasts in malignant testicular tumors. Lancet II:103, 1976.
77. Friedman M, Pearlman AW: Seminoma with trophocarcinoma: a clinical variant of seminoma. Cancer 26:46–64, 1970.
78. Javadpour N, McIntire KR, Walkmann TA: Human chorionic gonadotropin (HCG) and alpha-fetoprotein (AFP) in sera and tumor cells of patients with testicular seminoma: a prospective study. Cancer 42:2768–2772, 1978.
79. Mostofi FK: Pathology of germ cell tumors of testis. Cancer 45:1735, 1980.
80. Skinner DG: Nonseminomatous testis tumors: a plan of management based on 96 patients to improve survival in all stages by combined therapeutic modalities. J Urol 115:65, 1976.
81. Johnson DE, Bracken RB, Blight EM: Prognosis for pathologic stage I nonseminomatous germ cell tumors of the testis managed by retroperitoneal lymphadenectomy. J Urol 49:553, 1977.
82. Skinner DG: Advances in the management of nonseminomatous germinal tumours of the testis. Br J Urol 49:553, 1977.
83. Staubitz WJ: Surgical treatment of nonseminomatous germinal testis tumors. In: Cancer of the Genitourinary Tract. (Johnson ED, Samuels ML, Eds.) New York: Raven Press, 1979. (In press.9
84. Walsh PC, Kaufman JJ, Coulson WF, Goodwin WE: Retroperitoneal lymphadenectomy for testicular tumors. JAMA 217:309, 1971.
85. Staubitz WJ, Early KS, Magoss I, Murphy GP: Surgical treatment of nonseminomatous germinal testes tumors. Cancer 32:1206, 1973.
86. Whitmore WF Jr: Surgical treatment of adult germinal testis tumors. Semin Oncol (Accepted for publication)
87. Skinner DG: Management of nonseminomatous tumors of the testis. In: Skinner DG, DeKernion JB, (Eds). Genitourinary Cancer, Philadelphia WB Saunders Co, 1978, p. 470.
88. Skinner DG, Scardino Pt: Relevance of biochemical tumor markers and lymphadenectomy in management of nonseminomatous testis tumors: current perspective. J Urol 123:378, 1980.
89. Donahue JP, Perez JM, Einhorn LH: Improved management of nonseminomatous testes tumors. J Urol 121:425, 1979.

90. Staubitz WJ, Early KS, Magoss IV, Murphy GP: Surgical management of testis tumors. J Urol 111:205, 1974.
91. Van Der Werf-Messing B: Radiotherapeutic treatment of testicular tumors. Int J Radiat Oncol Biol Phys 1:325, 1976.
92. Hussey DH, Luk KH, Johnson DE: The role of radiation therapy in the treatment of germinal cell tumors of the testis other than pure seminoma. Radiology 123:175.
93. Javadpour N, Doppman JL, Bergman S, Anderson T: Correlation of computed tomography and serum tumor markers in metastatic retroperitoneal testicular tumor. J Comput Tomog 2:176, 1978.
94. Javadpour N: The role of biologic tumor markers in testicular cancer. Cancer 45:1755, 1980.
95. Javadpour N: Radioimmunoassay and immunoperoxidase of pregnancy specific beta-1 glycoprotein in sera and tumor cells of patients with certain testicular germ cell tumors. J Urol 123:514, 1980.

4. Surgical Management of High Stage Renal Cell Carcinoma

JEAN B. DE KERNION

1. INTRODUCTION

Renal cell carcinoma is not a common tumor and accounts for approximately 3% of adult malignancies. The tumor occurs more commonly among urban dwellers and is most commonly found in males (5.6 per 100 000 males and 4.1 per 100 000 females). Patients with polycystic kidney disease appear to have a predisposition to the development of renal carcinoma, and a definite increased incidence is noted in patients with von Hippel-Lindau's disease [1].

The anatomical location of the kidney makes renal carcinoma, though relatively an uncommon tumor, a major challenge to modern cancer therapy. The classic triad of pain, hematuria, and presence of a flank mass is actually found in relatively few patients, and almost invariably indicates far-advanced disease [2]. Frequently, the tumor is an incidental finding on examination for symptoms secondary to metastases or paraneoplastic syndromes produced by the primary tumor [3]. It is not surprising therefore that fully 30% of patients have metastases at the time of the original diagnosis, and many without metastases will have local tumor extension or involvement of the regional lymph nodes. As will be discussed later in this chapter, there is currently no effective management of renal cell carcinoma other than surgical excision. This factor has prompted the current philosophy of extended indications for radical surgery in the management of this tumor. A thorough understanding of the factors which influence prognosis is vital to an understanding of the current surgical philosophy and to a rational assessment of its therapeutic value.

Extension of tumor into the renal vein has traditionally been thought to be associated with a poor prognosis [4]. More recent studies have failed to show this correlation [5], perhaps due to the emphasis in recent years on

D.F. Paulson (ed.), Genitourinary Cancer 1, 101-120.

complete excision of the renal vein and on the identification of renal vein involvement preoperatively. Extension of tumor into the vena cava does not significantly compromise survival [6], provided tumor thrombus does not extend above the diaphragm.

Extension of tumor into Gerota's fascia and into the perinephric fat was a greater deterrent to survival prior to the widespread adoption of radical nephrectomy. Although considerable debate exists about the role of radical nephrectomy compared to simple nephrectomy in improving survival, it seems reasonable that complete excision of the perirenal fat will encompass tumor which extends through the renal capsule. However, even after radical excision of Gerota's fascia, extension of tumor into the perinephric fat decreases the five-year survival to approximately 45 %. Extension into adjacent contiguous organs is even a more dire prognostic sign, and few such patients are cured. The significance of inadequate excision of the tumor and persistence of tumor in the renal fossa is emphasized by the survival of only 5 % of such patients at 18 months [3].

An equally dire prognostic sign is the metastases of tumor to the regional nodes [7]. A continuing debate exists as to whether these nodes can practically be included in the field of surgical incision, and the results of lymphadenectomy will be discussed below. The presence of distant metastases is rarely associated with survival longer than two years. Systemic modalities have had little impact on this dire prognosis.

Faced with surgical management as the current sole effective therapeutic modality, it is not surprising that the surgical approach to renal carcinoma has been extended in attempts to encompass the tumor, Gerota's fascia, the regional lymph nodes, and in some cases, adjacent organs or vena cava. Similarly, the role of interventional radiology and radiotherapy has become a prominent part of management of high risk renal cell carcinoma. These surgical and radiologic approaches will be discussed, and their impact on survival will be analyzed.

2. TUMOR EXTENSION INTO INFERIOR VENA CAVA

Inferior vena cava involvement by renal carcinoma was traditionally felt to represent a hopeless clinical situation. Later, articles appeared attesting to the value of aggressive treatment of such patients and the significance of vena caval involvement was questioned [5, 6]. Isolated reports of removal of tumor thrombi from the entire inferior vena cava and right atrium represented the ultimate in aggressive surgery for renal carcinoma. Few such patients, however, were ultimately cured and important issues have been cystallized with respect to the indications and appropriate extent of such operations. First, an adequate work-up prior to surgical treatment of renal carcinoma must always include an inferior prior to surgical treatment of renal carcinoma must always include an inferior venacavagram. When extension above the diaphragm is suspected, retrograde filling of the supradiaphragmatic vena cava and right heart is essential. Secondly, excision of the vena cava is not always necessary. Most tumors appear as tumor thrombi extending from the vein into the cava, and can easily be removed from the lumen of the cava. Thirdly, extended excision of tumors involving the supradiaphragmatic vena cava appear to be palliative rather than curative. Fourthly, the extent to which excision of vena caval tumor thrombi will improve survival depends upon: 1) the extent of tumor involvement, and 2) whether the tumor represents a tumor thrombus or actually invades the wall of the vena cava.

In the excellent analysis by Clayman *et al.* [8] these parameters are clearly delineated and put into proper perspective. The authors suggest, on the basis of their observations and the published literature, that vena cava involvement be sub-classified, and that management of the patients should be tailored in cognizance of these prognostic factors. Classification according to this system will enable a more accurate and meaningful analysis of survival after surgical management of these patients.

2.1. Surgical Technique

The surgical approach depends to a great extent on the superior limit of the tumor extension into the cava, and on the laterality of the tumor. Often the tumor protrudes 1 or 2 cm from the renal vein into the vena cava, or the thrombus extends a few centimeters superiorly. Such tumors can usualy be managed in a straight forward fashion through the same incision used for standard radical nephrectomy. We prefer the supracostal 11th rib incision, which is extrapleural and extraperitoneal [9]. The vena cava is easily exposed through this incision to the point of the adrenal vein on the right, and proximal to the adrenal artery on the left. Tumors which extend almost to or near the diaphragm, especially tumor thrombi from the right renal vein, are best approached through a thoracoabdominal incision [9]. This incision is intrapleural, and may be extraperitoneal or intraperitoneal. We prefer to remain extraperitoneal unless the patient has had previous surgery and extensive adhesions and scarring. Subcostal, midline, or chevron incisions have also been employed with success, but often access to the upper portion of the infradiaphragmatic vena cava is difficult through these incisions. When the tumor thrombus extends to the diaphragm or above, access to the superior, para-cardiac portion of the inferior vena cava is essential. Either a high intrapleural, thoracoabdominal incision or, preferably, a midline sternotomy incision offer the needed exposure from the atrium to the origin of the inferior mesenteric artery. We have had no experience with the latter incision, though it has been advocated by others.

Extensive involvement of the vena cava often renders access to the renal artery difficult. Theoretically, although preoperative arterial embolization might devascularize the tumor thrombus resulting in embolization to the lungs, we have not seen this occurrence. We, therefore, feel it is appropriate to recommend peroperative embolization of the renal artery immediately prior to surgery. Although we do not advocate this as routine practice for all renal tumors, in this setting it often minmizes blood loss and facilitates early control of the renal vein and vena cava.

2.2. Infradiaphragmatic Caval Extension

When a small tumor thrombus extends from the renal vein into the lumen of the vena cava, a large partial occlusion clamp such as a Satinsky clamp is passed around the thrombus. A tennis racket type incision is made, circumscribing the insertion of the renal vein and extending superiorly in the vena cava to the upper extent of the thrombus. In this fashion, the tumor can be removed intact, and the vena cava is closed with two layers of running 4–0 nylon vascular sutures. The remainder of the radical nephrectomy is performed in the usual manner. Larger tumor thrombi, filling the lumen of the cava and extending more proximally, require isolation and control of the vena cava. The vena cava is incircled superior to the thrombus. This is most effectively done above the diaphragm. When the thrombus extends to the diaphragm or above, mobilization of the liver will provide access to the hepatic veins. The triangular and hepatic coronary ligaments are sharply divided and the entire liver is reflected medially off of the diaphragm. Small veins are encountered between the sulcus of the liver and the anterior surface of the vena cava. These are easily clipped or ligated and divided. After encircling the hepatic veins with vascular tapes, the contralateral renal vein is likewise controlled, and a tape is passed around the inferior vena cava below the level of tumor thrombus. An attempt is made to identify large lumbar veins and ligate them prior to opening the vena cava. If the artery was not embolized preoperatively, it is isolated and tied at this time. The vena cava is first occluded below the thrombus, after which the contralateral renal vein, hepatic veins, and proximal vena cava are occluded. A hockey stick incision is made to the superior aspect of the thrombus and it is removed intact. The cava is irrigated with saline and closed in two layers. Prior to completing the closure, air is flushed from the cava by releasing the occlusion of the proximal vena cava. The remainder of the nephrectomy is similar to the usual radical nephrectomy.

Excision of the vena cava surrounding the tumor thrombus has been previously advocated. Indeed, some tumors seem to invade the wall of the vena cava. In our experience, the outlook for such patients is extremely poor. When this phenomenon is encountered, it provides a justifiable basis for excision of the vena cava when possible. Preservation of flow from the right renal vein is essential, and limits the extents to which venacavectomy can be performed in the patients with invasion of the vena cava by a left renal tumor. When right renal tumors invade the vena cava, the cava can be sacrificed with relative impunity and the left renal vein can usually be ligated. An alternative approach is reanastomosis to the portal vein, though this is rarely, if ever, necessary. The anatomic basis for this phenomenon has been clearly outlined by McCollough *et al.* [10] and Clayman *et al.* [8]. Occasionally the tumor seems to be adherent to the inner wall of the cava at only one or two points, and limited or sleeve resection is possible.

2.3. Supradiaphragmatic Vena Cava Extension

Radical surgery for patients with extension of tumor to the base of the heart or into the right atrium must be construed as having a palliative role only. In practice, we have usually found that such patients have other poor prognostic indicators, including extension into the lymph nodes or involvement of adjacent organs. As noted above, the approach depends upon personal preference, but any approach must allow access to the vena cava from the right atrium to a point near its origin from the common iliac vessels. Invariably, the liver must be mobilized and the hepatic veins controlled. Small tributaries can be safely ligated and divided. The contralateral renal veins, proximal and distal vena cava must also be controlled. When the tumor extends to the atrium, cardiac bypass via the femoral vessels is an important adjunct to the operation. After occluding the tributaries, the patient is placed on bypass, and the vena cava is opened from the renal vein proximally to the base of the heart. With good fortune, the entire thrombus can then be delivered intact or at worst, in several segments. The vena cava should be thoroughly irrigated with sterile water prior to closure. We have, however, encountered situations in which tumor was thoroughly adherent to the inner wall of the vena cava for almost its entire length. These tumors have an oatmeal appearance and consistency, and cannot be excised, extracted, or suctioned from the cava. The outlook in this circumstance is hopeless, and in our experience, postoperative radiotherapy or chemotherapy have had little effect.

The results of surgery for vena caval extension of renal carcinoma, as stated above, depends upon several clearly defined factors. When the tumor extends as a thrombus into the vena cava below the diaphragm, the outlook for such patients appears to be approximately the same as patients without vena caval or renal vein involvement. The cure rate in such patients is more dependent upon other factors such as extension into Gerota's fascia or presence of lymph node involvement. When, however, the thrombus extends above the diaphragm, the prognosis is usually very poor, not markedly different from patients with metastases at the time of their original diagnosis. Extension of the thrombus into the right atrium offers a surgical challenge, and temporary triumphs have been anecdotally reported in the literature. Though most such patients return within several years with metastases, the procedure seems to have a palliative effect, and may increase survival in some cases. The validity of extensive surgery for supradiaphragmatic extension must be re-evaluated in light of our current knowledge. The rethinking of this principle will be influenced by the eventual identification of reasonable, effective surgical adjuvants.

3. LYMPH NODE METASTASES

Several prerequisites are important in recommending lymph node resection as a therapeutic measure. First, metastases to the regional nodes should occur with sufficient regularity to warrant their excision and the subsequent extension of an already major surgical procedure. Robson *et al.* [11] reported a 23% incidence of positive nodes in patients who underwent extensive lymphadenectomy along with radical nephrectomy. Other authors have reported similar incidence [12, 13] following extensive lymphadenectomy and this appears to be a true incidence of lymphatic metastases. Secondly, the presence of tumor in the lymph nodes must be a proven poor prognostic sign. This has been clearly demonstrated, and the ten-year survival of patients with regional lymphatic metastases is usually below 20% (see Table 1). Realizing that nodal metastases are a true reflection of systemic dissemination, this poor prognosis is not surprising. A third prerequisite is that the lymphatic metastases occur in a predictable and sequential fashion to allow exact definition of the extent of lymphadenectomy. Unfortunately, little is known about the pattern of lymphatic metastases. One of the few studies –

Table 1. Renal cell carcinoma: survival of patients with regional lymph node metastases

	5-Year (%)	10-Year (%)	Total Pts.
Flocks and Kadesky	16	16	21
Robson	35	35	88
Skinner et al.	14	3	29
Rafla	21	8	14
Petkovic *	5		22

* Most died within one year.

and perhaps the only one – on the distribution of lymphatic metastases from renal cancer was reported by Hülten [14]. In his study, most nodes were in the renal hilum or near the origin of the renal vessels from the vena cava and aorta. However, patients also had involvement on the opposite side of the great vessels or in isolated nodes in the iliac or supraclavicular regions. Although it appears that the lymph nodes near the renal hilum may be involved primarily, the profuse pattern of lymphatic metastases accompanying the neovascularity of renal tumors makes lymphatic dissemination possible at any point in the retroperitoneum and pelvis. Accordingly, re-examination of the impact of lymphadenectomy on survival and clarification of our current approach is in order.

The true influence of lymphadenectomy on survival of renal cancer patients is difficult to quantify. Rafla [15], and Skinner *et al.* [16] reported a 21% and 14% five-year survival respectively, in patients with lymphatic metastases. However, it is unclear whether all of these patients underwent lymphadenectomy and the extent of the lymphadenectomy is not uniform. The results of Flocks and Kadesky [17] were similar. The reports by Robson *et al.* [11], however, suggested that lymphadenectomy might indeed have therapeutic value since the five-year survival of their patients was 35% when regional nodes were involved. All of their patients had preoperative mediastinoscopy and node biopsy for staging and all had complete retroperitoneal lymphadenectomy.

These few reports represent the data as they currently exist supporting regional lymphadenectomy. Although the survival is poor, the implication of these reports is that an occasional patient might be benefited by excision of tumor bearing lymph nodes. Several points must be emphasized before conclusions can be based upon this published information.

First, in no report were the number or location of nodes specified. It is possible that survivors were patients who had one or several microscopically involved lymph nodes in or near the renal hilum. Such nodes would be removed by the standard radical nephrectomy, without extensive lymphadenectomy. Secondly, the potential for increased morbidity exists when the operation is extended to include the regional nodes. This must be evaluated in light of the admittedly meager improvement in survival reported in these series. The specifics regarding morbidity of lymphadenectomy are difficult to ascertain, but advocates feel that morbidity is not significantly increased. Extensive retroperitoneal dissection creates the potential for surgical morbidity above and beyond that imposed by a standard radical nephrectomy, no matter who performs the surgery. Admittedly, the extent of the morbidity will depend upon such diverse factors as patient selection, extent of dissection, extent of lymph node involvement, and skill of the surgeon.

A third, and often overlooked factor in the debate regarding lymphadenectomy is the degree to which lymphatic metastases truly reflect the extent of renal tumor dissemination. Non-choriocarcinoma germ cell tumors of the testes predictably metastasize first to the regional lymph nodes, and the presence or absence of retroperitoneal nodal metastases is an extremely reliable indicator of the true systematic extent of the disease. However, blood-borne metastases of renal carcinoma are at least as common as lymphatic metastases, and the status of the lymph nodes is thereby of limited importance in determining the extent to which the tumor has escaped from the renal fossa. Many patients with negative regional lymph nodes die of disseminated tumor, suggesting that blood-borne metastases may even be a more common cause of death than lymphatic metastases. This seriously mitigates against regional lymphadenectomy as a therapeutic maneuver. As alluded to above, another major argument against lymphadenectomy is the unpredictable distribution of lymphatic metastases from renal cancer. Large regional primary carcinomas frequently parasitize vessels from the omentum, small bowel mesentery, or other organs. Lymphatics which accompany these vessels may offer numerous avenues for haphazard tumor dissemination. It is therefore difficult to conceive how even the most meticulous retroperitoneal lymphadenectomy could remove all of these potential lymphatic deposits.

It is therefore difficult to support the routine practice of radical lymphadenectomy for renal carcinoma with therapeutic intent, for the numerous reasons stated above. However, we continue to practise regional lymphadenectomy with justification based on the literature experience and on our personal experience. If the major lymphatic flow from the renal tumor is indeed first to the renal hilar nodes and thence to adjacent paraortic or paracaval nodes in most patients, a patient with early lymphatic metastases to these nodes may occasionally be cured. Secondly, although not a proven fact, it is a reasonable assumption that patients might have done more poorly, had these sites not been excised. Thirdly, and most importantly, lymphadenectomy is a valuable staging maneuver. Although therapeutic adjuvants currently seem to offer little to patients with even limited node involvement, accurate knowledge of the extent of local and regional tumor spread will become important as new systemic adjuvant therapies are developed. Undoubtedly, interpretation of trials of postoperative adjuvant therapy is difficult and suspect when the status of the regional lymph nodes is unknown.

Extension of the surgical procedure in order to accomplish these limited goals can only be advocated if the morbidity and mortality are not thereby significantly increased. An extensive radical retroperitoneal dissection must increase morbidity to some extent even in the most skilled hands, and we have been unwilling to accept this morbidity in view of the limited gains of

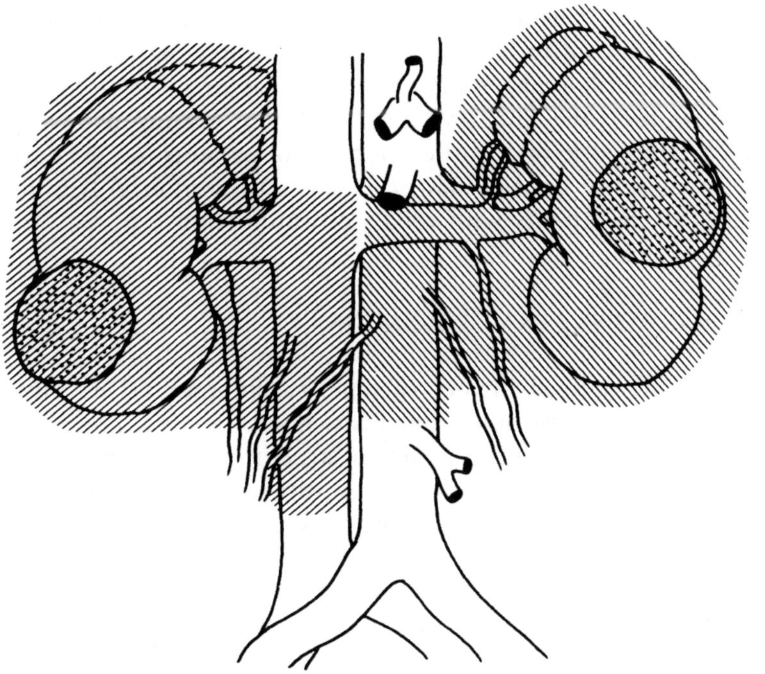

Figure 1. Extent of lymphadenectomy for renal carcinoma is indicated by shaded areas. The right radical nephrectomy is accompanied by removal of lymph nodes anterior and lateral to the vena cava; and left radical nephrectomy includes removal of lymph nodes anterior and lateral to the aorta. The distal extent of each is approximately the level of the origin of the inferior mesenteric artery. (From deKernion, J.B., Urologic Clinics of North America, 7:697, 1980.)

lymphadenectomy. We have therefore adopted an approach which adds little operative time and no detectable morbidity above and beyond the standard radical nephrectomy.

We prefer a supracostal, 11th rib incision, reserving the more painful and extensive intrapleural, extraperitoneal thoracoabdominal approach for patients with large upper pole tumors or large vena caval tumor thrombi (see above). After ligating the artery and dividing the main renal vein, dissection is begun along the aorta (for left-sided tumors) or vena cava (for right-sided tumors) beginning inferiorly at the level of the origin of the inferior mesentery artery. The dissection proceeds along the great vessel to the renal artery which is then re-ligated and divided flush with the aorta. Dissection then extends superiorly to ligate and divide the adrenal vessels. All lymphatic tissue is removed lateral and arterior to the ipsilateral great vessel. The medial extent of the dissection on either side are the interaorto-caval lymph nodes, but no attempt is made to dissect extensively between or behind the great vessels. The superior extent is the adrenal vein on each side (see Figure 1). Significant morbidity has not been noted following this approach. The addition of this unilateral lymphadenectomy requires fifteen to twenty minutes of operating time and provides important staging data and may be potentially therapeutic in a limited number of patients. At the current time, however, it does not appear that extensive retroperitoneal lymphadenectomy is justified in patients with renal cell carcinoma.

4. LOCALLY INVASIVE RENAL CARCINOMA

Because of the natural history of renal carcinoma and its propensity to grow and disseminate prior to diagnosis, many patients present with large primary tumors which invade adjacent structures. The most common presenting symptom in such patients is pain, usually from invasion of the posterior abdominal wall, paraspinous muscles and nerve roots. Extension into the liver is not common, and it is more common to find metastases to the liver rather than local invasion. The capsules of large tumors frequently indent and compress adjacent liver, but seldom actually grow into the hepatic tissue. Invasion of the duodenum and pancreas is an extremely poor prognostic sign, and this author knows of no such patients cured of their tumor. The small bowel mesentery and colon are not often invaded, although excision of these structures is often advisable when large tumors adhere to the bowel or mesentery.

The only treatment for the patient with local invasion by primary renal carcinoma is extensive excision. Since the tumors are usually encapsulated, they seldom directly invade the adjacent organs, except in the case of posterior abdominal wall muscles. Attempts should be made to excise the tumor completely, even if excision of bowel, spleen and muscle are required. En bloc partial hepatectomy is rarely curative, and this author knows of no patient cured of renal carcinoma which invaded the liver. However, an attempt to excise involved liver is preferable to leaving residual tumor. Extended excision, whenever possible, is mandated by the lack of any other effective means of treating renal cell carcinoma, and, as such, offers the only chance for cure. Partial excision of the primary lesion, or 'debulking', is seldom, if ever, indicated. In a series of patients with metastatic or recurrent renal carcinoma, only 12% of the patients who underwent incomplete excision of tumor were alive at 12 months [18]. Although surgery is the only effective treatment, the results of surgical excision when the tumor invades adjacent structures are very poor. Most reports indicate that less than 5% of patients with extension into adjacent viscera survive five years after surgery. However, it is unclear in these reports which patients underwent complete excision and the extent of involvement of the adjacent viscera is usually not stated [5, 11]. Therefore, it seems appropriate to individualize when selecting patients for extended radical nephrectomy. With the help of improved staging by use of computerized tomography, some patients may be spared an unnecessary partial excision of invasive renal tumors.

Attempted excision of tumors which invade the stomach, pancreas or duodenum seems imprudent. Local extension into the spine or paraspinous muscles is never resectable. We have, however, been able to extirpate tumors superficially involving the posterior abdominal wall muscles and occasionally such patients do well for extended periods. Most right renal tumors which are fixed to the liver do not directly invade the hepatic parenchyma. However, this is often difficult to ascertain at the time of surgery and excision of the adjacent hepatic tissue may be appropriate. Extension into the spleen and hepatic flexure of the colon should not deter the surgeon from attempting en bloc excision of the involved structures. It is of course imperative to recognize the colonic involvement preoperatively and institute proper bowel preparation. Involvement of the small bowel mesentery is very rare and is most common in tumors which recur in the renal fossa after nephrectomy. Excision of part of the small bowel mesentery and small bowel is feasible and should not deter one from attempting complete excision of a primary renal carcinoma.

The role of radiotherapy in locally extensive carcinoma has been much debated. Preoperative radiotherapy as a standard adjunctive modality is controversial, but several reports have indicated an increased survival [19, 20]. Two randomized studies have not shown a significant gain from routine preoperative radiotherapy. The Genitourinary Oncology Group under the direction of Claire Cox (personal communication) evaluated preoperative radiation therapy of 4500 rads followed by radical nephrectomy vs. radical nephrectomy alone. The findings suggest a slight impact on survival although the long-term follow-up has not been completed. The randomized study conducted by Werf-Messing [21] compared 3000 rads preoperative to non-preoperative therapy. The five-year survival was not influenced although the incidence of recurrence in the renal fossa was diminished. Little doubt exists that large renal tumors can sometimes be decreased in size by effective radiation therapy. Extensive large left-sided renal tumors can sometimes become resectable after such preoperative therapy, and it is our policy to consider this approach when the tumor appears adherent to adjacent structures. Delivery of radiotherapy to right-sided tumors, which often extend well under the liver, is more difficult. However, tumors which invade posteriorly can sometimes be rendered more easily resectable by preoperative therapy. The exact success rate of radiotherapy in such patients is unclear, and often the therapy seems to have no impact on the size of the tumor or involvement of the adjacent structures.

Postoperative radiotherapy has thus far not been shown to influence survival [22, 23]. However, the effect of postoperative radiotherapy on selected patients after excision of locally invasive tumors is not clearly understood. It seems reasonable that postoperative radiotherapy should be considered in certain instances. The fact that primary tumor sometimes partially regress following radiotherapy, and that the incidence of local recurrence was decreased in the series reported by Werf-Messing [21], suggests that radiotherapy may have some, if limited, effect on primary renal tumor. Therefore, when tumor is known to have been left behind in the renal fossa, or on adjacent structures, we have advocated use of postoperative therapy. The involved areas should be carefully marked with metal clips at the time of the surgery. Of course, this is more practical with left-sided tumors than with those on the right side due to potential liver damage by the radiation therapy.

Many tumors are not resectable by virtue of the extensive involvement of many areas in the retroperitoneum as well as adjacent viscera. As mentioned above, attempts at 'debulking' such tumors cannot be supported by the known outcome of such treatment. The use of hormonal or chemotherapeutic agents in such huge tumors has not been successful in any case of which I am aware. External radiotherapy may occasionally be palliative. However, tumors which are very extensive seldom respond sufficiently to radiotherapy to provide long-term palliation. The method of intra-arterial implantation of radioactive seeds may be a more effective method of management in these patients.

The development of sophisticated angiographic techniques, and the current availability of radioactive seeds have prompted renewed interest in this approach. Multiple tumor vessels can be selectively entered and embolized with the radioactive seeds. Currently, ^{125}I seeds appear to be the most effective since the low energy emission allows selective high dose irradiation to the tumor while sparing the adjacent normal tissues. Doses of 10 000 rads or greater can be safely delivered to large tumors, and the procedure can be repeated as often as necessary to achieve extensive tumor implantation. Fourteen patients with non-resectable or metastatic (Stage IV renal carcinoma) and eight patients with Stage III renal carcinoma were treated by this method. In patients treated early in the series, Radon seeds were used followed by 2500 rads of external beam therapy, and several patients had one or two doses of intra-arterial chemotherapy. The chemotherapy seemed to have no impact on the size of the tumor. Survival of the patients implanted with radioactive seeds was 59% at two years and 33% of patients at risk for five years. The tumor was not completely necrotic in the few patients in whom it was later excised or who subsequently had postmortem examinations, indicating that this is not a curative maneuver. Similarly, these metastases did not resolve. However, the survival of the patients is certainly greater than what had been previously observed, and, equally important, significant local palliation was achieved. Tumor size decreased in all patients. Pain control, weight gain and control of hemorrhage were achieved in approximately 80–85% of treated cases. The toxicity consisted of mild nausea or discomfort during the intra-arterial implantation procedure. This appears to be a reasonable approach to the patient with a large symptomatic nonresectable renal cell carcinoma [24].

Infarction of the renal artery with inert material in such patients also may be a consideration. However, infarction of large tumors by occlusion of the renal artery is associated with severe symptoms and may lead to tumor rupture or sepsis. Unless a nephrectomy can be anticipated as a feasible next step, inert infarction of these tumors does not seem to be a reasonable approach.

5. METASTATIC RENAL CARCINOMA

Approximately one-third to one-fourth of patients with renal carcinoma have metastases at the time the diagnosis is made. In the absence of effective methods of dealing with disseminated disease, surgeons have, for many decades, adopted the practice of palliative nephrectomy in such patients. The genesis of this practice is difficult to determine, but it seems to have been prompted by early observations that removal of the primary was sometimes associated with regression of metastases, and that this was an effective method of dealing with a symptomatic primary tumor.

Palliative nephrectomy for control of symptoms such as pain, hemorrhage, and endocrinopathy appears to be justified in the patient who has an expectation for a reasonable life span, perhaps six months or greater. The procedure, however, should not be commonly employed for the relief of symptoms. Although pain is a common problem, few patients have pain which cannot be easily controlled by narcotic analgesics, and the pain postoperatively and perioperatively is a poor trade-off for a minor complaint. The presence of severe pain generally indicates abdominal wall invasion which usually precludes complete surgical excision. When such tumors are incompletely excised, the patients rarely survive six months. Life threatening hemorrhage is a certain indication for palliative nephrectomy, but this is not a common occurrence. Other methods of dealing with hemorrhage are perhaps more practical. Percutaneous infarction of the bleeding vessels may be effective. Palliative radiotherapy is sometimes effective in controlling hemorrhage. In patients with very far-advanced disease, we have occluded the ureter with a bulb catheter and produced effective tamponade of the tumor and control of bleeding. An important factor when considering palliative surgery of any kind is the expected prospect for survival. The mean survival of patients with metastases at the time of diagnosis is approximately four months and only 10% of such patients survive one year [18]. Finally, in our experience troublesome endocrinopathy such as hypercalcemia is seldom significantly relieved by removal of the primary tumor, and the metastases continue to produce the parathormone-like substance. Nonetheless, an occasional patient may indeed be significantly benefited by relief of troublesome symptoms of various kinds with improvement of quality of life after palliative nephrectomy.

The practice of nephrectomy in patients who present with metastases at the time of diagnosis, in whom the primary tumor is not producing severe symptoms, was based mainly on the hope of inducing spontaneous regression of metastases, or prolonging survival. The literature reports continue to conflict, and no good studies have been made to firmly establish benefit following adjunctive nephrectomy. However, the practice continues to be advocated in some areas for a number of reasons. First, no other good therapy exists for such patients, many of whom are young and have an excellent performance status. Two, the unusual natural history of renal carcinoma suggests that intrinsical factors may be operative. From this was extrapolated the philosophy that removal of the primary might indeed improve the patient's ability to control the distant metastases. No firm evidence from experimental tumor growth kinetics lends support to this reasoning. Thirdly, regression of metastases has been observed after removal of the primary tumor [25, 26]. It is this phenomenon of regression of the tumor which has been most often inculcated to justify the practice of adjunctive nephrectomy, and the total clinical experience with this practice deserves careful scrutiny.

The exact number of patients with spontaneous regression is unknown and the literature is spotted with occasional single case reports. Several reviews have attempted to analyze this phenomenon. Bloom [26] reported approximately 43 cases of spontaneous regression of renal carcinoma and a number have been reported since that time. In all but two instances, regression occurred in patients who had pulmonary metastases and most patients were males. It must also be noted that most did not have histologic documentation of the nature of the metastatic lesion. Furthermore, regression in these patients was not necessarily equated with long-term cure. More recently, Freed *et al.* [25] presented 51 cases which seem to represent true regression of metastases. A similar observation was made, i.e., most regressions were of pulmonary metastases (45 of 51) and most occurred in males (38 of

51). Interestingly, although most tumors regress after the nephrectomy, some patients had no nephrectomy or had regression prior to nephrectomy. There can be little doubt that spontaneous regression of renal carcinoma does indeed occur, especially in males with pulmonary metastases. However, the incidence at which this occurs is more important than the absolute number of reported cases. Review of the literature suggests that this phenomenon occurs, either partially or totally, in approximately 0.4% of patients, or 1 in 250 [27]. This may even be an optimistic figure. In 533 patients reviewed from the Mayo Clinic [4], no incidence of regression of metastases was noted. Mostofi reported two survivors two years after the diagnosis in patients with metastases at the time of diagnosis for renal carcinoma. The incidence of regression of metastases following adjunctive nephrectomy is perhaps more germane to this discussion. In a collected review of a number of series from various institutions, the incidence of regression was approximately 0.8% [3]. It is also important to note that many of the metastatic lesions were not biopsied and that regression often occurred for brief periods of time. The mortality rate from the procedure varies, depending upon the patient selection, but is in the range of 2–15%. It, therefore, seems difficult to support the routine practice of palliative nephrectomy simply for the purpose of inducing regression of metastatic lesions, although this may occasionally occur.

Increase in survival is a legitimate goal of palliative surgery. However, little evidence suggests that adjunctive nephrectomy improves survival of patients with distant metastases. Johnson *et al.* [28] found no significant increase in survival after palliative nephrectomy except in patients whose metastases were confined to the skeletal system. This particular observation has not been confirmed by other authors and was perhaps a peculiarity of the patient population. In a series from this institution, a significantly greater survival of patients was noted after palliative nephrectomy [18]. However, this was based on patient selection and underscored the difficulty in assessing the impact on survival of such procedures. Only patients with good performance status were considered for surgery and therefore lived longer than those who did not undergo the adjunctive surgery. However, when the cumulative survival after adjunctive nephrectomy was compared to the survival of the entire population of patients with disseminated renal carcinoma, there was no difference in survival. This suggests that factors other than the nephrectomy were responsible for the survival pattern.

Based on the above review of the literature experience and upon personal experience, we have been reluctant to recommend adjunctive nephrectomy as a routine procedure. Palliative nephrectomy for relief of severe symptoms may occasionally be indicated. A second indication for nephrectomy in a patient with metastases is in the patient who presents with a single or several metastases which can be excised. The reported five-year survival rate following excision of pulmonary metastases is approximately 30% [29]. Admittedly, most such patients had previously had a nephrectomy. The removal of synchronous metastases cannot be expected to produce a similar survival rate, since other microscopic foci are likely to be present. However, in the absence of other treatment modalities, nephrectomy in the patient in good clinical condition, along with excision of limited metastatic foci seems to be a reasonable approach. A third indication is in the patient who has been shown to respond to a systemic modality. If, after several months of treatment, the metastases respond to chemotherapy or immunotherapy, it seems appropriate that the patient would benefit by the removal of a large primary lesion. A final indication is for the purpose of experimental therapy in the patient who gives proper informed consent. Removal of tumor with the intent of utilizing the tumor cells for experimental therapy protocols might be supported in the proper context. Similarly, removal of the tumor after infarction, as an experimental protocol, seems justified.

The practice of percutaneous infarction of primary renal carcinoma followed in several days by nephrectomy has been popularized by Johnson *et al.* [30]. The rationale for this approach can be found in clinical observations but patients seem to improve after palliative infarction of tumors, and experimental studies would suggest that destruction of tumors in situ may be associated with enhancement of the host immune response. In the most recent reports, 49 patients at M.D. Anderson were treated by percutaneous renal artery occlusion followed by nephrectomy and hormonal therapy. Of 36 evaluable patients, 6 patients had complete regression of tumor for 6–18 months, 5 patients had partial tumor regression, and 9 experienced some form of stabilization of growth of tumor for more than 12 months. The medium survival at the time of the report was 17 months for the treated population in contrast to an expected medium survival of 6 months. Both survival and response rate are impressive in view of the natural history of metastatic renal carcinoma. However, certain aspects of the study deserve careful evaluation. First, the authors treated 49 patients but evaluated 36, excluding the remainder on the basis that the response can be expected to occur 4.5 months after infarction. Therefore, patients who did not survive for that period were apparently excluded. Secondly, these patients all had pulmonary metastases. As noted above, most regressions of renal carcinoma are in patients with pulmonary metastases. Indeed, when one reviews reports of any form of treatment of this tumor, the vast majority of responders are those who have pulmonary lesions. Therefore this was an unusually favorable group of patients. Finally, the influence of hormone therapy is uncertain. Little evidence supports an active role of hormonal treatment in this tumor, although it has been advocated for decades, but it is difficult to segregate the importance of hormones from the significance of the infarction procedure. The evidence that infarction stimulates host immune response is scant. Delayed cutaneous hypersensitivity appeared to increase in most of the patients though lymphocyte blastogenesis response varied [31]. We have measured serum levels of antirenal carcinoma antibodies following infarction using the microcomplement fixation assay. Sera from 16 patients treated at our institution and at M.D. Anderson Hospital by Doctors Johnson, Swanson *et al.* were analyzed (unpublished data). In all but one instance, a significant increase (greater than $2 \log_2$) was noted within 48 hours following infarction. Levels then fell in most of the patients and levels varied following the subsequent nephrectomy. The significance of this finding in the small group of patients is unclear and does not unequivocally indicate a beneficial effect of the infarction with respect to tumor response or survival [32].

Our experience with infarction after nephrectomy is anecdotal, comprising 9 patients with various types of metastases. Though we have not noted any incidence of tumor regression, several patients with widely disseminated tumors and large retroperitoneal masses residual after nephrectomy have survived much longer than expected (8–16 months). The impact of this procedure on survival must await results of some ongoing prospective randomized trials. Meanwhile, the procedure should be used advisedly. Complications have occurred, including severe pain in every case, high fever, nausea, vomiting, paralytic ileus, and hypertension. One patient treated by this author developed a renal abscess followed by a gram negative septicemia and death. Unintentional embolization of peripheral vessels has also occurred.

A less disputed role of surgery in patients with disseminated renal carcinoma is in the management of the patient with a solitary metastasis. As noted above, the time of appearance of metastases in relation to nephrectomy is an important factor in determining outcome. The survival of patients who develop metastases more than two years after nephrectomy is considerably greater than those with synchronous metastases – a not surprising expression of the innate behavior of the tumor [18]. Regardless, excision of the solitary metastasis seems to be an effective treatment modality. Few patients (1–3%) will indeed present with a solitary metastasis and few more present with one or two lesions. Most of these are pulmonary lesions, although solitary osseous or soft tissue tumors can also often be excised. Excision of such lesions seems to be a worthwhile endeavor and is an effective palliative procedure. However, most such patients eventually develop other tumors and succumb to their disease. The palliation interval, however, may be extremely long. We have treated several patients who have had as many as five excisions of single lesions over a six- to eight-year period, with preservation of good functional status and apparent disease-free intervals between operations. Appearance of a new lesion within months after excision of a metastasis is an unhappy consequence of a palliative procedure. We, therefore, routinely treat the patient with some form of systemic therapy while observing the solitary metastasis for at least two or three months. In this fashion, the solitary nature of the metastasis is more certain.

6. CONCLUSIONS

The only effective treatment for renal carcinoma remains surgical excision. Until effective systemic modalities are identified, surgery is indicated whenever there is a reasonable prospect for cure or significant palliation (complete excision of locally extensive tumor, excision of infradiaphragmatic vena caval extension, excision of limited lymph node metastases, nephrectomy for relief of severe symptoms, and excision of solitary metastases). Ultimately, the clinical circumstances in which aggressive surgery is unlikely to produce cure or even significant palliation should be more carefully identified and should deter costly surgical management which produces undue morbidity and confines the patient to the hospital for extended periods ('debulking' of non-resectable tumors, excision of multifocal metastatic disease). Alternative approaches to provide palliation with less morbidity should be sought and tested in clinical trials. It is apparent, however, that all such approaches will have little impact on the natural course of renal carcinoma and on the survival of the population of renal cancer patients. Development of effective systemic management is essential to achieving this goal.

REFERENCES

1. Kantor AF, Meigs JV, Heston JF, Flannery JT: Epidemiology of renal cell carcinoma in Connecticut. J Natl Cancer Inst 57:495, 1976.
2. Skinner DG, Colvin RB, Vermillion CD *et al.*: Diagnosis and management of renal cell carcinoma. Cancer 28:1165, 1971.
3. DeKernion JB, Berry D: The diagnosis and treatment of renal cell carcinoma. Cancer 45:1947, 1980.
4. Myers GH, Fehrenbaker LG, Kelalis PP: Prognostic significance of renal vein invasion by hypernephroma. J Urol 100:420, 1968.
5. Skinner DG, Pfister RF, Colvin R: Extension of renal cell carcinoma into the vena cava: The rationale for aggressive surgical management. J Urol 107:711, 1972.
6. Schefft P, Novick AC, Strffon RA, Stewart BH: Surgery for renal cell carcinoma extending into the inferior vena cava. J Urol 120:28, 1978.
7. DeKernion JB: Lymphadenectomy for renal cell carcinoma: therapeutic implications. Urol Clin North Am, 1980.(In press.)

8. Clayman RV, Gonzalez R, Fraley EE: Renal cell carcinoma invading the inferior vena cava: clinical review and anatomical approach. J Urol 123:157, 1980.
9. de Kernion JB: Radical nephrectomy. In: Modern Techniques in Surgery: Urologic Surgery. (Ehrlich RM, ed.) Mount Kisco, NY: Future Publishing: 1980.
10. McCollough DL, Gittes RF: Ligation of the renal vein in the solitary kidney: effects on renal function. J Urol 113:295, 1975.
11. Robson CJ, Churchill B, Anderson W: Radical nephrectomy for renal cell carcinoma. J Urol 101:297, 1969.
12. Petkovic SD: An anatomical classification of renal tumors in the adult as a basis for prognosis. J Urol 81:618, 1959.
13. Angervall L, Carlstrom E, Wahlquist L: Effects of clinical and morphological variables on spread of renal carcinoma and in an operative series. Scand J Urol Nephrol 3:134, 1969.
14. Hülten L, Rosencrantz T, Wahlquist L, Ahren C: Scand J Urol Nephrol 3:129, 1969.
15. Rafla S: Renal cell carcinoma. Natural history and results of treatment. Cancer 25:26, 1970.
16. Skinner DG, Vermillion CD, Colvin RB: The surgical manegement of renal cell carcinoma. J Urol 107:705, 1972.
17. Flocks RH, Kadesky MC: Malignant neoplasm of the kidney: an analysis of 353 patients followed five years or more. J Urol 79:196, 1958.
18. deKernion JB, Ramming KP, Smith RB: Natural history of metastatic renal cell carcinoma: computer analysis. J Urol 120:148, 1978.
19. Cox CE, Lacy SS, Montgomery WG, Boyce WH: Renal adenocarcinoma: 28-year review, with emphasis on rationale and feasibility of preoperative radiotherapy. J Urol 104:51, 1970.
20. Riches EW: The place of radiotherapy in the management of parenchymal carcinoma of the kidney. J Urol 95:313, 1966.
21. Werf-Messing B: Carcinoma of the kidney. Cancer 32:1056, 1973.
22. Middleton RG, Presto AJ III: Radical thoracoabdominal nephrectomy for renal cell carcinoma. J Urol 110:36, 1973.
23. Lokich JJ, Harrison JH: Renal cell carcinoma: natural history and chemotherapeutic experience. J Urol 114:371, 1975.
24. Lang E, deKernion JB: Transcatheter embolization of advanced renal cell carcinoma with radioactive seeds. J Urol, 1981, (in press).
25. Freed SZ: Nephrectomy for renal cell carcinoma with metastases. Urology 9:613, 1977.
26. Bloom HJG: Hormone-induced and spontaneous regression of metastatic renal cancer. Cancer 32:1066, 1973.
27. Montie JE, Stewart BH, Straffon RA *et al.*: The role of adjunctive nephrectomy in patients with metastatic renal cell carcinoma. J Urol 117:272, 1977.
28. Johnson DE, Kaesler KE, Samuels MC: Is nephrectomy justified in patients with metastatic renal carcinoma? J Urol 114:27, 1975.
29. Middleton RG: Surgery for metastatic renal cell carcinoma. J Urol 97:973, 1967.
30. Johnson DE, Swanson DA: The management of renal carcinoma. Weekly Urology Update Series, Lesson 36, Vol 1:2, 1978.
31. Hersh EM, Wallace S, Johnson DE, Bracken RB: Immunological studies in human urological cancer. In: Cancer of Genitourinary Tract. (Johnson DE, Samuels ML, eds.) New York: Raven Press, 1979.
32. Wallace S, Chuang V, Green B, Swanson DA, Bracken RB, Johnson DE: Diagnostic radiology in renal carcinoma. In: Cancer of the Genitourinary Tract. (Johnson DE, Samuels ML, eds.) New York: Raven Press, 1979.

5. Health Risk and Management of Localized Prostate Cancer

CARL A. OLSSON and RALPH DEVERE WHITE

1. INTRODUCTION

Adenocarcinoma of the prostate gland is detected in 56 000 American men annually. In this same period of time, 20 000 men die of the disease. Prostate cancer is the third most common cancer death in men in this country, accounting for 25% of all adult male deaths by neoplasms.

This chapter will address various problems relating to adenocarcinoma confined to the prostate gland. These problems are in many respects unresolved. However, they may at least be clearly identified. We can define, by various staging parameters, cancers that are confined to the prostate gland. We can discuss methods of screening men for prostate cancers that may promise an improved rate of detection of localized disease. We can identify some of the characteristics of localized prostate cancer that correlate with a hazard to health and longevity.

Prior to initiating a review, it should be mentioned that the biologic potential of localized prostate cancer is difficult to determine, for a number of reasons. The disease occurs at an age when men are subject to death from a variety of other causes. Furthermore, prostate cancer is a slow growing neoplasm, so that long-term studies are required to judge the impact of localized disease on the host. Finally, both stage and histologic grade exert a profound impact on survival. However, in carrying out reviews such as this contribution, one must analyze and compare reports in which histologic grading may or may not be recorded and in which patients have been staged by substantially different techniques.

2. STAGING OF PROSTATE CANCER

The TNM system of staging of neoplasms adopted by the International Union Against Cancer (UICC) has not gained uniform acceptance in the

D.F. Paulson (ed.), Genitourinary Cancer 1, 121-142.

United States. In this country, workers traditionally employ variations of a system originally proposed by Jewett [1]. In recent years, numerous modifications of the Jewett system have been proposed in an attempt to further specify the extent of disease or characterize its biologic potential. There is no consensus on which of the proposed modifications are most appropriate. Furthermore, the staging system employed in this country suffers from the fact that many workers confuse clinical and surgical staging. For example, clinically staged C patients are apt to have lymph node metastases in 50% of cases, whereas surgically staged C patients, by definition, have undergone pelvic lymphadenectomy with no metastases found on histologic review of the resected nodes.

By definition, clinical stage A disease represents an error in diagnosis. In this instance, a patient undergoes prostatic resection for presumed benign prostatic hypertrophy and adenocarcinoma is found in the resected specimen. Further testing in such patients may reveal the presence of metastatic disease, so that the person initially assigned to clinical stage A frequently advances in stage as more parameters are tested (2-9). Due to its biological variations, there is general agreement that stage A disease consists of at least two sub-groups (with some workers suggesting three). Stage A-1 prostate cancer is the designation reserved for those patients in whom a small focus of well-differentiated adenocarcinoma of the prostate is found in the resected 'benign' specimen, and where repeat biopsy of the prostate (transurethral or perineal) reveals no residual cancer in the gland remnant. The classification of stage A-2 is assigned to patients in whom either numerous foci of well-differentiated cancer or any focus of less well-differentiated neoplasm is discovered on histologic examination.

Stage B prostate cancer is the classification assigned to individuals in whom a preoperative diagnosis of malignancy is established (by rectal examination and biopsy) and in whom the disease is felt to be clinically confined to the prostate gland. Based on the volume of disease as well as knowledge of worsening prognosis with increasing tumor volume, there is general agreement that stage B patients can also be subdivided into two groups. Stage B-1 is an assignment reserved for an individual in whom there is a solitary prostate nodule of less than 2 cm in diameter located in a single lobe of the prostate. Stage B-2 is the assignment conferred in those individuals who have more extensive disease (large nodules or involvement of both prostate lobes).

Clinical stage C disease is the assignment applied to patients who have obvious palpatory evidence of cancer extending beyond the confines of the prostate gland, usually penetrating the gland capsule and often involving the seminal vesicle. Stage D is a classification reserved for patients with demonstrated metastases to adjacent organs, lymph nodes, skeleton or other viscera. Various sub-groupings have been advocated to further define patients with both stage C and stage D prostatic cancer; these will not be discussed further in this presentation on localized disease.

Staging parameters leading to a decision that prostate cancer is confined to the prostate gland include rectal examination, analysis of serum acid phosphatase level, radioactive bone scanning and X-rays of the bony skeleton. At the time of diagnosis, these initial staging studies will confirm that metastases have occurred or that the disease has spread beyond the boundaries of the prostate in 80% of cases. Thus, in this discussion of adenocarcinoma confined to the prostate gland, we are limiting ourselves to an analysis of 20% of all patients with this disease. This number will be further reduced if surgical lymph node sampling is performed, because approximately one-fourth of patients with clinically presumed local disease have unsuspected lymph node metastases. The expectation that this significant percentage of understaging will adversely affect prognosis as well as potentially influence management has led to increasing popularity of surgical staging in patients with localized prostate cancer.

2.1. Pelvic Lymph Node Evaluation

Various techniques for evaluating the presence of metastases in the pelvic lymph nodes have been advocated in recent years. Lymphangiography carried out by means of bipedal injections results in correct estimation of metastatic disease relatively infrequently. Pertinent lymph nodes (obturator and hypogastric) may not be clearly outlined by bipedal lymphangiography. Furthermore, microscopic lymph node involvement is unlikely to be discovered by lymphangiography. Finally, fatty replacement of tissue is not uncommon in the pelvic lymph nodes and this may be misinterpreted as metastatic cancer. Some workers have advocated carrying out lymphangiography with percutaneous thin needle biopsy of suspicious nodes to avoid this latter confusion. Most workers, however, feel that lymphangiography is not sufficiently accurate to confirm the presence or absence of prostate cancer metastasis [9, 10].

The best means of accurately establishing the presence or absence of lymph node metastases appears to be surgical lymphadenectomy or lymph node sampling. This operation is carried out in the retroperitoneum through either a midline or extended Pfannenstiel abdominal incision. The lymph nodes sampled or removed in the course of staging patients with prostate cancer include the external iliac, hypogastric and obturator node groups.

As stated above, the overall percentage of understaging in patients with clinically presumed stage A or B prostate cancer is approximately 25%. Generally speaking, the worse the histologic grade and the more extensive the tumor within the prostate, the more likely lymph node metastases will be found. Since by definition, patients with stage A-1 disease have well-differentiated, small foci of adenocarcinoma, it is rare to find a patient in this clinical stage category demonstrating pelvic lymph node metastases, and surgical lymph node staging is not routinely recommended for such patients [11]. In contrast, patients with stage A-2 prostate cancer will be found to have lymph node metastases in nearly 30% of cases [7, 11]. The reason for this is not surprising, for, by definition, stage A-2 prostate cancer is either more diffuse or composed of a worse histologic grade (or both). The incidence of positive lymph nodes in patients with stage B-1 prostate cancer is approximately 10–15%. In contrast, the patient with the more diffuse stage B-2 lesions is likely to have lymph node metastases found approximately 20% of the time (though figures up to 45% have been reported) [12].

The significance of pelvic lymph node metastases has been clearly established in recent years. As reported by Whitmore, 85% of patients with pelvic lymph node metastases demonstrated disease progression within a five-year follow-up interval. In contrast, patients with negative lymph nodes experienced only a 25% chance of demonstrating overt metastatic disease in the same time period [6]. In a smaller series of 112 patients undergoing lymphadenectomy for prostatic cancer, we found 37 men with lymphadenopathy, of whom 16 experienced disease progression (5 died of metastatic cancer) within an average time interval of 13 months. In the 75 patients with negative lymph nodes observed over the same period of time, only 5 had progressed and there were no cancer deaths [7]. Because of these observations, there is increasing consensus that surgical intervention is warranted in order to determine the presence or absence of pelvic lymph node metastases in localized prostate cancer. Knowledge of the pelvic lymph node status is not only important form a prognostic point of view, but may exert a profound influence on the selection of therapy for patients with localized disease. For example, one is unlikely to select radical prostatectomy in patients who have already demonstrated lymph node metastasis. On the other hand, one may be willing to elect aggressive adjuvant treatment in such patients because of the associated poor prognosis.

A final point should be made about pelvic lymph node dissection. While it is not absolutely certain that this procedure is devoid of therapeutic benefit, it is most likely that its therapeutic value in most patients will be minimal. It would therefore be a significant contribution if the presence or absence of lymph node metastasis could actually be ascertained without surgical intervention. Whether or not computed axial tomography will prove advantageous in this regard remains to be seen.

3. HISTOLOGIC GRADE

More and more it appears that histologic grade exerts a profound influence on clinical prognosis in patients with localized prostate cancer. Of great concern to the urologist, however, is the fact that there is no unanimity regarding the grading systems presently advocated for this disease. Prostate cancer is a neoplasm in which it is difficult to judge histologic grade because of the heterogeneity of the cells contained within the tumor. These cells demonstrate different ultrastructural features as well as differing architectural patterns of growth. The situation is further complicated by the fact that histologic grading in some instances is confined to an analysis of small tissue specimens (as obtained by needle biopsy of the prostate). It is possible that cellular and architectural growth patterns in small tissue samples may differ from similar measurements in the entire tumor. Furthermore, when comparing the histologic grade of the primary tumor with that of a metastasis, there is, at times, little correlation between the two, employing the grading systems that have already been described.

A variety of recent techniques have been developed to analyze the individual prostate cancer cell. Employing light microscopic morphometry or stereology to analyze nuclear/cytoplasmic ratios, presence of prominent nucleoli and the like, efforts are made to identify cellular characteristics that correlate with tumor aggressiveness. One of the potential drawbacks of this cellular analysis rests with the question of whether the aggressiveness of a prostate cancer is dependent on its most malignant component or an average of all the cells contained within the tumor. The answer to this question is dependent upon a comparison of selective and randomized measurements of prostate cancer cells, and remains to be seen.

The most popular grading system in this country is that reported by Gleason [13]. Histologic grading in this system is based on an evaluation of the overall pattern of growth of the tumor when examined at relatively low magnification (40–100×). Five patterns of growth are identified and are assigned values of 1–5 with increasing histologic appearance of agressiveness. Observations of two separate patterns of growth in each tumor are recorded, assigning both the primary and secondary pattern values of 1–5, resulting in a final histologic grade varying between 2 and 10. Gleason grading is helpful in predicting the likelihood that a patient with localized disease has pelvic lymph node metastases at the two extremes of the scoring range. In patients with a histologic grade of 2–4, the chances are no more than 16% that pelvic lymph nodes will be involved; tumors with a histologic grade of 8–10 will be associated with pelvic lymph node metastases in 60–100% of cases [6, 9]. However, the majority of patients with prostate cancer will demonstrate histologic scores in the mid-range (5–7), and in this range, Gleason grading has no predictive value in determining that lymph node metastasis has occurred.

Even prior to the establishment of the Gleason grading system, there was certainly an awareness of the prognostic importance of histologic grading. Many workers had observed that patients with poorly differentiated stage A prostate cancer fared significantly worse than patients with well-differentiated stage A disease. For example, Bauer showed a 47% ten-year survival in well-differentiated stage A patients, compared with a 14% ten-year survival in poorly differentiated stage A prostate cancer [14]. Hanash, employing a grade I/grade IV system of histologic scoring reported 75% of patients with grade I, stage A prostate cancer were alive after ten years, whereas only 36% of patients with grade III or IV disease were alive after a similar period [15]. These were among the observations that led to our understanding of the distinction between stage A-1 and A-2 prostate cancer. The impact of histologic grading on survival in stage B disease is also well known. Culp reviewed the results of radical prostatectomy and concluded that, even when dealing with the same stage lesions, patients with grade I cancer experienced a 50% better survival than those with grade II lesions [16].

4. SCREENING FOR LOCALIZED PROSTATE CANCER

Because of the small percentage of prostate cancer patients who remain assigned to low clinical stages (localized disease) after clinical and surgical staging studies have been completed, there has been increasing interest in the development of a screening test for adenocarcinoma of the prostate in men over 45–50 years old. In order for a screening test to be cost-effective, the general population should show a relatively common disease incidence. One must assume that early disease undergoes progression and that advanced disease competes as a cause of death in the general population under review. Finally, one must assume that early disease, if detected, may be cured. These premises for cost-effective screening have not been totally resolved in the case of adenocarcinoma of the prostate. Prostate cancer is a relatively common disease (34 per 100 000 males). Untreated early prostate cancer usually undergoes progression (provided one removes stage A-1 cancer from consideration and analyzes patients with stages A-2, B-1 and B-2 prostate cancer). Advanced disease certainly competes as a cause of death in individuals who, if cancer-free, have a life expectancy that is greater than 10–15 years. It is still unclear, however, whether localized disease can be thoroughly cured.

Methods advocated for the screening of prostate cancer (other than rectal exam and biopsy) include studies of urinary and plasma levels of carcinoembryonic antigen, serum levels of creatine kinase-BB and serum levels of prostatic acid phosphatase. Carcinoembryonic antigen studies in the plasma and urine are of little value in screening for localized prostate cancer, as patients with stages A and B disease have not shown an elevation of this tumor marker in either body fluid [17]. Silverman reported that 3 of 4 patients with stage B prostate cancer showed an elevation of creatine kinase-BB in the serum. With additional studies of this enzyme by other workers, the ability to detect localized disease with this serum marker has not been borne out [18, 19]. Enzymatic assays for the measurement of prostatic acid phosphatase will be elevated in 75% of patients with metastatic disease. However, it is generally agreed that enzymatic assays are sufficiently insensitive to elevations of prostatic acid phosphatase to allow detection of disease confined to the prostate capsule. In an effort to increase the sensitivity of assays for prostatic acid phosphatase, a number of immunoassay techniques have been developed, all relying on the immunologic specificity of anti-prostatic acid phosphatase antibodies. The quality of the antibodies employed in these immunoassays depends upon the purity of the antigen against which the antibody is raised as well as the monospecificity of the resultant antiserum.

Foti and Cooper reported a solid phase radioimmunoassay in 1975 [20]. Their initial report stated that this radioimmunoassay was able to detect 33% of patients with stage A disease and 79% of patients with stage B prostate cancer. This significant advance, compared to the results obtained with enzymatic assays for prostatic acid phosphatase, led to an initial burst of enthusiasm for the screening potential of immunoassays for prostatic acid phosphatase. However, close analysis of the patients studied in this initial report demonstrated that 51% of the total cancer population was composed of patients with stage A and stage B disease. This observation suggested a significant degree of understaging in the population studied and this would imply that many of the patients classified as stage A and B actually had more advanced disease, in which case an elevated serum prostatic acid phosphatase would not be surprising. The immunoassay reported by Foti and Cooper also suffered from the fact that there was a 6% false positive rate.

Counterimmunoelectrophoresis is a simpler technique for the immunoassay of prostatic acid phosphatase. It can be conducted in a matter of hours vs. days and requires neither specialized equipment nor radioisotopes for determination. Originally reported from Roswell Park Memorial Institute, this technique demonstrated elevations of serum prostatic acid phosphatase in only 30% of patients with stage A or B disease [21]. Wajsman, in 1979, summarized the results obtained from a number of cooperating institutions using the counterimmunoelectrophoresis technique for assaying prostatic acid phosphatase. The study was positive in 38% of patients with stage A disease and 35% of patients with stage B disease [22]. These figures are close to the percentage of expected lymph node metastases in these two disease stages so that it is possible that the immunoassay was detecting patients with metastatic disease only. Thus, while immunoassays for prostatic acid phosphatase are more sensitive than enzymatic assays, they do not appear to be reliable for the detection of prostate cancer confined to the prostatic capsule.

Whenever discussing screening tests for any disease, one must analyze the test according to its sensitivity (freedom from false negative assays), specificity (freedom from false positive assays) and the prevalence of the disease sought. For example, if there were a disease that was extremely common (1 per 1000 population), and there was a screening assay that was sufficiently sensitive to detect 100% of patients with the disease with a 99% specificity, one could anticipate carrying out 1000 assays to obtain 11 positive results, only 1 of which would be indicative of the presence of the disease. In the case of prostate cancer, the figures are far worse than those suggested in the example just given. Prostate cancer has a prevalence of 34 per 100 000 men. Radioimmunoassays for the detection of serum prostatic acid phosphatase have no better than 70% sensitivity to the disease and no better than 94% specificity. These figures, reflecting the 'state of the art' in immunoassays for prostatic acid phosphatase suggest that many thousands of tests would have to be conducted to find 244 individuals with elevations of prostatic acid phosphatase, only 1 of whom would be shown to have prostatic adenocarcinoma.

A newer immunoassay for prostatic acid phosphatase has been developed by Chu and Wajsman [23]. It is a solid phase immunofluorescent assay, utilizing the immunologic specificity of anti-prostatic acid phosphatase antibody in a solid phase support, along with the fluorescent properties of alpha naphthol. The sensitivity of this test appears to be several hundred-fold greater than either radioimmunoassay or counterimmunoelectrophoresis in measuring prostatic acid phosphatase. In initial clinical evaluations at Roswell Park Memorial Institute, this solid phase immunofluorescent assay detected an elevated acid phosphatase in almost all untreated patients with stage A prostate cancer and in 60–70% of patients with stage B or C lesions who were undergoing standard treatment. The data leading to this initial report was derived from a small patient sampling. This test appears to be the most sensitive method developed to date for the detection of elevations of prostatic acid phosphatase, but we will have to await further evaluation to see if it can be made applicable to screening large populations of patients for localized prostate cancer.

It may be unrealistic to presume that studies of body fluids will lead to early detection of prostatic adenocarcinoma. The most proximate fluid to the prostate gland, of course, is the prostate exprimate (expressed prostatic secretions). Grayhack and co-workers have conducted a number of studies of the prostatic exprimate in benign and malignant prostatic disease. They have found that the ratio between LDH isoenzyme 5 and isoenzyme 1 is reversed in patients with prostate cancer, regardless of the stage of the disease. An initial difficulty encountered with this assay was that white blood cells expressed in the prostatic fluid led to similar reversals of the LDH 5 to 1 ratio. However, by additionally analyzing the prostatic exprimate for levels of transferrin (a marker unaffected by the presence of white blood cells) Grayhack and his colleagues have reported that they can detect 80% of patients with localized disease with great accuracy [24].

From the above discussion it is apparent that we have no screening test for cancer of the prostate that will reliably detect the disease when it is confined to the prostatic capsule. The expectation that we will be able to utilize a combination of prostatic fluid studies as well as more sensitive measurements of serum levels of prostatic acid phosphatase to detect cancer confined to the prostate remains to be confirmed in additional clinical trials. At the present time, the best means for the detection of early disease appears to be rectal examination and early biopsy of the prostate glands that are palpably abnormal. Urologists are occasionally reluctant to conduct prostatic biopsy if their level of suspicion is low, fearing that the complications of prostatic biopsy are not warranted with a low index of suspicion. However, it should be recalled that in every series analyzed, only 50% of nodules palpated in the prostate represent malignant disease, while the remaining nodules are indicative of benign prostatic hypertrophy, prostatitis, calculi and granulomatous disease [25]. With this in mind, the urologist should anticipate no better than a 50% yield of confirmation of malignant process in his personal series of prostatic biopsies. If one's personal yield of cancer is higher than 50% on prostate biopsy, one is probably not carrying out a sufficiently aggressive biopsy program.

5. MANAGEMENT OF LOCALIZED PROSTATE CANCER

Few, if any, prospectively randomized studies of the management of localized prostate carcinoma have been reported. Therefore, one must resort to historical controls and comparison series when discussing the options for management of this neoplasm. Such historical comparisons, however, are subject to a number of limitations. Many series reporting treatment response in stage A and stage B prostate cancer failed to distinguish patients with stage A-1 versus A-2 neoplasms. A similar statement can be made regarding reports that fail to recognize the difference between B-1 and B-2 prostatic adenocarcinoma. Even when tumor stage is accurately reported, other important prognostic variables, such as grade of neoplasm, are not mentioned in some series available for historic comparison. Since prostate cancer is a slowly progressive lesion, a follow-up period of 10–15 years is required to judge the effect of the disease and its management; many of the series are reported with considerably shorter observation intervals. In many series where a fifteen-year follow-up is available, the data must be reinterpreted in terms of the utilization (or lack thereof) of some of the staging tests now recognized as important but simply not available during the period of patient accession. For example, the majority of patients reported in some series were staged without the benefit of serum acid phosphatase determinations, radioactive bone scans, and the like. Information regarding the presence or absence of pelvic lymph node metastasis is usually lacking in reports of management of localized prostatic adenocarcinoma. As we have seen above, as many as 45% of patients with clinically staged B-2 disease will have pelvic lymph node metastases, so that an article that reports the results of management of clinical stage B-2 prostatic adenocarcinoma will, in fact, be describing a group of patients of whom nearly half have experienced metastasis beyond the confines of the prostate capsule. Finally, in some series there has been relatively haphazard use of endocrine manipulation in an adjuvant fashion to the primary treatment modality under comparison.

As pointed out by Whitmore, the natural history of localized prostatic cancer may not follow an orderly progression from stage A to stage B and from these stages to stages C and D [25]. If there were an orderly progression, one could assume that all patients with stage A disease would eventually progress to stage D and one would simply have to know the length of time to progression to calculate whether or not the disease was a sufficient risk to length and quality of life to warrant therapeutic intervention. As had been pointed out above, however, at least some patients with stage A disease will not experience progression.

5.1. Radical Prostatectomy

The treatment modalities available for localized prostatic cancer consist of radical prostatectomy or irradiation. The assumptions one makes in choosing radical prostatectomy is that cure can be achieved if the entire cancer load is excised and that no other form of therapy provides equally effective disease control.

Even if radical prostatectomy were the best form of therapy, it should be chosen with the realization that there are complications associated with this operation. Nearly all patients undergoing radical prostatectomy will be rendered impotent. Although the use of penile implants is now recognized as a means of overcoming the problem of impotence, the potential for urinary incontinence continues to be a consideration. However, we agree with Walsh's observation that urinary incontinence should be experienced in less than 2–3% of cases, provided the procedure is performed by an experienced surgeon [27].

After the publication of Jewett's early series of radical prostatectomy, demonstrating a 50% ten-year survival and 35% fifteen-year survival, it became apparent that some individuals managed with radical prostatectomy were not cured [28]. Soon after the publication of the Jewett series, Bagshaw and Ray reported their ten-year experience with external beam radiation therapy in patients with localized prostate cancer, demonstrating a ten-year survivability precisely the same as Jewett had accomplished with radical surgery [29]. Because of this report, and the complications associated with radical surgery, many workers advocated radiation therapy as the preferred treatment technique for adenocarcinoma confined to the prostate gland.

5.2. Radiotherapy

Two general techniques for delivering radiation therapy to the prostate have been popularized. External beam irradiation is usually accomplished utilizing a high energy source (cobalt 60 or betatron). The majority of treatment protocols are designed to deliver 5000 rads to the entire pelvis, encompassing the site of pelvic lymph node drainage. An additional 2000 rads is delivered by a smaller portal to the porstate region selectively, resulting in a total administration of approximately 7000 rads delivered to the prostate gland.

An alternative method of delivering radiation to the prostate employs interstitial implantation of radioemitters. Although the technique of interstitial implantation of the prostate dates back to 1917, the use of radioemitters in the treatment of prostate cancer was popularized by Flocks in 1952 [30]. He utilized combinations of surgery, external beam irradiation and collidal gold^{198}. Modern techniques of interstitial irradiation employ gold^{198}grains or encapsulated iodine^{125}, as advocated by Carlton and Whitmore, respectively [6, 31].

Gold^{198} is a high energy emitter with a short half-life and large radius of tissue penetrance (6 cm). Iodine^{125} is a low energy emitter with a narrow range of tissue penetrance and a half-life of two months. These different characteristics of radioisotopes of iodine and gold present advantages and disadvantages in comparison [32]. Since radioactive gold has a greater tissue penetrance, fewer particles must be implanted into the prostate to result in reasonable isodose configuration. Of course, the potential for radiation scatter to contiguous tissues (bladder and rectum) is higher. Furthermore, the higher energy emitted by gold^{198} increases the danger of radiation exposure to hospital personnel and the patient's family. Finally, the short-life of gold^{198} requires that the isotope be produced near the institution conducting the implantation. In contrast, iodine^{125} is a safer isotope to use. Its longer half-life allows for a reasonable period of shelf-life prior to implantation. This long period, however, makes it difficult to judge the need (if any) for a boost of external beam therapy in patients implanted. Finally, its short radius of tissue penetrance requires that numerous separate needles must be implanted into the prostate gland in order to achieve a reasonable isodose configuration.

Generally, patients undergoing interstitial irradiation with gold receive an external beam boost to improve the distribution of radiation in the prostate gland. Dosages of approximately 4000 R are usually employed. In contrast, interstitial irradiation accomplished with iodine^{125} is usually conducted without an external beam radiation plan. When external beam therapy *is* advocated in addition to interstitial iodine, it is wise to postpone the external boost until at least the first half-life is over (60 days) so that the initial results of interstitial therapy alone (with its side effects) may be judged. Furthermore, it is wise to reduce the amount of external beam irradiation to level no higher than 2000 R in order to avoid severe radiation proctitis.

Interstitial irradiation is usually conducted along with surgical pelvic lymphadenectomy. Therefore, one advantage of interstitial irradiation is the resultant excellent (surgical) staging of the patient with localized prostate cancer. This information is not only important from a prognostic point of view, but some workers also use the presence of lymph node metastasis as an indication for additional adjuvant therapy [7, 33]. On the other hand, since interstitial irradiation requires that surgery be carried out, there is the potential for postoperative complications. The overall complication rate following surgery of this sort is approximately 10–15%. The most common complications are wound infection or separation, pelvic phlebitis, lymphocele and pulmonary embolus [7].

External beam irradiation of the prostate is associated with a decrease in erectile potency in as many as 40% of patients, while the incidence of impotence following interstitial irradiation is extremely low [6, 34, 35]. Nearly half the patients administered external radiotherapy will experience at least some degree of transient bladder or bowel irritability during therapy. Unrelenting proctitis may be anticipated in as many as 5% of patients treated with external beam irradiation.

The effectiveness of radiation therapy in the control of localized prostatic adenocarcinoma has come under increasing scrutiny in recent years. As evidenced by clinical examination and postirradiation prostatic biopsy, approximately 40% of patients treated with radiotherapy fail to demonstrate local control of disease. Hulick reported 147 patients with stage A to stage C prostate cancer who were treated with external irradiation (6500–7000 rads) [35]. Local tumor control, as judged by clinical examination, was achieved in 91 patients, of whom 71 were alive and free of disease after a three-year observation period. However, of the 62 patients whose primary disease was not palpably controlled, 45 had died. Regardless of the method by which radiation therapy is delivered, posttreatment biopsies of the prostate will continue to show apparently viable malignant cells in nearly half the patients [10, 31, 36, 37]. Carlton reported 37% positive biopsies stage B patients treated with interstitial gold and an external beam irradiation boost [31]. Rhamy reported 87% positive biopsies in patients treated with external beam irradiation [36]. Sewell conducted a survey of post-irradiation biopsies and found an overall incidence of persistent malignancy in 38% of cases [37]. Finally, Lytton demonstrated a 50% incidence of persistent malignancy following interstitial irradiation employing iodine^{125} [10].

While it was initially claimed by some workers that the malignant cells shown on posttreatment biopsies had no biological potential, both Hadley and Kiesling demonstrated that these cells maintain the electron microscopic features of nonirradiated cancer cells [38, 39]. Bruce demonstrated that irradiated cancer cells continued to show the potential to produce acid phosphatase [40]. Finally, Paulson showed that irradiated human prostate cancer cells were capable of establishing viable explants in the nude mouse [41].

With these preliminary remarks regarding the management of localized prostatic carcinoma, we can now address specific points related to the disease in each of its localized stages.

5.3. Stage A Prostate Cancer

Occasional patients undergoing prostatic resection for presumed bening prostatic hypertrophy will demonstrate adenocarcinoma of the prostate in the resected specimen. It is now clear that we can differentiate which of such patients require additional treatment. We have already discussed the contributions of Bauer and Hanash to our understanding of the influence of histologic grade on patient survival in stage A prostate cancer. Schoonees found that prostate cancer was the cause of death in 14.3% of his stage A patients; all deaths occurred in patients who had poorly differentiated tumors [42]. Similarly, Green analyzed 83 cases of stage A disease, 86% of whom had grade I lesions. In these individuals there was no alteration of life expectancy, whereas 8 cancer deaths occurred in individuals who had other than well-differentiated carcinoma found in the resected specimen [43]. The extent of neoplastic involvement of the resected prostate also influences prognosis. For example, Barnes found that, when less than 25% of the resected prostate chips were involved by adenocarcinoma, a ten-year survival of 56% and fifteen-year survival of 35% was recorded. In contrast, when more diffuse disease was present in the resected specimen, ten- and fifteen-year survival statistics fell to 26% and 14%, respectively [44].

With this information, we now realize that patients with stage A prostate cancer should be separated into two categories, depending upon histologic grade of the unsuspected carcinoma as well as extent of involvement of the prostate. Patients in whom any amount of cancer is discovered with less than well-differentiated grade should be classified as stage A-2. Patients with diffuse disease, regardless of histologic grade should also be characterized as stage A-2. These patients warrant additional therapy, provided they can be anticipated to enjoy otherwise a ten-year life expectancy.

On the other hand, patients with 1–3 foci of well-differentiated adenocarinoma discovered on histologic examination of the resected prostate apparently enjoy normal life expectancy. The responsibility of the urologist, in dealing with these patients, is to insure that the initial report of only a few foci is accurate. Two means by which he can make this assurance are: a) additional histologic examination of the resected tissue, and b) repeat biopsy of the prostate remnant.

Since the ability to detect small foci of prostatic adenocarcinoma increases with the thoroughness of histologic examination, step-sectioning of the resected tissue should be performed to confirm that the foci initially seen on routine sections were indeed all that were present. For example, Emmet demonstrated a 13% incidence of prostate cancer with the use of routine sectioning techniques in an autopsy series conducted on men over the age of 50. However, when step-sectioning of the prostate was carried out, this figure rose to 24% [45]. Denton analyzed 500 men over the age of 50 who underwent transurethral resection of the prostate. Stage A prostate cancer was found in 6% of the specimens analyzed by routine sectioning. However, an additional 15% of prostates were found involved after step-sectioning the resected tissue [46].

If step-sectioning reveals no additional well-differentiated adenocarcinoma beyond the 1–3 foci initially reported, the patient should undergo rebiopsy of the prostate biopsy two to three months following the initial resection. McMillen reported the results of repeat biopsy in 27 patients with a single focus of adenocarcinoma of the prostate found at transurethral resection. In 10 of 27 patients, a repeat resection demonstrated residual cancer [47]. Whether or not the repeat biopsy must be carried out by resection of the prostatic fossa or whether the same information can be obtained by perineal needle biopsy remains to be seen.

Based on historical reports cited above, patients with 1–3 foci of well-differentiated adenocarcinoma of the prostate found in tissue resected for presumed benign disease experience a normal life expectancy, and the chance of the disease having an influence on survival is extremely small. Presumably, in these cases, the transurethral resection or enucleation prostatectomy has removed whatever cancer was present in the gland. On the other hand, patients with stage A-2 prostate cancer, as defined by more extensive disease or any histologic grade other than well-differentiated will require additional attention. Since the incidence of lymph node metastases in this group of patients is anticipated to be approximately 30%, these patients should probably undergo surgical staging, as advocated by Donohue. In his report, 18 patients with stage A-2 prostatic adenocarcinoma underwent pelvic lymphadenectomy and 4 of the 18 showed lymph node metastases [48]. Our own experience with surgical staging in stage A-2 disease showed that 28% of patients are understaged unless surgical lymphadenectomy is performed [7].

As we have already discussed, patients with stage A-2 disease, upstaged by the discovery of pelvic lymph node metastases, experience poor prognosis. These patients should be considered to have systemic disease and they probably warrant systemic therapy in addition to local management techniques. Radical prostatectomy is not justified in the presence of systemic disease. Irradiation can be employed for local control and this may be achieved by either external beam therapy or by an interstitial approach, although interstitial implantation is made more difficult by the previous prostatic resection. After the use of irradiation to secure local control of cancer remaining in the prostate remnant, a number of workers would advocate adjunctive systemic treatment [7, 33]. Such systemic therapy could consist of either cytotoxic agents or endocrine manipulation.

If, on the other hand, the patient with stage A-2 disease is found to have no lymph node metastases, selection of therapy is more controversial. Because radical prostatectomy is a more difficult procedure after prior resection, many workers feel that extirpative surgery is not a good choice. Furthermore, since stage A-2 prostate cancer, by definition, consists of either diffuse tumors or lesions that are poorly differentiated, some authorities feel that this disease has already progressed beyond the point where radical prostatectomy is useful [27]. However, these sentiments leave the urologist in a therapeutic dilemma. As pointed out above, interstitial irradiation is difficult to achieve following prostatic resection. Furthermore, there is no good evidence that stage A-2 disease can be controlled by external beam irradiation. If, after having carried out all the routine clinical staging studies as well as surgical lymphadenectomy, one finds that there is no evidence of metastatic disease, radical prostatectomy might well be justified, regardless of its difficulty. Indeed, Heaney reported 8 cases of stage A prostate cancer treated by radical prostatectomy. No patient in this small series died of cancer [49]. Nichols reported an experience with radical prostatectomy in 33 patients with multifocal stage A prostatic adenocarcinoma [50]. Residual cancer was found in 27 of the removed glands. Sixty percent of the patients lived ten years or longer (100% age-adjusted survival). This excellent experience may be explained partly by the fact that the majority of the cancers in this series were histologically well-differentiated. At the present time, however, unless one adopts an attitude of therapeutic nihilism in patients with surgically staged A-2 adenocarcinoma of the prostate, radical prostatectomy would appear to be a not unreasonable course of action provided one ensures that systemic spread has not already occurred. Although Nichols reported significant morbidity associated with radical surgery in this circumstance, others, including ourselves, have not seen operative morbidity in these patients to be substantially different from that experienced in the previously unoperated radical prostatectomy candidate.

5.4. Stage B Prostate Cancer

As previously mentioned, there as been a waning interest in radical prostatectomy as a therapeutic choice in patients with stage B adenocarcinoma of the prostate. The experience of Bagshaw and Ray, in achieving a 50% ten-year survival in such patients with the use of external beam radiotherapy matched the ten-year survival statistics achieved in the 'bellweather' prostatectomy series of Jewett [28, 29]. Furthermore, it appeared that, in the hands of most urologists, radical prostatectomy was indeed associated with the morbidity of impotence and with at least some degree of incontinence. Radiation therapy delivered by external beam techniques, could be achieved with a substantial decrease in the likelihood of incontinence and at least a 50% improved capacity to maintain erectile potency. A more intensive review of these two series, however, shows that they are not really comparable. In favor of the prostatectomy series is the fact that Jewett tried to restrict surgical candidacy to patients with stage B-1 nodules, whereas the radiotherapy group included both patients with stage B-1 and B-2 cancer. As an aside, at this point, it should be emphasized that nearly one-third of Jewett's patients were discovered to have stage B-2 or higher stage disease on histologic review. A second point that should be emphasized in considering the comparability of the Bagshaw and Jewett experiences is that a number of the radiotherapy patients received various forms of hormone treatment, which might have worked to an overall improved outlook in these patients. The third, and most significant feature interfering with the comparability of the ten-year survival achieved with Bagshaw's radiotherapy vs. Jewett's radical prostatectomy has to do with the era in which patients were accessed to each study. The Bagshaw article, reporting a ten-year follow-up, described a group of patients, the last of whom were accessed in the early 1960s. In contrast, the Jewett article, published in

Table 1. Survival following external beam radiation therapy for stage B prostate cancer

Series	Treatment	Stage	5-year survival	5–10 year survival	10-year survival
Bagshaw [34]	ERT	B	75%		50%
Taylor [51]	ERT	B	58.8%		
Perez [52]	ERT	B	70%		
	Au^{198} ERT^{+}				
Carlton [31]		B		74.5%	
Whitmore [6]	I^{125}	B/C	79.0%		

1969, included a group of patients, the last of whom was accessed in 1953. In fact, the first radical prostatectomy in this series was carried out in 1909. It is obvious that the patients in these two reports were staged by different means, since many patients were entered into therapy (particularly radical surgery) prior to the development of some of the staging studies now available to us today. Furthermore, it is clear that advances in treatment of infections, cardiac disease management and the like during the first half of the 20th century exerted a profound influence on life expectance in the American male, rendering historic comparisons between these two reports patently inappropriate.

Table 1 demonstrates survival data achieved with both external beam irradiation and interstitial radiotherapy in stage B adenocarcinoma of the prostate [6, 31, 34, 51, 52]. It is immediately apparent that most studies report survival rates after five years of follow-up. Carlton's data reflects survival after a five- to ten-year interval. This method of reporting survival is difficult to compare with other reports where survival statistics are cited for specific intervals of time (five-year survival and ten-year survival, respectively). Bagshaw's data is the only series reflecting a ten-year survival statistic thus far, and the significance of this statistic has already been discussed. As has been previously pointed out, localized adenocarcinoma of the prostate is a slow growing lesion, requiring a ten- to fifteen-year interval to judge the impact of the disease (and its management), so that it may well be premature to state that radiotherapy achieves as good control of localized prostate cancer as does radical prostatectomy. Furthermore, we must bear in mind the incidence of persisting neoplasm found on biopsies of irradiated prostate cancers. Heretofore, there has been confusion as to whether the positive biopsy (seen in 30–50% of irradiated prostates) exerted any prognostic significance. It is now clear, however, that patients with positive posttreatment biopsies fare much worse than patients in whom the postirradiation biopsy shows no evidence of neoplasm [53]. Since many of the survivors at 5 years in all of the radiotherapy series have (or are suspected

Table 2. Survival following radical prostatectomy for stage B prostate cancer

Series	Stage	No. of patients	10-year survival	15-year survival
Jewett (early) [28]	B	103	50%	27%
Culp [16]	A/B	115	72%	54%
Gilbertson [56]	A/B	22	69%	
Correa [57]	B	67	79%	62%
deVere White [58]	B	25	64%	
Boxer [59]	B	200	62%	
Jewett-Walsh [55]	B	57	64%	51%

to have) persistent malignancy, it can be anticipated that the initial apparent success of radiation therapy will be lost as the observation period following therapy becomes longer. Indeed, this phenomenon has already been reported. Bagshaw presented a fifteen-year follow-up on 348 patients of stage B prostate cancer recently. Although the ten-year survival was 58% in this large series, by 15 years there were only 20% survivors [54].

In contrast, the long-term survival following radical prostatectomy for localized prostate cancer is shown in Table 2 [16, 28, 55–59]. Other than the initial Jewett series, it can be seen that radical prostatectomy can result in ten-year survivals of 60–80% and fifteen-year survivals are in the range of 50–60% [16, 55–59]. Excluding the original Jewett series from consideration for the time being, the difference in percentage of survival reported at ten and fifteen years in these studies is probably not significant, when considered in terms of the average age of the patient treated and the era in which treatment was rendered. In fact, most of the statistics approach 100% survival at the ten-year and fifteen-year interval when interpreted in terms of actuarial survival curves [55–57].

Of particular interest is the Jewett-Walsh series, reported in 1979 [55]. Simply by analyzing patients from a more modern era (1951-1963) the fifteen-year survival from radical prostatectomy was 51%, compared to the 27% previously reported from the same institution. Since the institution, the surgeons, the treatment criteria and the management principles were precisely the same, it must be inferred that the patient population differed because of improved staging of the disease as well as better control of associated disease processes.

In fairness, it should be pointed out that both the Culp and Jewett series attempted to restrict radical prostatectomy to patients with B-1 adenocarcinoma. Even with this effort, nearly one-third of patients in each series were found to have diffuse prostatic disease and/or seminal vesicle involvement. When analyzed as subgroups, these patients fared much worse than the overall patient population. For example, of the 39 patients with microscopic evidence of extra-prostatic extension in the original Jewett series, only 15% lived ten years and no patients survived fifteen years. Furthermore, four patients in the original Jewett series had tumors of high histologic grade and none lived to fifteen years.

Because of these observations regarding diffuse disease and high grade stage B prostate cancer some workers have suggested that radical prostatectomy is inappropriate in these circumstances [27, 55]. However, it should be emphasized that none of the radical prostatectomy series available for survey at this time represent patient groups wherein surgical staging has been conducted. Patients with high grade lesions or patients with more diffuse lesions are precisely those in whom pelvic lymph node metastases would be more likely to occur. It may well be that the associated pelvic lymph node metastasis determines the poor prognosis in patients with histologically undifferentiated stage B-1 and/or stage B-2 prostatic adenocarcinoma. Thus, statements regarding the appropriateness (or lack thereof) of radical prostatectomy in the management of these patients may be premature and should probably be withheld until further information regarding results of extirpatory surgery in surgically staged patients is available.

6. CONCLUSION

From the evidence available it is apparent that stage A-1 prostate cancer influences neither the patient's life expectancy nor the quality of his life. Therefore, stage A-1 prostate cancer needs no further treatment.

In contrast, it has been clearly established that stage A-2, B-1 or B-2 prostate cancer does influence both life expectancy and quality of life in individuals with a greater than ten- to fifteen-year life expectancy. Although there is continued confusion regarding the efficacy of radical prostatectomy vs. radiation therapy in these treatment stages, certain facts should be kept in mind when selecting treatment. The growth of localized prostate cancer is sufficiently slow so that there will not be a substantially different outlook at five years in the patient managed with either form of therapy. The number of patients treated by radiation therapy in whom a ten-year follow-up is available for review is still too small to judge the effectiveness of this treatment modality. Certainly, available data on fifteen-year survivals achieved with external beam radiation therapy is poor. On the other hand radical prostatectomy has enjoyed a long-term follow-up in many series. Although subgroups in these series with higher grade and more diffuse lesions apparently do poorly, the impact of surgical staging on better patient selection remains to be seen. Until all this information is available for comparative review, the authors feel that radical prostatectomy is the most effective means available for managing the patient with localized prostate cancer.

REFERENCES

1. Jewett HJ: The present status of radical prostatectomy for stages A and B prostate cancer. Urol Clin North Am 2:105, 1975.
2. McCullough DL, Prout GR Jr, Daley JJ: Carcinoma of the prostate and lymphatic mestastases. J Urol 111:65, 1974.
3. McLaughlin AP, Saltzstein SL, McCullough DL, Gittes RF: Prostatic carcinoma: Incidence and location of unsusprected lymphatic metastases. J Urol 115:89, 1976.
4. Flocks Rh, Culp D, Porto R: Lymphatic spread from prostatic cancer. J Urol 81:194, 1959.
5. Hilaris BS, Whitmore WF Jr, Batata MA, Grabstald H: Radiation therapy and pelvic node dissection in the management of cancer of the prostate. Am J Roentgenol 121:832, 1974.
6. Barzell W, Bean MA, Hilaris BS, Whitmore WF, Jr: Prostatic adenocarcinoma: Relationship of grade and local extent to the pattern of metastases. J Urol 118:278, 1977.
7. Babayan RK, deVere White R, Austen G, Jr, Krane RJ, Feldman M, Olsson CA: Benefits and complications of staying pelvic lymph node dissection in prostatic adenocarcinoma. The Prostate 1:315, 1980.
8. Prout GR Jr, Heaney JA, Friffin PP, Daly JJ, Shipley WA: Nodal involvement as a prognostic indicator in patients with prostatic carcinoma. J Urol 124: 223, 1980.
9. Kramer SA, Spahr Jr, Brendler CB, Glenn JF, Paulson DF: Experience with Gleason's histolpathologic grading in prostate cancer. J Urol 124:223, 1980.
10. Lytton B, Collins JT, Weiss RM *et al.*: Results of biopsy after early stage prostatic cancer treatment by implantation of 125-I seeds. J Urol 121:306, 1979.
11. Golimbu M, Schinella R, Morales P *et al.*: Stage A-2 prostatic cancer: Clinical pathological, and prognostic differences from A-1 and B disease. J Urol 119:618, 1978.
12. Wilson CS, Dahl DS, Middleton RG: Pelvic lymphadenectomy for the staging of apparently localized prostatic cancer. J Urol 117:197, 1977.
13. Gleason DF, Mellinger GT, The Veterans Administration Cooperative Urological Research Group: Prediction of prognosis for prostatic adenocarcinoma by combined histological grading and clinical staging. J Urol 111:58, 1974.
14. Byar DP, The Veterans Administration Cooperative Urological Research Group: Survival of patient's with incidentally results of a clinical trial of conservative treatment. J Urol 108:908, 1972.
15. Hanash KA, Utz DC, Cook En N, Taylor WF, Titus JL: Carcinoma of the prostate: A 15-year follow-up. J Urol 107:450, 1972.
16. Culp OS: Radical perineal prostatectomy: Its past, present and possible future. J Urol 98:618, 1968.
17. Reynoso G, Chu TM, Guinan P, Murphy GP: Carcinoembryonic antigen in patients with tumors of the urogenital tract. Cancer 29:1, 1972.
18. Silverman LM, Dermer GB, Zweig MH, Van Steirleghem AC, Tokes ZA: Creatinine kinase BB: A new tumor associated marker. Clin Chem 25, No. 8:1432, 1979.
19. Feld RD, Witte DL: Presence of creative kinase BB isoenzyme in some patients with prostatic carcinoma. Clin Chem 23, No. 10:1930–1932, 1977.

20. Foti ACG, Cooper JF, Herschman H, Malvaez RR: Detection of prostatic cancer by solid-phase radioimmunoassay of serum prostatic acid phosphatase. N Engl J Med 297:1357, 1977.
21. Chu TM, Wang MC, Scott WW, Gibbons RP, Johnson DE, Schmidt JD, Loening SA, Prout GR, Murphy GP: Immunochemical detection of serum prostatic acid phosphatase. Methodology and clinical evaluation. Invest Urol 15:319, 1978.
22. Wajsman Z, Chu TM, Saroff M, Slack N, Murphy GP: Two new direct and specific methods of acid phosphatase determination: National field trial. Urol 13:8, 1979.
23. Wajsman Z, Lee C, Chu TM, Murphy GP: A new fluorescent immunoassay for human prostatic acid phosphatase in prostate cancer (SPIF). Surgical Forum 30:568–69, 1979.
24. Grayhack JT, Lee C, Kolbusz W, Oliver L: Detection of carcinoma of the prostate utilizing biochemical observations. Cancer 45:1896, 1980.
25. Jewett HJ: Significance of palpable prostatic nodule. JAMA 160:838–9, 1956.
26. Whitmore WF Jr: The natural history of prostatic cancer. Cancer 32:1104, 1973.
27. Walsh PC: Radical prostatectomy for the treatment of localized prostatic carcinoma. Urol Clin North Am 7:3, 1980.
28. Jewett HJ: Significance of palpable prostatic nodule. JAMA 160:839–9, 1956.
29. Ray GR, Cassady JR, Bagshaw MA: Definitive radiation therapy of carcinoma of the prostate. Radiology 106:407–18, 1973.
30. Flocks RH, Kerr HD, Elkins HD, Culp D: Treatment of carcinoma of prostate by intestinal radiation with radioactive gold: Preliminary report. J Urol 68:510, 1952.
31. Carlton CE Jr: Radiactive Isotope Implantation for Cancer of Prostate. In: Genitourinary Cancer. (Skinner DS, deKernion JB, eds.) Philadelphia: W.B. Saunders, 1975, p. 380.
32. Herr Harry W: Iodine-125 implantation in the management of localized prostatic carcinoma. Urol Clin North Amer 7:3, 1980.
33. Loewing S, Narryana A: Adjuvant chemotherapy to definitive treatment of prostate cancer. The Prostate 1:321, 1980.
34. Bagshaw MA, Ray GR, Pristenna DA, Catellino RA, Mears EM, Jr: External beam radiation therapy of primary carcinoma of the prostate. Cancer 36:723, 1975.
35. Hulick PR: A review of 147 cases of adenocarcinoma of the prostate treatment with radiation therapy at wilmington Medical Center, 1967–1975. Del Med J 50, No. 9:477, 1978.
36. Rhamy RK, Wilson SK, Caldwell WL: Biopsy-proved tumor following definitive irradiation for respectable carcinoma of the prostate. J Urol 107:627.
37. Sewell RA, Braren V, Wilson SK, Rhamy rk: Extended biopsy followup after full course radiation for respectable prostatic carcinoma, 113:371, 1975.
38. Kiesling VJ, Friedman HI, McAninch JW *et al.*: The ultrastructural changes of prostate adenocarcinoma following external beam radiation therapy. J Urol 122:633, 1979.
39. Hadley MA: Radiotherapy of prostatic carcinoma. Proceedings of The 22nd Annual ASTR Meeting.
40. Mahan DE, Bruce AW, Manley PN, Franchi L: Immunohistochemical evaluation of prostatic carcinoma before and after radiotherapy. J Urol 124:488, 1980.
41. Mickey DD, Wunderli H, Vollmer R, Sanders A, Paulson DF: Radiation and chemotherapy studies of human urogenital tumors maintained in nude mice. Presented AUA, Washington, DC, May 21, 1978.
42. Schoonees R, Palma LD, Gaeta JF, Moore RH, Murphy GP: Prostatic carcinoma treated at categorical center: Clinical and pathological observations. NY State J Med 72:1021, 1972.
43. Greene LF, Simon HB: Occult carcinoma of the prostate: Clinical and therapeutic study of eighty-three cases. JAMA 158:1494–1498, 1955.
44. Barnes R, Hirst Albert and Rosenquist R: Early carcinoma of the prostate: Comparison of stages A and B. J Urol 115:404–5, 1976.

45. Emmett JL, Barker KW Jr, Jackman RJ: Transrectal biopsy to detect prostatic carcinoma: A review and report of 203 cases. J Urol 87:460–474, 1962.
46. Denton SE, Choy SH, Valik WL: Occult prostatic carcinoma diagnosed by the step-section technique of the surgical specimen. J Urol 93:296–298, 1965.
47. McMillen SM, Wettlaufer: The role of repeat transurethral biopsy in stage A carcinoma of the prostate. J Urol 116:759, 1976.
48. Donohue RE, Pfister RR, Weigel JW, Stonington OG: Pelvic lymphadenectomy in stage A prostatic cancer. Urol 9:973, 1977.
49. Heaney JA, Chang HC, Daly JJ, Prout GR, JR: Prognosis of clinically undiagnosed prostatic carcinoma and the influence of endocrine therapy. J Urol 118:283–287.
50. Nichols RT, Barry JM Hodges CV: The morbidity of radical prostatectomy for multifocal stage I prostatic adenocarcinoma. J Urol 117:83–84.
51. Taylor WJ, Richardson RG, Haffermann MD: Radiation therapy for localized prostate cancer. CA 43:1123, 1979.
52. Perez CA, Walz B, Zivnuska FR, Pielepich M, Prasad K, Royce R, Bauer W: Radiation therapy in the treatment of carcinoma of the prostate localized to the pelvis (Abstract), 4 (Suppl 2): 129–130, 1978.
53. Carlton CE Jr: Personal Communication.
54. Bagshaw MA: Radiotherapy of prostatic carcinoma: Proceedings of The 22nd Annual ASTR Meeting, presented at Stanford University, 1980.
55. Jewett HJ: Radical perineal prostatectomy for palpable clinically localized, non-obstructive cancer: Experience at Johns Hopkins Hospital, 1909–1963. J Urol 124:492, 1980.
56. Gilbertsen VA: Cancer of the prostate gland: Results of early diagnosis and therapy undertaken for cure of the disease. JAMA 215:81–84, 1971.
57. Correa RJ, Gibbons RP, Cummings KB, Mason JT: Total prostatectomy for stage B carcinoma of the prostate. J Urol 117(3):328–329, 1977.
58. de Vere White R, Paulson DF, Glenn JF: The clinical spectrum of prostate cancer. J Urol 117:323-327, 1977.
59. Boxer RJ, Kaufman JJ, Goodwin WE: Radical prostatectomy for carcinoma of the prostate: 1951–1976, Review of 329 patients. J Urol 117:208, 1977.

6. Chemotherapy of Superficial Bladder Carcinoma

GEORGE R. PROUT, JR. and I. KATHLEEN HAGEN

1. CHEMOTHERAPY OF SUPERFICIAL BLADDER CARCINOMA

Superficial bladder carcinoma (O, A, B_1 [1]; TIS, Ta, T1 [2]) is probably one of the most commonly diagnosed carcinomas, leaving skin tumors aside, in the United States. About 30 000 new patients will be diagnosed annually [3]. Data obtained from September 1974 through August 1976 by National Bladder Cancer Collaborative Group A (CGA) indicated that patients with and without prior history of bladder tumors were distributed in the way as shown in Table 1 [4].

The conceptual problems presented by these patients with superficial carcinoma are several. The disease is polychronotopic, a neoplastic diathesis prone to recur with increasing frequency in many patients but without becoming lethal. Hence, large numbers of patients experience repeated, nonlethal tumor events, some over many years, before an invasive lesion develops or some competing cause for mortality intervenes. Thus, patients with low-stage bladder carcinoma represents a major problem in cancer control.

The heterogeneity of bladder carcinoma makes no single definition accurate. Further, in many patients the process of neoplasia is a dynamic event, constantly continuing and changing. With biopsies and cytology we can witness some of the end results of the process, but we remain disadvantaged in understanding the simplest processes that initiated these results [5–13]. For instance, in Table 2 are survival rates for patients with superficial carcinoma. In Table 3 are recurrence rates reported by several authors. We cannot answer definitively high priority [14–22] questions such as: what were the signalling events that indicated impending disaster for the patients in Table 1 who failed to survive, and: in Table 2, did the superficial recurrences arise from a field of abnormal urothelium or did implantation of tumor cells play a major role in recurrence? Or, in the latter instances, were both factors

Table 1. Distribution of bladder cancer in 682 patients

	Without previous history	With previous history	Total patients accessioned
Bladder carcinoma confirmed histologically	354	328	682
Extension of extravesical cancer	0	41	41
Extent of disease:			
Extension beyond the bladder	41	58	99
Muscle invasion (T2, T3)	84	56	140
Lamina propria invasion (T1):			
Muscle tissue in specimen	55	40	95
No muscle tissue	40	25	65
Mucosa only (Ta)	124	103	227
Unknown	10	5	15

functioning in varying degrees in different patients? Before proceeding to intravesical treatment of low stage carcinoma, these topics need some brief examination.

Melicow [23] reported on TIS as an intraepithelial neoplastic process in bladders where invasive carcinoma was also present. Eight years later Eisenberg *et al.* [24] reported on tumors and associated proliferative lesions. They did not isolate TIS but included it with other lesions that were not clearly neoplasms. This was the first report of superficial papillary carcinoma existing with TIS and one third of these patients died of invasive, metastatic carcinoma. There then appeared a spate of reports which suggested that the urothelium [25–32] was often the site of diffuse changes that finally led to

Table 2. Five-year survival rate for superficial bladder tumor [79]

	No.	Survival (%)	Invasion (%)	Recurrence (%)
Deming, 1950 [5]	109 (p)		7.3	69
Nichols & Marshall, 1956 [6]	86	84 (T1)		
Pyrah *et al.* 1969 [7]	207 (p)		6.6	54
Lerman *et al.*, 1970 [8]	125 (p)	88	9.6	31 (s), 66 (m)
Williams, 1977 [9]	167	72 (T1)	7.8	50 (s), 70 (m)
Greene *et al.*, 1973 [10]	100	80 (T1)	10.0	73
O'Flynn, 1975 [11]	126	62 (T1)		
Barnes, 1977 [12]	64	73		
Althausen, 1976 [13]	129	81	30	85

p = papilloma; s = single tumor; m = multiple tumors.

Table 3. Intravesical Thio-Tepa for Definitive Therapy of superficial bladder tumor

	Number patients	Complete (%)	Partial (%)	None (%)
Jones & Swinney 1961 [14]	13	–	85	15
Esquivel *et al.* 1965 [15]	13	3	4	3
Abbassian & Walker, 1966 [16]	13	23	38	38
Veenema *et al.*, 1962 [17, 18]	46	37	35	28
Edsmyr & Bowman, 1970 [19]	19	41	41	17
Pavone-Malcaluso, 1971 [20]	25	32	32	36
Nieh *et al.*, 1978 [21]	27	56	–	44
Koontz *et al.*, 1981 [22]	95	47	–	39

the appearance of some morphological type of transitional cell carcinoma. For instance, Althausen *et al.* [13] followed 129 patients for five years who had at least one papillary tumor (Grade I, II, Ta, T1). In this retrospective review, all but 20 had a recurrence. Adequate mucosa surrounding the tumor was available for histological examination in 78 patients. Upon review, 12 had TIS. Of these, one patient was well seven years later, having had seven recurrences, one was lost to follow-up, two died from myocardial infarction and one of gangrene. The remainder died of invasive carcinoma. In addition, 26 patients had atypia in the gratuitously resected mucosa. Nine of these patients died of invasive carcinoma. This is a retrospective review and possibly overstates the case for progressive disease. Prospectively collected data is currently being analyzed by various segments of CGA.

The concept which has been convincingly presented to the medical community is that bladder carcinoma arises from cells that have probably been injured by some carcinogen. The injury is diffuse in nature, affecting many populations of cells and these cells ultimately display preneoplastic and, finally, neoplastic characteristics. This is known as a field change disease, having features in common with skin malignancies, lung, bowel and buccal mucosa.

There is another process by which recurrent tumors may arise in the bladder that has always been considered a possibility but until recently there has been little experimental or clinical evidence that proves the case. However, Boyd and Burnand [33] found a 50% recurrence at the first cystoscopy, and the tumors were much more commonly on the dome; Page *et al.* [34] made similar observations and the prospective data collected from new patients by Heney *et al.* [35] strongly support the observations that recurrences of the dome, anterior and posterior walls are far in excess of what might be anticipated, considering the site of the initial lesion. Actually, the frequency of dome recurrence was statistically significantly higher when compared to the incidence of lesions on the posterior and anterior walls.

Experimentally, Soloway described using a subcarcinogenic intravesical dose of methyl nitrosourea (MNU) into C3H mice [36]. This produces an extreme cystitis. When a single cell suspension of the mouse TCC cell line was introduced, extensive implantation occurred. Later, the procedure was modified extensively by transurethral introducing a polyethylene tube with a small stainless steel wire through the tube. A tiny burn resulted when the wire received a low voltage charge and when suspensions of the C3H TCC line were introduced about 60–70% of the animals sustained takes. A more basic nature of inquiry has been conducted by Sandberg *et al.* and Falor and Ward [37, 38] who, in short, studied karyotypic characteristics of TCC in humans. While it is possible that the process of karyotyping may have selected out certain clones of cells that displayed particular chromosomal abnormalities, both groups found that the same marker chromosome was often found in each of several tumors found within the patient's bladder, indicating a monoclonal origin for each of the tumors present. They also found that recurrent tumors would commonly have a marker chromosome that was identical to the one found in the original tumor.

Thus, it would appear that, in some patients, a field change process is occurring, in others implantation is the cause for recurrences, and in some segment of the population with bladder tumors, both processes take place simultaneously. Some simple means of determining a monoclonal vs. a polyclonal origin would be of great help in classifying these patients and their tumors differently. One group may have an inexorably progressive, relapsing disease and the other a disease that may be readily treated by intravesical therapy.

A last comment about implantation. It has always been difficult to reconcile our actual observations with the field change hypothesis. An individual may live for decades and never have a bladder tumor. Suddenly, after a bout of hematuria, a tumor is found and treated. Then the patient has a 30–50% chance of having other tumors within a year and when further tumors are produced then the likelihood for further tumor growth is even greater. This was thought to be due to the field change process, even though it is at considerable variation with what occurred in the patient's life until the first tumor was identified and treated, and it is with some reluctance that, in the absence of positive cytology and/or selected mucosal biopsies, one accepts the proposition that the promotor has suddenly fine tuned the susceptible cells to blossom forth into papillary tumor at three-, six- or twelve-month intervals. Until better evidence is produced, teleology suggests implantation as a cause for rapid recurrences.

2. INTRAVESICAL CHEMOTHERAPY

It is axiomatic that any agent instilled in the bladder must rid a significant proportion of the patients' bladders of tumor without producing unacceptable toxicity, either locally or systemically. Further, one might expect a reasonably long tumor-free, post-therapy period – one that might extend for years. The fact that relapse is the rule, even after excellent therapeutic treatment, strongly supports the field change process. One may be able to kill all the tumor cells present, but one must have a tumor cell or a cell very much like a tumor cell before topical therapy is effective. Biopsies taken after chemotherapeutic agents have been instilled suggest that some forms of atypia are not particularly affected.

One would also expect the agent to contribute in no way to the production of tumors, an event that may not be so remote in view of the nature of some of the compounds being employed. As a corollary to this, when the agent is effective, then one would hope to be able to continue its use prophylactically and still be free of the threat of drug-induced tumor and/or unacceptable levels of toxicity.

3. ABLATIVE, DEFINITIVE TREATMENT OF SUPERFICIAL TUMORS

The many reports concerning the results of surgical therapy for superficial tumors are testimony to the firmly established therapeutic attitudes of Urologists. Only within the past decade have new data and concepts emerged that might alter these attitudes. These newer concepts are the result of the acquisition of further biological information concerning the course of the treated disease over a period of years.

Chemotherapeutic agents have been important in this regard, though study designs have not always been precise in their aims nor have the data always been of the highest order. It is extremely difficult to conduct *any* retrospective study on the effect of cytotoxic agents instilled intravesically and draw valid conclusions.

The agent used most extensively in the U.S.A. in patients with superficial TCC has been an alkylating agent, thio-TEPA (TTPA), (N, N′, N″-triethyline thiophosphoramide). It was introduced in 1953 for use as a systemic agent for neoplastic processes. Jones and Swinney [14] were the first to report on its intravesical effectiveness in destroying low stage TCC. Some relevant results from a number of reports are shown in Table 3. The data from Nieh *et al.* [21] and Koontz *et al.* [22] were the results of a prospective protocol produced by the members of National Bladder Cancer Collaborative Group A (CGA). It is very likely that different criteria were used in the selection of patients for each of the studies reported. The dose and periodicity of treatment varied widely as well. Unhappily, these data are largely empiric and are the result of clinical testing, in the broadest sense.

The study reported on by Koontz *et al.* [22] consisted of two parts, the first of which was to determine the ablative effect of 60 mg vs. 30 mg of TTPA, and to determine the toxicity associated with both dosages, each of which was instilled into the dehydrated patient once a week for four weeks, followed by a rest of four weeks, by cystoscopy, and then by another four weeks of treatment. Next came a four-week rest and then cystoscopy, followed by another four weeks of treatment, a four-week rest and then cystoscopy, to reach a final decision. Biopsies of bladder mucosa and tumor(s) were stipulated before and after therapy.

Because no report contained equivalent data, the responses to the different doses of TTPA and the response after the first and second course are shown in Table 4. These data indicate that there was no difference in

Table 4. Thio-tepa treatment: response to first and second courses of therapy. According to dose [a]

Dose and course	Tumor response							
	Success		Failure		Unknown [b]		Total	
	No.	(%)	No.	(%)	No.	(%)	No.	(%)
30 mg Thio-tepa								
1st course	35	(70.0)	13	(26.0)	2	(4.0)	50	(100)
2nd course	24	(68.5)	5	(14.3)	6	(17.2)	35	(100)
Combined	24	(48.0)	18	(36.0)	8	(16.0)	50	(100)
60 mg Thio-tepa								
1st course	26	(57.8)	15	(33.3)	4	(8.9)	45	(100)
2nd course	21	(80.8)	4	(15.4)	1	(3.8)	26	(100)
Combined	21	(46.7)	19	(42.2)	5	(11.1)	45	(100)
All patients								
1st course	61	(64.2)	28	(29.5)	6	(4.3)	95	(100)
2nd course	45	(73.8)	9	(14.8)	7	(11.4)	61	(100)
Combined	45	(47.4)	37	(38.9)	13	(13.7)	95	(100)

[a] Response to 1st course:
Success = slight or moderate reduction of tumor, or complete remission
Failure = appearance of new tumor(s); tumor larger or unchanged
Response to 2nd course:
Success = Complete remission
Failure = Histological evidence of remaining or new tumor

[b] Includes 4 patients who refused first course of therapy and 8 patients who refused or did not receive the full second course. Exclusion of these 12 patients from the analysis increases the overall success rate to 54%, 57% for the 30 mg dose and 51% for the 60 mg dose.

(From Koontz *et al.* [22]).

Table 5. Thio-tepa treatment: summary of response to treatment, according to visible tumor characteristics at entry

Tumor characteristics	Tumor response [a]							
	Success		Failure		Unknown [b]		Total	
	No.	(%)	No.	(%)	No.	(%)	No.	(%)
No. of tumors								
1	11	(61.1)	5	(27.8)	2	(11.1)	18	(100)
2	7	(58.3)	4	(33.3)	1	(8.4)	12	(100
3	6	(67.7)	2	(22.2)	1	(11.1)	9	(100)
more than 4	16	(36.4)	21	(47.7)	7	(15.9)	44	(100)
none visible	5	(41.7)	5	(41.7)	2	(16.6)	12 [c]	(100)
Total	45	(47.4)	37	(38.9)	13	(13.7)	95	(100)
Size of largest tumor								
less than 1 cm	11	(45.8)	9	(37.5)	4	(16.7)	24	(100)
1–2	19	(57.6)	11	(33.3)	3	(9.1)	33	(100)
3–4	6	(46.2)	5	(38.5)	2	(15.3)	13	(100)
greater than 4	3	(27.3)	6	(54.5)	2	(18.2)	11	(100)
none visible	6	(42.9)	6	(42.9)	2	(14.2)	14 [c]	(100)
Total	45	(47.4)	37	(38.9)	13	(13.7)	95	(100)
Shape								
flat	2	(50.0)	2	(50.0)	0	(0.0)	4	(100)
sessile	8	(57.2)	3	(21.4)	3	(21.4)	14	(100)
papillary	20	(43.5)	19	(41.3)	7	(15.2)	46	(100)
combination	8	(47.0)	8	(47.1)	1	(5.8)	17	(100)
none visible	7	(50.0)	5	(35.7)	2	(14.3)	14 [c]	(100)
Total	45	(47.4)	37	(38.9)	13	(13.7)	95	(100)

[a] Response to total course of treatment, including patients who failed on the first course.
[b] See footnote, table 3.
[c] In addition to 11 patients without visible tumor at entry to study, the following number of patients with unreported descriptive information are included:
No. of tumors 1
Tumor size 3
Tumor shape 3
(From Koontz *et al.* [22]).

response between the two doses. Table 5, also taken from Koontz *et al.* demonstrates that successful therapy was more likely to result when no more than three tumors were evident and when the tumors were not greater than 3–4 cm in size. Tumor shape demonstrated no relationship to response.

Table 6 also provides data not previously available. The tumors res-

Table 6. Thio-tepa treatment: summary of response to treatment, according to the central pathology laboratory's diagnoses of stage and grade

CPL stage	Tumor response [a]							
	Success		Failure		Unknown [b]		Total	
	No.	(%)	No.	(%)	No.	(%)	No.	(%)
Carcinoma-*in-situ* (TIS)	11	(55.0)	5	(25.0)	4	(20.0)	20	(100)
Stage O (Ta)	20	(45.5)	19	(43.2)	5	(11.3)	44	(100)
Stage A (T1)	11	(47.8)	8	(34.8)	4	(17.4)	23	(100)
Stage A plus TIS	1	(25.0)	3	(75.0)	0	(0.0)	4	(100)
No CPL report	2	(50.0)	3	(50.0)	0	(0.0)	4	(100)
Total	45	(47.4)	37	(38.9)	13	(13.7)	95	(100)
CPL pathologic grade								
I	16	(51.6)	13	(41.9)	2	(6.5)	31	(100)
II	13	(39.4)	14	(42.4)	6	(18.2)	33	(100)
III	14	(51.9)	8	(29.6)	5	(18.5)	27	(100)
No CPL report	2	(50.0)	2	(50.0)	0	(0.0)	4	(100)
Total	45	(47.4)	37	(38.9)	13	(13.7)	95	(100)

[a] See footnote, table 4.
[b] See footnote, table 3.
(From Koontz *et al.* [22]).

ponded about the same, regardless of grade and stage. What is significant is the 55% response seen in patients with TIS.

From these several reports it is evident that TTPA is effective in destroying tumors in about 50% of the patients treated. It is important at this juncture to recognize that many of the patients treated were treated only after multiple TUR's and only TTPA stood between the patient and cystectomy. As will be noted later, much more may be learned from patients with less superficial tumors – information that provides for the generation of important hypotheses relative to the pathogenesis of tumor recurrence.

4. TOXICITY OF DEFINITIVE THERAPY

Most investigators have reported relatively little toxicity. This may be due, in part, to the experience of Abassian and Wallace [16] which clearly defined the upper limits of dosage. They instilled 90 mg of TTPA in 50 ml of water in the bladders of 15 patients with tumors at four-day intervals until 360 mg had been administered. Nine patients had increased frequency, two had hematuria, two had fever and may have had urinary tract infec-

Table 7. Thio-tepa treatment: frequency of observed toxicity, by Dose

	Observed protocol toxicity								Subtotal				Total	
	Leukopenia		Thrombo-cytopenia [a]		Urinary tract symptoms [b]		Combination [c]		Observed toxicity		No reported toxicity			
	No.	(%)	No.	(%)	No.	(%)	NO.	(%)	No.	(%)	No.	(%)	No.	(%)
30 mg Thio-tepa	1	(2.0)	3	(6.0)	1	(2.0)	3	(6.0)	8	(16.0)	42	(84.0)	50	(100.0)
60 mg Thio-tepa	6	(13.4)	0	(0.0)	1	(2.2)	1	(2.2)	8	(18.8)	37	(82.2)	45	(100.0)
Total	7	(7.4)	3	(3.2)	2	(2.1)	4	(4.2)	16	(16.9) [d]	79	(83.1)	95	(100.0)

[a] Reported toxicity
Leukopenia: WBC < 3000/mm^3
Thrombocytopenia: Platelets <100 000/mm^3

[b] Includes: 1 patient with pyuria, hematuria, urinary tract infection
1 patient with hematuria.

[c] Includes: 1 patient with a low hemoglobin and a urinary tract infection
1 patient with lower back pain, mild hematuria
1 patient with leukopenia and a low hemoglobin
1 patient with hematuria, CVA.

[d] Of the 16 patients with reported protocol toxicity, treatment was terminated for 4 patients and interrupted for the other 12.

(From Koontz *et al.* [22]).

tions. Dysuria occurred even though the urine was sterile. Seven patients had significant suppression of the white blood cell county, six had a severe depression and two of these died with stomatitis, enteritis, fever, hemorrhage and pancytopenia. Aside from these disturbing complications, no authors have reported such events with the same frequency and/or severity. Toxicity is clearly dose-related, but it is probably also related to the extent of inflammation, necrosis and amount of tumor present in the bladder. Leenglmayer and Czech [39] found that when 60 mg of TTPA in 60 ml of distilled water was instilled, 19% was absorbed from normal bladders in one hour, while disseminated tumors, whether small or large, and necrosis after TUR increased absorption to nearly 100% within an hour. Further, the levels remained for four hours after instillation.

These observations are somewhat in keeping with the experience of Esquivel *et al.* [15] who treated 20 patients with TTPA (60 mg/60 ml). Half of the patients were in stages greater than T1. Five patients developed leukopenia or thrombocytopenia severe enough to cause cessation of treatment. The complication occurred after the later doses (third and fourth) had been given. In each patient treatment was resumed after one week. Age may add to toxicity, though this has not been proven. One death occurred in a 74-year-old women who might predictably have developed some complication since her bladder contained a necrotic tumor (T1) with 'satellite metastases'. She developed pancytopenia after four instillations of TTPA (60 mg/60 ml). A similar case was reported by Watkins *et al.* [40].

Perhaps the most precise estimate of toxicity may be obtained from the prospective study of CGA [22]. In testing the two doses of TTPA, 60 mg vs. 30 mg, it was found that 16 patients developed toxicity according to the treatment protocol. In four, treatment was terminated; in 12 patients it was interrupted and then resumed. The details are shown in Table 7.

From this review, one may conclude that the therapeutic response depends on the number and size of the tumors being treated. One may anticipate a complete response in at least one-third of the patients and a partial response in another third. In selected patients, the response rate may be higher. Clearly, the incidence and severity of toxicity make the agent worthy of use in destroying tumors.

5. PROPHYLLAXIS - THIO TEPA

While tumor destruction is a requisite of any agent purported to be cytotoxic when instilled intravesically, the tumor-free period enjoyed by the host is nearly equivalent in importance. Should recurrences appear within a few months, then a search for better agents should be conducted.

So that tumor-free periods might be prolonged with a minimum of risk and discomfort to the patient, prophylactic TTPA has been instilled into the bladders of thousands of patients on dozens of dosage regimens. Only some of these have been reported because of the difficulty in conducting such studies. Veenema *et al.* [18], using 30 patients as their own controls (incidence of tumor recurrence before and after therapeutic TTPA: 8 instillations, cystoscopy, 4 instillations each 1–2 weeks followed by instillations at 4–6 weeks for one year; dose, either 30 or 60 mg at each instance), reported that 15 patients had no recurrence over a three-year period and the actual recurrences were reduced to about one-third of those observed before therapy.

Drew and Marshall [41] reported on a small group of carefully studied patients who were treated with TTPA for long periods of time (24–207 weeks). These patients, all having had multiple tumors resected in the past, were tumor-free between 92 and 190 weeks. None of these patients exhibited toxicity of any type.

Wescott [42], after an induction period of weekly instillations of 60 mg intravesically for four to six weeks, treated 14 patients who had had tumors previously with monthly instillations. While the total observation times are not clear in the article, the data indicate that some of these patients were tumor-free for over two years.

There are other recorded experiences [43] which indicate that prophylatic TTPA has an effect on the recurrence rate. Again, the design of the studies frustrates one in reaching a definite estimate. The patients are not well categorized, the dosage schedules flexible and the tumors poorly characterized. The EORTC study, prospective and randomized between TTPA, VM26 and no therapy, is of assistance in clarifying some of these issues. Patients with their first tumor had a median time recurrence of 45 weeks while, in sharp contrast, those patients who had had previous tumors had a median time of 23 weeks for recurrence. It made no difference in either group whether the patient received either drug, or no therapy at all. However, there proved to be a statistically significant advantage for the TTPA-treated patients regarding the *number* of recurrences experienced when compared to the VM26 and control groups. Toxicity is not discussed in this chapter.

Koontz *et al.* [22] have set down specific details for eligibility for the prophylactic group. It proved to have important implications for future trials. The patients were randomized to either no therapy, or 30 or 60 mg of TTPA. The characteristics of the patient–tumor relationship are shown in Table 8. Investigator's option included patients with previous tumors, patients who had had large tumors resected and patients with tumor extending to the lamina propria. The 'post-therapy' patients shown in the table were

Table 8. Thio-tepa prophylaxis: distribution of patients by type of eligibility according to assignment

Prophylaxis type	Assignment							
	Prophylaxis							
	30 mg		60 mg		Control		Total	
	No.	(%)	No.	(%)	No.	(%)	No.	(%)
Regular								
Three tumor events in past 18 months	5	(21.7)	3	(13.0)	5	(10.6)	13	(14.0)
Multi-focal tumors	5	(21.7)	4	(17.4)	10	(21.3)	19	(20.4)
Invesitigator's option	5	(21.7)	9	(39.2)	17	(36.2)	31	(33.3)
Subtotal	15	(65.2)	16	(69.6)	32	(68.1)	63	(67.7)
Post-therapy	8	(34.8)	7	(30.4)	15	(31.9)	30	(32.3)
Total	23	(100.0)	23	(100.0)	47	(100.0)	93	(100.0)

(From Koontz *et al.* [22]).

those who had responded to TTPA therapy. All were cystoscopically free of tumor upon accession.

One year after accession (Table 9) there was a clearcut advantage for patients in the prophylactic group and no difference between doses of drugs. However, if one removes the 'treatment group' from each arm, the curves are not significantly different ($p = 0.20$) (Figure 1). Regardless, more patients in the prophylactic group were tumor-free for a longer period. The most impressive comparison resulted when the patients previously treated successfully with TTPA and who then received TTPA prophylactically were

Table 9. Thio-tepa prophylaxis: percentage of patients disease-free at 12 months, by assignment and cytology status

Cytology status	Number of patients		Disease-free at 12 months [b]	
	Prophylaxis	Control	Prophylaxis	Control
Positive [a]	10	12	56%	40%
Negative	35	35	69%	40%
Total	45 [c]	47	66%	40%

[a] Cancer cells present.
[b] Calculated by the Modified Life Table method.
[c] Excludes one patient who had two disease-free weeks after randomization.
(From Koontz *et al.* [22]).

Table 10. Thio-tepa prophylaxis: frequency of observed toxicity, by dose

Prophylaxis assignement	Observed protocol toxicity						Subtotal		Total
	Leuko-penia [a]	Thrombo-cyto-penia [a]	Low hemo-globin [a]	Urinary tract symptoms [b]	Other	Combi-nation [c]	Observed toxicity	No reported toxicity	
	No. (%)	No. (%)	No. (%)	No. (%)	No. (%)	No. (%)	No. (%)	No. (%)	No. (%)
30 mg Thio-tepa	0 (0.0)	0 (0.0)	1 (4.3)	0 (0.0)	0 (0.0)	0 (0.0)	1 (4.3)	22 (95.7)	23 (100.0)
50 mg Thio-tepa	1 (4.3)	1 (4.3)	0 (0.0)	4 (17.4)	1 (4.3)	2 (8.8)	9 (39.1)	14 (60.9)	23 (100.0)
Control	0 (0.0)	0 (0.0)	0 (0.0)	0 (0.0)	0 (0.0)	0 (0.0)	0 (0.0)	47 (100.0)	47 (100.0)
Total	1 (1.1)	1 (1.1)	1 (1.1)	4 (4.3)	1 (1.1)	2 (2.0)	10 (10.7) [d]	83 (89.3)	93 (100.0)

[a] Reported toxicity
Leukopenia: WBC <3000/mm^3
Thrombocytopenia: Platelets <100 000/mm^3
Low hemoglobin: Hgb <10 gm.

[b] Includes: 2 patients with urinary tract infections
1 patient with irritative symptoms: frequency, dysuria, urgency
1 patient with moderate dysuria, frequency, severe urgency.

[c] Includes: 1 patient with low blood values, pain and abdominal tenderness
1 patient with low WBC, low hematocrit.

[d] Of the 10 patients with reported protocol toxicity, prophylaxis was terminated for 6 patients and interrupted for the other 4.
(From Koontz *et al.* [22]).

compared to the control group (Figure 2). The difference was significant at 12 months and beyond ($p = 0.05$). At one year no patient had a recurrence while the post-therapy control group experienced a 60% recurrence rate.

This experience suggests that if seeding of viable cells occurs, intensive TTPA therapy destroys tumors in about half the patients and prophylaxis in those patients is effective for a year and longer. If invisible areas of truly neoplastic cells are scattered about the field of urothelium, the same probability exists. These are destroyed by TTPA therapy in half the patients and prophylaxis is effective in those. The likelihood of both circumstances existing simultaneously seems fairly high, from what is now known about superficial tumors.

As a corollary, we have left a discrete papillary tumor behind after biopsy. This has been used as an index lesion. If the tumor is destroyed by definitive TTPA, there is adequate justification for prophylaxis to be used. If not destroyed by TTPA, the lesion is again biopsied and then fulgurated or resected. There seems little to be gained in repeating the TTPA, either therapeutically or prophylactically.

Toxicity experiences for these patients is shown in Table 10. Of the 93 patients accessioned, 46 received prophylactic TTPA. Treatment was interrupted in four ptients and terminated in six. Irritative symptoms and infection were the more commonly encountered problems. Conjecturally, if the patients and investigators had known the rewards of continuation, efforts to correct matters might have been more diligently pursued and therapy recommenced.

All the experiences recorded indicate that TTPA has a definite role in controlling superficial bladder carcinoma. In the past, TTPA was used only in those cases where the quantitative aspects of the tumor diathesis exceeded the ability of the resectionist to remove visible tumor. If one recalls the recurrence rates, then it is evident that the risk/benefit ratio is easily satisfied by adding adjuvant intravesical cytotoxic agents to surgical destruction of tumors, even when there are only a few superficial lesions present and this is the patient's first or second recurrence. Currently, we have no way of knowing what course each patient will follow, but if intravesical TTPA will alter events in terms of prolonging the tumor-free period, then there seems every reason to proceed. Ample precedence exists, of course. The real problem is deciding when to give the agent and how much. Ideally, one would prefer to instill TTPA immediately after biopsy/fulguration/TUR. Burnand *et al.* [44] have done this, using 90 mg instilled for 30 min once. Little toxicity and a significant decrease in recurrences resulted. Gravell *et al.* [45] used 30 mg BID for three days or weekly for six weeks after surgical treatment. Again, toxicity was low and a significant decrease in recurrences resulted.

Table 11. Epodyl: triethylene glycol diglyceridyl ether

Author	No. of patients	Dose	Response			Comment
			Complete	Partial	None	
Abassian, Wallace [16]	15	100 mg/day for 2 weeks	5	3	7	Dysuria – 12 patients Leukopenia – 8 patients
Riddle, Wallace [46]	56	100 ml of 1 % solution daily for 2 weeks		26		All failed within a year; occasional frequency and strangury
Recurrent, multiple tumors	40	100–200 ml of 1 % solution q wk × 12 then monthly for 1 year				
		at 3 months	20	17	3	Minimal local effects
		at 6 months	11	8	0	(19 patients)
		at 12 months	6	2	1	(9 patients)
Riddle [47]	32	Same, at 24 months	15 47 %	6 19 %	11 34 %	If fulguration is necessary, do not give Epodyl for 3 weeks.
Riddle *et al.* [48]	4	Same	4 – No tumor			Pts had TIS; 7 patients with dysuria,
Hannestad *et al.* [51]	13	Same	3/4 – No tumor for 2 years			strangury; 3 patients with positive
Robinson *et al.* [52]	51	Same	15 No long follow-up	20	11	culture; decreased bladder capacity.
Nielsen, Thybo [53]	44	Same	19 C or P (43 %)			7 patients irritative symptoms, therapy stopped
Popa *et al.* [54]	25	Same	13 'seldom had recurrence during next year'			Cystis – therapy stopped – 2 patients
Smith *et al.* [55]	16	Same	12 4/5 tumor-free after 3 years	3		2 patients did not tolerate therapy
Fitzpatrick [49]	64	Same	39			20/39 recurrences
Riddle *et al.* [50]	64	Same	11/20 recurrences after 2 years			5 patients experienced dysuria and frequency; treatment stopped

Currently, the CGA is planning to test single against multiple instillations of TTPA after surgical therapy. This issue needs resolving. If immediate therapy is equally effective and has no greater toxicity, this would clearly be the choice.

6. OTHER INTRAVESICAL AGENTS

None of these agents has been adequately tested in the U.S.A. though evaluation of Mitomycin-C (MMC) is now being conducted.

6.1. Epodyl (Triethulene glycol diglyceridyl ether)

This agent has been used in England and elsewhere but the manufacturer has not seen fit to confront the expense and other rigors of the American bureaucracy so that it might be tested and used in the U.S.A. Contacts with officials of ICI Americas, Inc. have not been productive.

Some of the relevant references are shown in Table 11. The last reference summarizes the results of 64 patients with multiple, superficial papillary bladder tumors which had ceased to be controlled by endoscopic resection and diathermy. They were treated before July 1972, with 100 ml of 1% Epodyl in distilled water which was left in the bladder for one hour. This was given weekly for 12 weeks, then monthly for a year, and then every three months. All were followed to December 1978.

After one year 39 patients were free of disease and 25 had recurrences. Of the 38 free after one year, 20 patients later developed recurrences, in 11 cases not until two years after starting the drug. Of the 25 patients who had recurrences after one year, 24 never became free of tumor, but one did become free two years later. The side effects of treatment included a systemic allergic reaction in one patient and severe dysuria and frequency in five patients which caused the treatment to be stopped. Initially, frequency and urgency were noted for the first week or two in several other patients, but the symptoms subsequently subsided and treatment continued. If the initial response was favorable, the prognosis was good. On failure to clear the bladder by the twelfth month or if histology changed 'from PIS to Pla or Plb' while on treatment, the prognosis became poor and indicated immediate need for radical treatment [49, 50].

Thus, this agent deserves a Phase III trial in comparison with TTPA.

6.2. Doxorubicin (See Table 12)

This agent has been very well tolerated and it has a response rate equivalent to or greater than that of TTPA, according to European investigators. The agent will be studied by the EORTC and Collaborative Group A, as well.

Table 12. Doxorubicin

Author	No. of patients	Dose	Response (%)	Comment
Pavone-Macaluso [56] review	98	10, 20, 40 mg/wk for 4 wks, then monthly 50–150/mg	CR: 34 [a] PR: 43 [b]	Noc., 12, 30 and 33% PRs response
Prophyllaxis	10 mg/wk for 4 wks then monthly		Recurrence rate at 6 months = 30%	
Niijima [57]	Unknown	20, 30, 50, 60 mg 3×/wk for 2 wks	CR+PR: 56, 72, 74%	Absorption minimal
coop. study	194	Same	More than 50% in 31, 68, 69%	Irritative symptoms in 30–40% of patients
Edsmyr *et al.* [58]	8 TIS 9/18 T1 5/18	80 mg/100 ml once a month for 5 or more months Same	CR: 100 (1 with + cytol.) CR: 100 PR: 5 patients	Irritative symptoms in 3 patients No myelosuppression
Jacobi *et al.* [59]	15	40 mg/30 ml started 3–4 wks after endoscopic therapy	10 no tumor (mean 22 months) 13 recurrences	
Banks *et al.* [60]	13	50 mg/150 ml/30 min for T1 tumors	8 free of tumor (median range remission 10 months)	No toxicity

[a] CR, complete response.
[b] PR, partial response.

6.3. Mitomycin C

Mitomycin C (MMC) has been available for clinical trials since 1958 [58], and was FDA-approved for general cancer chemotherapeutic use in the United States in 1974 [59].

This antibiotic was isolated from *Streptomyces caespitosus* and functions as a bi- or possibly a tri-functional alkylating agent. The three potentially active moieties are the quinone, aziridine, and urethrane groups. The drug must be activated *in vivo* by NADPH-dependent reduction of quinone which allows Mitomycin C to form cross-links in DNA, thus inhibiting mammalian DNA synthesis. It is most effective in cell phases late G_1 or S. The drug also plays a role in DNA degradation by cleavage [60].

Histologically, both light and electron microscopic cytotoxic changes have been described in normal and malignant transitional cell epithelium following intravesical Mitomycin C in the rat. The cells have lucid nuclei and hypervacuolated cytoplasm. Ultrastructurally, both tumor and normal bladder cells are denuded of microvilli, and there is an increase in intercellular spaces. These changes may be focal and are compatible with drug-induced cellular necrosis [61]. Mitomycin C may also enhance tumor necrosis secondary to fibrinoid degeneration of the underlying interstitial tissue and vessels [62].

The liver is believed to be the major site of biotransformation although most tissues have a similar capability. Metabolism yields an unstable, reactive moiety which alkylates and then cannot react further. When Mitomycin C is administered systemically, severe cumulative myelosuppression may ensue and cellulitis or necrosis can occur if there is extravasation at injection sites. However, this agent is poorly absorbed through intact urothelium [63]. This is perhaps related to the fact that Mitomycin C is a relatively large molecule with a molecular weight of 334 (nearly twice that of TTPA).

In the late 1960s, following several reports in the Japanese literature on the benefits of intravesical Mitomycin C in treating bladder cancer, Mishina *et al.* [62] corroborated these findings in a study of 50 patients with all stages of bladder cancer (88% were Stage A or B_1) treated over a period of seven years. The dose of Mitomycin C was 20 mg, which was diluted with sterile distilled water to a concentration of 1 mg/ml and instilled into the bladder three times weekly for 20 doses. The patients restricted fluid intake for 12 h prior to treatment and until they voided, usually two to three hours later. Complete response (all residual tumor disappeared) was obtained in 44% and partial response in 32%. There was no systemic toxicity and only three patients (6%) had mild local reactions which did not prevent completion of the chemotherapeutic course.

Of the variables evaluated (stage, grade, form, number and size of tumors), only number showed no correlation with response. A complete remission was obtained in 67% of the patients with Stage A disease, whereas less complete and partial responses occurred with increasing stage. Simularly, a lower grade correlated with an increased effectiveness in both complete and partial responses. Papillary pedunculated tumors responded better than papillary sessile or non-papillary sessile. Response decreased as individual tumor size was greater than 1 cm, but there was no correlation between number of tumors and effectiveness of Mitomycin C.

A multi-institutional study of intravesical Mitomycin C in 63 patients with Grade I-II, Stage O-A bladder carcinoma reported an overall response rate of 67% with 45% complete responders [67]. Doses from 20–60 mg diluted to a final concentration of 1–2 mg/ml were instilled weekly for eight weeks. The instillation was held for two hours and pre-treatment/treatment fluid restriction was used. Median complete remission interval for the two lowest dose groups was 14.5 months (range 1-36+ months). No myelosuppression or other significant systemic toxicity was detected, and there were infrequent local irritative effects. Three patients experienced a transient rash on their hands. Serial serum samples were analyzed using microbiological inhibition assays and no Mitomycin C could be detected. If a transurethral resection had taken place, intravesical Mitomycin C was begun no sooner than three weeks postoperatively.

There was no statistical difference in dose response in 55 evaluable patients, although there was a trend toward increased effectiveness at higher doses. Two patients who experienced recurrent tumors after Mitomycin C were retreated; one achieved a complete response and the other a partial following a second Mitomycin C course. There was no correlation in response with prior chemotherapy or radiotherapy or to the extent of the bladder surface involved in the neoplastic process. A correlation in response with prior chemotherapy or radiotherapy or to the extent of the bladder surface involved in the neoplastic process. A correlation between response and size of individual tumors was not reported. Partial response in 22% of the patients often allowed decrease of tumor burden to permit transurethral resection of all residual disease.

A separately analyzed subset from the foregoing study consisted of 43 patients from one institution [68]. In these patients, the best responses occurred at doses of 30 mg or more, with a complete response of 49% and a partial response of 30%. This study showed a better response if the tumor was less than 1 cm, regardless of burden of disease.

Continued investigation with this agent is needed specifically to optimize treatment schedules and to evaluate the effect in carcioma *in situ* and the effect of maintenance therapy, as well as to provide long-term follow-up in those patients who have received a known carcinogen, Mitomycin C, particularly when they may have a urothelium which is potentially predisposed to neoplastic degeneration.

7. RADIOTHERAPY

External beam therapy has been unsatisfactory in destroying superficial tumors, in providing for tumor-free periods of significance after therapy, and for improving survival [69–73]. Intracavitary radioactivity in contained carriers has likewise failed [74] and Co beads [72] sewn through tumors has also been unsuccessful in controlling tumor growth and regrowth.

Perhaps the most remarkable results have been those of Van der Werf-Messing, who, after discarding external beam and then cobalt seeds for the treatment of superficial carcinoma, started using radium needles implanted transvesically. Only tumors of 5 cm or less are treated in this fashion and they must be solitary. Whether the tumors are resected transurethrally or transvesically is not clear from the publication [75]. The needles are withdrawn after high local doses of irradiation have been delivered. The five-year recurrence rate after such therapy is about 10%. The explanation for this dramatic difference is lacking. Seeded tumor cells may be killed by irradiation, the patients may be selected by virtue of the single lesion, the disease may be different in Holland and/or the field change disease may be irradiated coincidentally. The answer may never be known.

8. IMMUNOTHERAPY

It has long been proposed that bladder carcinoma would be one of those neoplastic processes that would respond to some form of immunotherapy, since the disorder was likely to be carcinogen-induced and therefore possibly more antigenic and since the patients with low-stage carcinoma were immuno-competent. Thus, the appropriate combinations of agents might yield a remarkable advance.

Olsson *et al.* [76], while studying the immuno-competence of patients with TCC, used key hole limpet antigen and other agents to make estimates of this quality. In follow-up, the patients who had received nonspecific immuno-stimulation were found to be more reactive, but less patients had recurrences and those that did had lesser numbers of recurrence. These observations have not been tested further. The hypothesis remains attractive.

Animal studies indicate that injections of bacillus Calmette-Guerin (BCG) elicit anti-TCC responses. Human studies using BCG seem to have an effect on local tumor growth and recurrences. The therapeutic plans used by both Morales *et al.* [77, 78] and Lamm *et al.* [79, 80] included the use of the Pasteur strain of BCG administered intravesically and percutaneously weekly for six weeks. Treatment was started one or two weeks after TUR or fulguration of tumors: 120 mg of BCG was instilled in the bladder and 5 mg ($5 \times 10 >$ organisms) were given percutaneously into alternate upper thighs using a Heaf gun. Lamm *et al.* have reported the results of a prospective study involving 37 patients followed three to twelve months. The data indicate that, within the time limits of the study, the treated patients had significantly longer tumor-free periods. The follow-up period is brief and further observation is necessary.

9. THE FUTURE

Because of the mix of implanted cells and the wide range of preneoplastic lesions, the problems will be very difficult to separate. Regardless, there should be a continued search for agents that have the capability of preventing preneoplastic cells from giving rise to neoplastic progeny. Our trial with 13-*Cis*-retinoic acid yielded unsatisfactory results [81] but this should not deter further investigation.

Single agents need to be tested further in Phase II studies and then to be studied in Phase III trials. Epodyl needs to be studied in the U.S.A., as does Doxorubicin. When levels of activity have been established, limited trials of sequential agents should be employed. The highest priority should be given to reparative processes in the vesical mucosa of several species after single cytoxic agent exposure, so that DNA synthesis and other phases of the cell cycle can be estimated after insult. Thus, strategy based on data rather than empiricism can be developed for sequential drug therapy.

Reliable non-invasive techniques that are more accurate than cytology would be extremely cost-effective. These require high priority in any funding scheme for they would decrease cost and save far more than they cost, in terms of dollars and of morbidity.

Until these techniques are available, it is essential for the proper evaluation of all patients with bladder carcinoma who are to be treated conservatively to have good cytological facilities at their disposal. These are not available across the United States; only a fraction of the patients with bladder carcinoma have this essential service available to them. It would be entirely appropriate for some agency, private or Federal, to establish an adequate number of centers, possibly five to seven, for this purpose.

REFERENCES

1. Marshall VF: The relation of the preoperative estimate to the pathologic demonstration of the extent of vesical neoplasms. J. Urol 68:714, 1952.
2. American Joint Committee for Cancer Staging and End-Results Reporting: Manual for Staging of Cancer 1978. Chicago, Whiting, 1978, p.113.
3. American Cancer Society: Estimated new cancer cases by sex for all sites - 1980. In: Ca - A Cancer Journal for Physicians 30:30, 1980.
4. Cutler SJ, Heney NM, Friedell GH: Longitudinal study of patients with bladder cancer: factors associated with disease recurrence and progression. In: AUA Monographs. (Bonney WW, Prout GR Jr. eds.) Vol. 1. Baltimore: Williams & Williams, 1981, p.35.
5. Deming CL: The biological behavior of transitional cell papilloma of the bladder. J Urol 63:815, 1950.
6. Nichols JA, Marshall VF: Treatment of histologically benign papilloma of the urinary bladder by local excision and fulguration. Cancer 9:566, 1956.
7. Pyrah LN, Raper FP, Thomas GM: Report of a follow-up of papillary tumors of the bladder. Br J Urol 36:14, 1964.
8. Lerman RJ, Hutter RVP, Whitmore WF JR: Papilloma of the urinary bladder. Cancer 25:333, 1970.
9. Williams JL, Hammonds JC, Saunders N: T1 bladder tumors. Br J Urol 49:663, 1977.
10. Greene LF, Hanash KA, Farrow GM: Benign papilloma or papillary carcinoma of the bladder. J Urol 110:205, 1973.
11. O'Flynn JD, Smith JM, Hanson JS: Transurethral resection for assessment and treatment of vesical neoplasms. Urology 1:38, 1975.
12. Barnes RW, Dick AL, Hadley HL Johnston OL: Survival following transurethral resection of bladder carcinoma. Cancer Res 37:2895, 1977.
13. Althausen AF, Prout GR Jr, Daly JJ: Non-invasive papillary carcinoma of the bladder associated with carcinoma in situ. J Urol 116:575, 1976.
14. Jones HC, Swinney J: Thio-tepa in the treatment of tumors of the bladder. Lancet 2:615, 1961.
15. Esquival EL, Mackenzie AR, Whitmore WF: Treatment of bladder tumors by instillation of thiotepa and 5-fluorouracil. Invest Urol 2:381, 1965.
16. Abbassian A, Wallace DM: Intracavitary chemotherapy of diffuse non-infiltrating papillary carcinoma of the bladder. J Urol 96:461, 1966.
17. Veenema RJ, Dean AL Jr, Roberts M, Fingerhut B, Chowdhury BK, Tarassoly H: Bladder carcinoma treated by direct instillation of thio-tepa. J Urol 88:60, 1962.
18. Veenema RJ, Dean AL Jr, Uson AC, Roberts M, Longo F: Thiotepa bladder instillations: therapy and prophyllaxis for superficial bladder tumors. J Urol 101:711, 1969.
19. Edsmyr F, Bowman J: Instillation of thio-tepa (Tifosyl) in vesical papillomatosis. Acta Radiol (Ther) (Stockh) 9:395, 1970.
20. Pavone-Macaluso M: Chemotherapy of vesical and prostatic tumors. Br J Urol 43:701, 1971.
21. Nieh PT, Daly JJ, Heaney JA, Heney NM, Prout GR Jr: The effect of intravesical thio-tepa on normal and tumor epithelium. J Urol 119:59, 1978.
22. Koontz WW, Jr, Prout GR, Jr, Smith W, Frable WJ, Minnis JE: The use of intravesical thio-tepa in the management of non-invasive carcinoma of the bladder. J. Urol. 125:307, 1981.
23. Melicow MM, Holowell J: Intra-urothelial cancer: Carcinoma-insitu, Bowen's disease of the urinary system: Discussion of 30 cases. J Urol 68:763, 1952.
24. Eisenberg RB, Roth RB, Schweinsberg MH: Bladder tumors and associated proliferative mucosal lesions. J Urol 84:544, 1960.

25. Schade ROK, Swinney J: Pre-cancerous changes in bladder epithelium. Lancet 2:943, 1968.
26. Koss LG, Tiamson EM, Robbins MA: Mapping cancerous and pre-cancerous bladder changes. A study of urothelium in ten surgically removed bladders. JAMA 227:281, 1974.
27. Utz DC, Hanash KA, Farrow GM: The plight of the patient with carcinoma-in-situ of the bladder. J Urol 103:160, 1970.
28. Melamed MR, Grabstald H, Whitmore WF Jr: Carcinoma-in-situ of the bladder: Clinicopathologic study of a case with suggested approach to detection. J Urol 96:466, 1966.
29. Moloney PJ, Elliott GR, McLaughlin M, Sincleir AB: In situ transitional cell carcinoma and the non-specifically inflamed contracting bladder. J Urol 111:162, 1974.
30. Hultengren N, Orell SR: Widespread in situ carcinoma of the bladder with multifocal early invasion: report of a case subjected to total cystectomy. Scand J Urol Nephrol 5:273, 1971.
31. Yates-Bell AJ: Carcinoma-in-situ of the bladder. Br J Surg 58:359, 1971.
32. Utz DC, Zincke H: The masquerade of bladder carcinoma-in-situ as interstitial cystitis. Trans Am Assoc Genitourin Surg 65:64, 1973.
33. Boyd PJR, Burnand KG: Site of bladder tumor recurrence. Lancet 3:1290, 1974.
34. Page BH, Levison VB, Curwen MP: The site of recurrence of non-infiltrating bladder tumors. Br J Urol 50:237, 1978.
35. Heney NM, Nocks, BN, Daly JJ, Prout GR, Jr, Newall JB, Griffin PP, Perrone TL, Szyfelbein WM: Ta and T1 bladder cancer: location, recurrence and progression. J. Urol (In press.).
36. Soloway MS: Intravesical and systemic chemotherapy of murine bladder cancer. Cancer Res 37:2918, 1977.
37. Sandberg AA: Chromosome markers and progression in bladder cancer. Cancer Res 37:2950, 1977.
38. Falor WH, Ward RM: Prognosis in well differentiated non-invasive carcinoma of the bladder based on chromosomal analysis. Surg Gynec & Obstet 144:515, 1977.
39. Leenglmayer G, Czech K: Absorption studies on intraluminal thio-tepa for topical cytostatic treatment of low-stage bladder tumors. J Urol 106:72, 1971.
40. Watkins WE, Kozak JA, Flanagan JJ: Severe pancytopenia associated with the use of intravesical thio-TEPA. J Urol 98:470, 1967.
41. Drew JE, Marshall VF: Effects of topical thiotepa on the recurrence rate of superficial bladder cancers. J Urol 68:740, 1968.
42. Wescott JW: The prophylactic use of thiotepa in transitional cell carcinoma of the bladder. J Urol 96:913, 1966.
43. Byar D, Blackard C: Comparisons of placebo, pyridoxine and topical thiotepa in preventing recurrence of stage I bladder cancer. Urology 10:556, 1977.
44. Burnand KG, Boyd PJR, Mayo ME, Shuttleworth KED, Lloyd-Davies RW: Single dose intravesical thiotepa as an adjuvant to cytodiathermy in the treatment of transitional cell bladder carcinoma. Br J Urol 48:55, 1976.
45. Gavrell GJ, Lewis RW, Meehan WL, LeBlanc GA: Intravesical thiotepa in the immediate postoperative period in patients with recurrent transitional cell carcinoma of the bladder. J Urol 120:410, 1978.
46. Riddle PR, Wallace DM: Intracavitary chemotherapy for multiple non-invasive bladder tumors. Br J Urol 43:181, 1971.
47. Riddle PR: The management of superficial bladder tumors with intravesical thiotepa. Br J Urol 45:84, 1973.
48. Riddle PR, Chisholm GD, Trott PA, Pugh RCB: Flat carcinoma in situ of the bladder. Br J Urol 47:829, 1976.

49. Fitzpatrick JM, Khan O, Oliver RTD, Riddle PR: Long-term follow-up in patients with superficial bladder tumors treated with intravesical Epodyl. Br J Urol 51:545, 1980.
50. Riddle P: Survival in patients treated with epodyl (1968–1978). In: Bladder Tumors and Other Topics in Urological Oncology. (Pavlone-Macaluso M, Smith PH, Edsmyr F, eds.) Vol. 1, p. 33, 1980.
51. Hannestad R, Otnes B: Epodyl in the treatment of bladder cancer. Tidsskr Nor Laegeforen 96:25, 1976.
52. Robinson MRG, Shetty MB, Richards B, Bastable J, Glashan RW, Smith PH: Intravesical Epodyl in the management of bladder tumors: combined experience of the Yorkshire Urological Cancer Research Group. J Urol 118:972, 1977.
53. Nielsen HV, Thybo E: Epodyl treatment of bladder tumors. Scand J Urol Nephrol 13:59, 1979.
54. Popa G, Peters HJ, Potempa J: Conservative treatment of bladder papillomas with Epodyl. Therapiewoche 28:2013, 1978.
55. Smith JF, Lane V, O'Flynn JD: Epodyl in management of invasive vesical neoplasms. Urol 11:474, 1978.
56. Pavone-Macaluso M: Intravesical treatment of superticial (T1) urinary bladder tumors. A review of a 15-year experience. In: Diagnostics and Treatment of Superficial Urinary Bladder Tumors. Stockholm: Montedison Lakemedel, A.B., 1979, p. 21.
57. Niijima T: Intravesical therapy with adriamycin and new trends. In: Diagnostics and Treatment of Superficial Urinary Bladder Tumors. Stockholm: Montedison Lakemedel, A.B., 1979, p. 37.
58. Edsmyr F, Burlin T, Boman J, Duchek N, Esposti PL, Gustafson H, Wilkinson H: Intravesical therapy with adriamycin in patients with superficial bladder cancer. In: Diagnostics and Treatment of Superficial Urinary Bladder Tumors. Stockholm: Montedison Lakemedel, A.B., 1979, p. 45.
59. Jacobi SH, Kurth KH, Klipper KF, Hohenfeller R: On the biological behavior of T1 transitional cell tumors of the urinary bladder and initial results of the prophylactic use of topical adriamycin under controlled and randomized conditions. In: Diagnostics and Treatment of Superficial Urinary Bladder Tumors. Stockholm: Montedison Lakemedel, A.B., 1979, p. 83.
60. Banks MD, Pontes JE, Izbicki RM, Pierce JM Jr: Topical instillation of doxorubicin hydrochloride in the treatment of recurring superficial transitional cell carcinoma of the bladder. J Urol 118:757, 1977.
61. Wakaki S, Muramo H, Tamora K, Shipmpizu G, Kato E, Kamada H, Kudo S, Fujimoto Y: Isolation of new fractions of antitumor mitomycins. Antibiot Chemother 8:228, 1958.
62. Personal communication, Bristol Laboratories, 1980 (IKH).
63. Lown JW: The molecular mechanism of antitumor action of the mitomycins. In: Mitomycin C – Current Status and New Developments. (Carter SK, Crooke ST, eds.) New York: Academic Press, 1979, p. 5.
64. Daskal Y, Crooke ST: Morphological effects of Mitomycin C on cellular fine structure. In: Mitomycin C – Current Status and New Developments. (Carter SK, Crooke ST, eds.) New York: Academic Press, 1979, p. 41.
65. Mishina T, Oda K, Murata S, Ooe H, Mori Y, Takashi T: Mitomycin C bladder instillation therapy for bladder tumors. J Urol 114:217, 1975.
66. Reich SD: Clinical pharmacology of Mitomycin C. In: Mitomycin C – Current Status and New Developments. (Carter SK, Crooke ST, eds.) New York: Academic Press, 1979, p. 243.
67. DeFuria MD, Bracken RB, Johnson DE, Soloway MS, Merrin CE, Morgan LR, Miller HC, Crooke ST: Phase I-II study of Mitomycin C topical therapy for low-grade, low-stage tran-

sitional cell carcinoma of the bladder: an interim report. Cancer Treat Rep 64:225, 1980.
68. Bracken RB, Johnson DE, von Eschenbach AC, Swanson DA, DeFuria D, Crooke S: Role of intravesical Mitomycin C in management of superficial bladder tumors. Urology 16:11, 1980.
69. Caldwell WL: Radiotherapy: Definitive, integrated and palliative therapy. Urol Clin North Am 3:129, 1975.
70. Caldwell WL, Bagshaw MA, KaplanHS: Efficacy of linear accelerator X-ray therapy in cancer of the bladder. J Urol 97:294, 1967.
71. Goffinet DR: Radiotherapy for invasive carcinoma. Presented at Stanford University Medical Center Second Annual Symposium on Disease of the Urinary Tract, March, 1974.
72. Van der Werf-Messing B: Cancer of the bladder treated with intracavitary application of Cobalt 60 beads. Clin Radiol 22:101, 1971.
73. Buschke F: Supervoltage irradiation: prophylactic versus therapeutic use for transitional cell carcinoma of the bladder, Group I. JAMA 206:2724, 1968.
74. Hewitt CB, Kiser WS, Antunez AR, Chernak ES: Intracavitary radiation in the treatment of bladder tumors. J Urol 107:603, 1972.
75. Van der Werf-Messing B: Carcinoma ofthe bladder treated by suprapubic radium implants. The value of additional external irradiation. Eur J Cancer 5:277, 1969.
76. Olsson CA, Chute R, Rao N: Immunological reduction of bladder carcinoma recurrence rate. Trans Am Assoc Genitourin Surg 65:66, 1973.
77. Morales A, Ersil B: Prophylaxis of recurrent bladder cancer with bacillus Calmette-Guerin. In: Cancer of the Genitourinary Tract. (Johnson, Samuels, eds.) New York: Raven Press, 1979, p. 121.
78. Morales A: Adjuvant immunotherapy in superficial bladder cancer. Nat Cancer Inst Monogr 49:315, 1978.
79. Lamm DL, Thor DE, Harris SC, Reyna JA, Stogdill VD, Radwin HM: BCG immunotherapy of superficial bladder cancer. J Urol 124:38, 1980.
80. Lamm DL: Personal communication, 1980 (GRP, Jr).
81. National Bladder Cancer Collaborative Group A: Unpublished data, 1980.
82. Soloway MS: The management of superficial bladder cancer. Cancer 45:1856, 1980.

7. Immunology of Genitourinary Tumors

WILLIAM J. CATALONA, TIMOTHY L. RATLIFF and ROBERT E. McCOOL

In this presentation, we review some of the experimental evidence that bears on the relationship between urologic cancer and host immunity.

1. BRIEF OVERVIEW OF TUMOR IMMUNOLOGY

1.1. Antigens

Most naturally occurring antigens, including cell-surface antigens, are protein or carbohydrate molecules or combinations of the two (glycoproteins). Transplantation antigens are cell-surface antigens that are expressed on nearly all cells of the body. The expression of transplantation antigens is coded for by genes located in the HLA complex on the sixth chromosome in humans. In many experimental systems, tumor cells behave as foreign tissue grafts because their membranes express antigens that are either lacking or masked on normal cells. During the process of malignant transformation tumors not only gain new tumor-associated antigens, but also often lose normal tissue antigens. For example, some human tumors have been shown to express less HLA antigen than normal cells [122]. In addition some tumor cells lose blood group antigens which are normally expressed on most epithelial cells [60]. This latter phenomenon has been shown to be of potential clinical importance in some tumors because it reflects a state of undifferentiation that is not always detectable morphologically [133].

Tumor-associated antigens can be classified into three general groups. *Unique* antigens are characteristic of carcinogen-induced tumors and are strongly immunogenic in the host. *Oncogenic viral-induced* antigens are shared antigens that exhibit specificity for the virus, the tumor, and all tumors induced by that particular virus; viral-induced tumor antigens are also immunogenic in the host. *Fetal* antigens are normally produced during fetal life but not in large quantities after birth, presumably because the genes controlling their production are inactivated by then. These genes become

D.F. Paulson (ed.), Genitourinary Cancer 1, 169-214.

derepressed in some tumor cells and thus fetal antigens can be produced again. Fetal antigens are not usually immunogenic in the host because tolerance to them develops during neonatal life, but they can be useful as tumor markers.

Most adequately studied experimental tumors – i.e., the viral- and carcinogen-induced tumors – have been found to express strong tumor-associated antigens. However, naturally occurring tumors generally have been found to be weakly antigenic, and some are apparently not antigenic at all. Thus it remains unclear whether tumor-associated antigens are very often characteristic of cancers occurring in nature.

1.2. Immune Response

It has been known since the early 1960s that there are two fundamental types of lymphocytes: B lymphocytes and T lymphocytes. Both arise from a common stem cell in the bone marrow. B lymphocytes differentiate into antibody-producing plasma cells, but their proliferation and differentiation is regulated by T lymphocytes. T lymphocytes can become effector cells for cell-mediated immune responses and as such can destroy tumor cells, reject foreign grafts, and activate macrophages by producing soluble substances. T cells also have a major regulatory function: they can become helper cells or suppressor cells. T cells express a variety of differentiation antigens on their surfaces that are lacking on B cells. These differnetiation antigens are differentially expressed on T helper cells and on T suppressor cells. Indeed, tumor regression was induced recently in a mouse tumor system by selectively eliminating T suppressor cells through administering antibodies directed against differentiation antigens expressed exclusively on the suppressor T cells [83].

Macrophages also are important cells in immune responses. These are large, phagocytic cells that help process antigen in the induction of antibody responses; they can also be armed by T cells specifically to destroy tumor cells or can be activated by various means to kill tumor cells nonspecifically.

Killer cells (K cells or NK cells) are a subpopulation of lymphocytes, presumably of T cell lineage, that are operationally defined as those cells that mediate spontaneous (NK) and antibody-dependent cell mediated cytolysis (ADCC). There is some evidence to suggest that K cells may be importnt in restricting tumor growth.

1.3.. Immune Response Genes

Genes in the major histocompatibility complex, called immune response (IR) genes, are located on the sixth chromosome in humans, and play a key role in regulating the responses of lymphocytes to many antigens.

1.4. Historical Perspectives of Tumor Immunology

Tumor immunology had to await the development of transplantation immunology and the availability of inbred strains of mice. In 1933, Gross [84] showed that it was possible to immunize a mouse against a tumor that arose in the same inbred strain of mice, but this observation initially was received with scepticism. In 1957, Prehn and Main [182] demonstrated that tumor-immune mice could reject a tumor and accept normal skin from the same inbred mouse. In 1960, Klein [123] showed that an experimental animal could be immunized to reject a graft of his own chemically induced tumor, and that resistance to the tumor graft could be transferred to another mouse of the same strain by transferring lymphoid cells but not antibody. In 1961, Sjogren [203] demonstrated that the polyoma virus induced tumors only in mice which had impaired immunity but once the tumor was induced it could then be transplanted to normal adult mice. Sjogren further demonstrated that immunization of normal mice with the polyoma virus conferred protection against any tumor induced by the polyoma virus.

Subsequent studies confirmed that with few exceptions tumor immunity in experimental animals is mediated by lymphocytes and not antibodies. Immune sera have been effective against some leukemias and lymphomas, but in most other tumors systems antibody blocks tumor immunity.

The hypothesis of immune surveillance, which originated with Ehrlich in 1909 [70] and was later made popular by Thomas [216] and Burnet [33], was a proposal that cell-mediated immunity destroyed tumor cells that arose spontaneously before they could grow to a critical mass, and that cancer resulted from a failure of this immunologic surveillance mechanism. Currently this hypothesis does not very well explain the occurrence of most cancers. Although many cancer patients are found to have impaired immune systems, many others do not.

1.5. Evidence for Tumor Immunity in Humans

The transplantation techniques used in animals obviously are not directly applicable to humans; therefore, *in vitro* immunologic techniques have been widely applied to the study of human cancer. One of the most popular of these is the cytotoxicity assay. In cytotoxicity assays tumor cells are cultured in the presence of lymphocytes, and lymphocyte-mediated tumor cell destruction is evaluated by measuring the amount of isotope released from dying tumor cells (or remaining in surviving tumor cells, depending upon the assay used). The early results of cytotoxicity studies in human tumors suggested that human tumors expressed histologic type-specific antigens that cross-reacted: that is, bladder cancer patients' lymphocytes were thought to be cytotoxic to bladder cancer cells from other patients but not to other types of tumor cells such as melanoma, breast cancer, etc. These early observations seemed to suggest that human tumor-associated antigens behaved in a manner similar to cross-reacting viral or fetal antigens rather than unique tumor antigens. Subsequent and more carefully controlled studies of tumors in humans showed, however, that many normal controls have lymphocytes that are cytotoxic to a variety of tumor cells and also that many cancer patients exhibit cytotoxicity to tumor cells of different histogenetic types. The explanation for these findings is that tumor cells can express a variety of cell surface antigens that also include fetal and viral antigens. In this regard both fetal and viral antigens have been associated with a number of different tumor cells including urologic cancers.

At the present time our understanding of human tumor antigens remains quite fragmentary; however, a preponderance of evidence shows that both animal and human tumors express antigens that elicit immune responses in the host. Despite these, the tumor continues to grow and often causes the death of the host. It is believed that this paradox can be explained by immunologic escape mechanisms.

1.6. Immunologic Escape Mechanisms

There is no single satisfactory explanation for the success of tumors in the face of an active immune response. A multitude of immunologic escape mechanisms have been demonstrated, but their relative biologic importance is unknown. A general impairment of host immunity accompanies a number of tumors and this impairment usually increases as the tumor grows. T cell functions are generally more impaired than B cell functions and macrophage activity may be either reduced or heightened. Impaired immunity has been attributed variously to immunoregulatory proteins, fetal antigens such as alpha fetoprotein or human chorionic gonadotropin (HCG), which are known to have immunosuppressive properties, and suppressor cells and their products.

Anti-cancer treatments such as radiation therapy and chemotherapy can suppress, sometimes selectively, certain lymphocyte functions. Some tumor responses, such as cytotoxic responses, are harmful to the tumor, while others, like the production of blocking antibody or the generation of suppressor cells, actually protect the tumor. Thus immunosuppressive anti-cancer treatments can alter the balance between the host and the tumor for better or for worse.

Another potential immunologic escape mechanism is the blocking of the effector limb of the immune response. This can be produced by free antibody that coats the tumor cell and covers its antigenic determinants, by free antigen that binds to receptors on the effector cells and thus precludes their cytotoxic potential, and by antigen-antibody complexes that can work at either the tumor cell or the effector cell level. Clinical studies have shown that enhancing antibody activity is present in the sera of many patients with progressive tumors, but not in the sera of patients who are tumor-free [102].

Other immunologic escape mechanisms include loss of clones of tumor cells expressing strong antigens by immunoselection, antigenic modulation in which the tumor cells temporarily cease to express antigens in certain environments but will re-express them in other environments, uneven distribution of cytotoxic cells in the body, and the generation of suppressor cells and their products.

1.7. Immunotherapy

Immunologic manipulations have been used in attempts to control tumor growth for decades. Immunotherapy logically can be characterized as active or passive. In passive immunotherapy, immunologic reagents such as serum, cells, or cell products are administered to the tumor-bearing host in the hope that they will act to destroy tumor. Passive immunotherapy with serum or cells has been generally unsuccessful, except against a few virus-induced experimental tumors. Passive immunotherapy with subcellular fractions such as immune RNA or transfer factor has not been adequately studied, but there is little convincing data so far to justify much enthusiasm about this approach.

In active immunotherapy the host is stimulated to produce an immune response that causes tumor cell death. Bacterial products are known to have profound effects on immunologic reactions. They can increase antibody production, increase graft rejection, and increase resistance to viral and bacterial infections. The most commonly used bacterial products are Bacille-Calmette-Guerin (BCG) and *Corynebacterium parvum* (*C. parvum*). The use of BCG in certain animal tumors has been found to increase resistance to tumor growth. BCG can also activate macrophages to kill selectively certain tumor cells. BCG has been used in many clinical studies, and has been shown to be most effective when injected directly into the tumors. This has been referred to as systemic immunotherapy; however, the question has been raised about whether this is really a systemic immune response or merely an example of tumor not growing well in sites of delayed cutaneous hypersensitivity reactions.

Newer models for immunotherapy have been aimed at selectively eliminating suppressor cell function and augmenting host immune responses with interferon, a biologic response modifier. These studies are in their initial phases, and much more work will be necessary before their clinical value is known.

2. CARCINOMA OF THE PROSTATE

2.1. *Evidence for Tumor-Associated Antigens in Prostatic Cancer*

There is very limited evidence to suggest that human prostatic carcinomas express tumor-associated antigens. In a study primarily of bladder cancer, Bubenik and coworkers [30] showed that primary culture tumor cells from a patient with prostatic carcinoma were killed in an *in vitro* cytotoxicity assay by the patient's own leukocytes, but not by leukocytes from bladder cancer patients.

In 1975, Avis and coworkers [7] reported *in vitro* cell-mediated cytotoxicity studies in nine patients with carcinoma of the prostate and ten control patients (patients with benign prostatic hypertrophy (BPH)). In addition 16 other control patients were studied, including normal men, normal women, patients with renal carcinoma, and women with benign breast disease. Peripheral blood lymphocytes from patients with BPH or prostatic cancer were cytotoxic to primary culture cells from either prostatic cancer or BPH, but not to normal fibroblasts or cultures from other tumors. Lymphocytes from normal control patients or from patients with nonprostatic cancers were not cytotoxic to either the prostatic cancer or BPH-derived cells. The authors suggested that antigens expressed on both BPH and carcinoma of the prostate were not present on nonprostatic cells. However, one weakness of the study is that occult prostatic carcinoma might have been present in the BPH patients, and there is no way this could have been ruled out.

More recently, Okabe and coworkers [167], using a ^{51}Cr-release assay, examined cell-mediated cytotoxicity against the prostatic cancer cell line EB 33 in 29 patients with carcinoma of the prostate. Their controls included 10 women and nine patients with BPH. They found that lymphocytes from patients with stage B prostatic carcinoma produced almost total killing of target cells, while lymphocytes from patients with stage C and D produced far less cytotoxicity against EB 33 cells. Moreover, lymphocytes from pelvic lymph nodes of prostatic cancer patients produced less cytotoxicity than did peripheral blood lymphocytes. Finally, many of the control patients including women exhibited some cytotoxicity against prostatic cancer cells. This study suggested that cell-mediated cytotoxicity was not absolutely specific for prostate cancer associated-antigens.

Brannen and coworkers [22] tested for delayed cutaneous hypersensitivity reactions to potassium chloride (KCl) extracts of prostatic carcinoma and BPH. Four of ten patients with carcinoma of the prostate had positive skin test responses to their own tumor extract and one also exhibited a positive response to a prostatic cancer from another patient. Only one of ten patients with prostatic carcinoma had a positive skin test response to an extract of BPH. Nine of ten patients with BPH had negative responses to BPH extracts, while one had a positive response to his own BPH extract. This patient was subsequently found to have prostatic carcinoma as well. These results were interpreted as suggesting that carcinoma of the prostate expresses cell-surface antigens that are not found in BPH and that these antigens are capable of inducing delayed cutaneous hypersensitivity reactions in tumor-bearing patients.

Ablin and coworkers [1, 3] presented data from assays of leukocyte migration inhibition and leukocyte adherence inhibition (LAI) suggesting that prostatic cancers express tumor-associated antigens that can be solubilized by potassium chloride. Subseqeuntly, a number of other investigators [15, 17, 118] have found positive LAI assay results in many patients with prostatic cancer. For example, Bhatti and coworkers [15], using a tube dilution assay system, reported that 77% of prostatic cancer patients had positive LAI responses to prostatic cancer extracts. In their study lymphocytes from prostate cancer patients were either incubated with or without a prostatic cancer antigen. In another study, reported by Evans and coworkers [78], 89% of patients with prostatic carcinoma had positive LAI reactions to prostatic cancer extracts. From the results of studies like these has arisen the suggestion that perhaps the LAI assay could be used as a screening test for prostatic cancer.

Kaneti, Thompson and Reid [118] examined antitumor immunity to prostatic carcinoma with a tube LAI assay. In their study peripheral blood lymphocytes from 37 prostatic cancer patients and 128 control patients (normal and BPH) were incubated separately with saline extracts from prostatic carcinoma or an unrelated cancer extract. Five of 37 (14%) of the patients with prostatic carcinoma had positive LAI responses compared with 2 of 128 (1.5%) of control subjects. The investigators postulated that there were relatively few positive reactions among their prostatic cancer patients because most of these patients had advanced disease. Interestingly, *in vitro* treatment of lymphocytes with prostaglandin E_2 resulted in positive LAI responses in 61% of prostatic carcinoma patients, but in only 3% of controls. The investigators suggested that this response may indicate a functional defect in the antitumor response of the peripheral blood lymphocytes, perhaps caused by an excess of circulting tumor antigen.

A number of investigators [86] have reported that many prostatic cancer patients have elevated serum and urinary levels of the fetal antigen known as carcinoembryonic antigen (CEA), and human prostatic epithelial cells have been shown to produce CEA in tissue culture [230]. Broder and coworkers [23] also reported the presence of another fetal antigen, human chorionic gonadotropin (HCG), in one patient with prostatic cancer; however, production of HCG by prostatic cancer patients is an unusual occurrence. Guinan [85] evaluated serum samples from 47 prostatic cancer patients for the fetal antigen alpha fetoprotein (AFP) and found positive titers in none.

Viral particles and viral antigens have been associated with prostatic cancer cells [166]. Moreover, it has been clearly shown that normal prostatic epithelium can be induced by viruses to undergo malignant transformation [174].

Normal, BPH, and malignant prostatic epithelial cells also produce an antigenically distinctive form of acid phosphatase that can be detected by radioimmunoassay and demonstrated by immunocytochemistry [180]. Moreover, a number of investigators [149, 173, 225] demonstrated the presence of another antigen distinct from acid phosphatase, called the prostatic antigen, in both benign and malignant prostatic tumors. This prostate differentiation antigen was extensively characterized by Wang and coworkers [225] and was demonstrated to be present in prostatic tissues exclusively. It was purified to homogeneity and was found to have a molecular weight of about 33 000. In subsequent studies [173] this antigen was detected in the serum of only 9% of prostatic cancer patients, but was not found at all in the serum of patients with BPH.

Only a small number of investigations have been conducted on the antigenicity of experimental prostatic carcinoma in animals. In 1970, Mondal and coworkers [150] observed that mouse prostatic cell clones that were transformed *in vitro* with the carcinogen methylcholanthrene were strongly antigenic in 11 of 12 cases. There was no antigenic cross reactivity between these clones of transformed cells. This study showed that chemically transformed prostatic cancer cells have the capacity to develop tumor-associated transplantation antigens, at least in mice.

In 1977, Lopez and Voight [138], studying the spontaneous adenocarcinoma of the prostate in the Copenhagen rat (R3327), reported proliferative responses in mixed lymphocyte-tumor cell cultures by lymphocytes from tumor-bearing animals but not lymphocytes from normal animals. Moreover, lymphocytes from tumor-bearing animals did not respond to normal prostate cells, muscle cells, kidney cells, or cells from the squamous cell variety of the R3327 tumor. The investigators also used an assay based on tumor antigen-induced nonspecific cytotototoxicity directed against chicken red blood cell targets, and reported that extracts from prostatic cancers, but not control extracts, induced non-specific cytotoxicity. Similar studies were also reported by Claflin and coworkers [50].

White and coworkers [229] reported that electrodesiccation of the canine prostate altered the prostatic tissue and created new antigens that remained in the prostate. These antigens could be identified by fluorescent antibody techniques.

At the present time our understanding of prostatic carcinoma-associated antigens remains incomplete and many more studies need to be done.

2.2. Impairment of Host Immune Mechanism in Prostatic Cancer

Although prostatic carcinomas may express antigens that can elicit immunologic responses in the host, the tumors often continue to grow nonetheless and in many instances cause the death of the patient. This paradox has been explained by a variety of different potential immunologic escape mechanisms whereby the hosts' immunologic responses could be either subverted or suppressed.

There is much evidence that host cell-mediated immunologic activity is depressed in many patients with prostatic carcinoma. Robinson and coworkers [191] reported that lymphocyte proliferative responses to the mitogen phytohemagglutinin (PHA), a nonspecific stimulator of T lymphocytes, were significantly impaired in patients with metastatic prostatic cancer compared with either control patients or patients with BPH. Robinson found that responses of patients with local prostatic cancer were not significatnly different from those of control patients with BPH; however, in some patients with focal carcinoma infiltration, PHA responses were actually greater than normal.

We studied delayed cutaneous hypersensitivity responses to dinitrochlorobenzene (DNCB), another test of T lymphocyte function, in 25 patients with prostatic carcinoma [39] and found that DNCB responses could be impaired both in patients with local carcinoma and in those with metastases. However, not all patients with advanced prostatic carcinoma showed impaired DNCB reactivity; in fact, some patients with widely disseminated cancer manifested normal DNCB reactivity. Our results were subsequently confirmed by Elhilali and coworkers [72] and by Schellhammer and coworkers [198] in a study of patients who were surgically staged. However, results at variance with ours were reported by Decenzo and coworkers [61], by Huus and coworkers [114] and by Brosman and coworkers [26], all of whom reported that DNCB reactivity was more severely impaired in patients with metastatic disease. Williams and Castro [233] found that all 21 prostatic cancer patients they tested, seven of who. . had metastatic disease, had positive DNCB responses; however, in their study extraordinarily high doses of DNCB were used for skin testing.

McLaughlin and coworkers [140] reported on impaired lymphocyte responsiveness to PHA when lymphocytes were cultured in the patients' own serum. In 42 prostatic cancer patients, most of whom were surgically staged, McLaughlin found no correlation between the extent of tumor and the PHA response. McLaughlin also reported that clinical remission of prostate cancer induced by orchiectomy resulted in an improved PHA response in only one of six patients. In subsequent studies, McLaughlin and Brooks [139] reported that the impaired lymphocyte response to PHA was in fact caused by a circulating alpha-2 globulin in the plasma. In our laboratory, we studied lymphocyte responses to PHA among prostatic cancer patients and found similarly impaired reactivity in patients with local and with metastatic cancer and significantly more of the plasma factors that inhibited PHA response among patients with metastatic disease [46]. Moreover, we found that the impairment was not entirely attributable to plasma factors, but was due at least in part to a deficiency in the proportion of T lymphocytes in the peripheral circulation [42].

Menon and Stefani [141] also evaluated prostatic cancer patients for plasma blocking factors, but found no evidence of them in any of their patients. Although they did find a slight elevation of the alpha-2 globulin fraction in patients with metastases, this did not correlate with inhibitory blocking activity of the serum.

More recently, Herr and associates [110] reported suppressor macrophages in the serum of prostatic cancer patients that caused an impaired lymphocyte proliferative response to PHA and other mitogens. In Herr's study removal of macrophages restored PHA response while addition of adherent cells back to cultures again produced the impairment.

Herr [109] also found that in prostatic cancer patients lymph nodes with normal, lymphocyte-depleted or hyperplastic appearances on histologic examination produced progressively less lymphocyte proliferation. The depletion histologic pattern occurred in patients with lymph node metastases in five of eight cases studied. Previous studies by Barzell *et al.* [8] in patients undergoing pelvic lymphadenectomy and ^{125}I implantation had demonstrated that the depleted pattern was more common in patients with high stage B_2 or C prostatic cancer, high-grade cancer, patients with positive nodes, patients with tumors that did not respond to radiation therapy, and patients who developed subsequent metastases.

In our laboratory we found that the cytolytic activity of K cells, which are effector cells that mediate antibody-dependent cell-mediated cytotoxicity, and of natural killer (NK) cells, which mediate spontaneous cytotoxicity, are also impaired in many prostatic cancer patients [44]. The mechanisms underlying this impairment are not entirely clear.

Cells of the macrophage-monocyte series also have shown perturbed function in patients with prostatic cancer. Monocyte chemotactic responses were reported to be depressed in patients with prostatic carcinoma [24]; however, in our studies macrophage-mediated cytotoxic function was actually enhanced [44]. Similarly, Sanford and coworkers [197] found that patients with prostatic cancer exhibited enhanced cytotoxic reactivity against virally transformed cells.

Information on B lymphocyte function in prostatic cancer patients is both limited and conflicting. Gursel and coworkers [89] reported a tendency toward increased IgG levels and decreased IgM levels in patients with advanced prostatic cancer. Ablin and coworkers [2] found that both IgG and IgM levels were in the low normal range but that IgA levels and levels of C′3 were increased. Schmidt and coworkers [200] found no significant differences in the IgG, IgA, IgM or IgE levels between prostatic cancer patients and control (normal) patients. Studies measuring antibody responses to specific antigens in prostatic cancer patients have not been reported to our knowledge.

Ablin and coworkers [1] reported evidence for 'blocking antibodies' as an immunologic escape mechanism in prostatic cancer patients. In their leukocyte adherence inhibition (LAI) assays, serum factors blocked LAI responses, but these factors were not characterized biochemically. Mikulsky and coworkers [140] presented evidence based on inhibited antibody-dependent cell-mediated cytotoxicity (ADCC) that patients with prostatic cancer, particularly advanced stages of disease, have circulating antigen-antibody complexes. These complexes, if bound to Fc receptors on K cells or NK cells, could explain the impaired ADCC and NK activity observed in some prostatic cancer patients.

Nonspecific suppressor T cell precursors that can be activated by mitogens have been demonstrated both in the peripheral blood and in regional lymph nodes of prostatic cancer patients [43]. However, the role of these suppressor cells remains to be determined.

Whitmore and Gittes [230] examined the prostate as a potential immunologically privileged site. They found that the survival of skin allografts in the prostate was somewhat prolonged. Animals immunized with sheep red blood cells by injection of these cells into the prostate developed hemolytic antibody titers that were comparable to those induced by injection of sheep erythrocytes at other sites. However, delayed cutaneous hypersensitivity reactivity to sheep red cells was less when the red cells were injected into the prostate at 21 days after skin allografting than when they were injected into other organs. These studies suggested that the prostate may be somewhat of an immunologically privileged site in terms of cell-mediated immune responses, but not in terms of humoral immunity.

2.3. Prognostic Significance of Host Immune Competence

In a number of tumors impaired host immunity correlates with subsequent death of the host. One interpretation of this finding has been that impaired immunologic responses cause rapid progression of tumors. Another interpretation has been that the immunologic impairment is simply a secondary manifestation of advanced malignancy.

There is only limited evidence that bears on the prognostic significance of host immunocompetence in patients with prostatic carcinoma. In a study we conducted [45], DNCB reactivity was correlated with the subsequent clinical course one year after skin testing in 38 patients with prostatic carcinoma. In this study, we found no correlation between DNCB reactivity and the development of metastases in patients who at first had only local disease, nor did we find a significant correlation between DNCB reactivity and further tumor progression in patients who had metastatic disease at the time of testing and who later received endocrine therapy. Similar results were reported by Decenzo and coworkers [61]. The correlation we did observe was between impaired immunologic reactivity and tumor progression among patients who did not receive endocrine therapy. Thus, the androgen-dependence of the tumor may be a more important determinant of clinical course than host immunocompetence. However, in patients having either androgen-independent tumors or patients not receiving endocrine therapy, host immunologic factors may play a role in the clinical evolution of the disease.

2.4. *Immunotherapy*

Two studies of cryo-immunotherapy for prostatic carcinoma have been reported. In 1970, Soanes and coworkers [205] reported on three prostatic cancer patients whose metastatic lesions regressed several months following transurethral cryotherapy of the prostate. These investigators cited, as the basis for cryotherapy, previous animal studies suggesting that such a procedure could induce the production of antibodies directed against prostatic antigens. In 1972, Gursel and coworkers [90] reported on the results of transperineal cryotherapy in 11 patients who were in relapse of metastatic prostatic cancer following endocrine therapy. Eight of these patients reported relief of pain; however, there was no correlation between pain relief and changes in acid phosphatase activity. One patient had evidence of regression of skeletal metastases on bone scan while 10 exhibited no change. Ten of the eleven patients died within one year of treatment.

These results were interpreted as suggesting at least a temporary systemic therapeutic benefit from cryosurgery; however, controlled clinical studies to confirm such a benefit have not been done. Moreover, other investigators have not found a measurable immunologic effect following cryodestruction of the prostate.

There are a number of early studies of nonspecific active immunotherapy of prostate cancer including anecdotal reports of patients treated with Coley's toxin. The data from these studies are essentially uninterpretable.

A clinical trial of nonspecific active immunotherapy for prostatic carcinoma with BCG was first reported by Merrin and coworkers in 1975 [143]. They studied 17 patients with histologically proven stage D carcinoma of the prostate. Patients were stratified according to their skin test reactions to purified protein derivative (PPD). Those with positive skin tests were treated with intraprostatic injections of BCG, 1 mg per week (type and number of organisms not specified) for four weeks or, alternatively, 1 mg of BCG the first week, 2 mg the second week, 4 mg the third week, and 6 mg the fourth. Patients with negative PPD skin tests were given 50 mg of BCG by mouth in an attempt to sensitize them; however, none of these patients' skin tests converted to positive and, therefore, they were not included in the results of this trial.

Of the seven patients with positive BCG skin tests, five (71%) were reported to have objective responses to BCG therapy as indicated by a 50% decrease in the size and induration of the prostate. There were no changes in measurable metastases, and biopsies taken after BCG therapy showed necrosis of the tumor in three patients but no change in the others' tumors. The general condition of the seven patients after receiving BCG injections was described as worse in four, stable in two and improved in one patient. Although the initial injections of BCG were well tolerated, later injections produced fever in all patients. Two patients had anaphylactoid reactions to BCG and one patient developed a rectoprostatic fistula. As a phase I trial this study provided only limited information, but the authors did document measurable evidence of tumor regression in five patients.

In a similar uncontrolled phase I trial of BCG immunotherapy, Robinson and coworkers [193] reported on two sequential trials of prostate cancer treated with multiple intraprostatic injections of BCG. These investigators used Galaxo BCG (number of organisms not stated) at weekly intervals beginning with a 1 cc dose and increasing the dose by 1 cc each successive week for a total of six weeks. In their initial clinical trial six patients who were in relapse of prostatic carcinoma after endocrine therapy were treated. Four of the six were reported to have improved micturition and general medical condition, but all died within two years of treatment. There was no clinical or postmortem evidence of tumor destruction and the complications of therapy were minimal.

Robinson's second clinical trial [192] included eight similar patients, six of whom had stage C disease and two of whom had stage D disease. All had previously been treated with endocrine therapy and six of the eight had positive skin tests to PPD. In the second trial, unlike the first, complications of treatment were substantial. All six patients developed fever, three developed gastrointestinal bleeding and autopsy studies revealed diffuse widespread granulomas in many organs of the body. Accordingly, Robinson recommended against administering more than three intraprostatic BCG injections. Four of the six patients who had positive PPD tests were reported to be alive six months to one year after therapy. As a phase I trial, this study provided only minimal useful information on dose-toxicity relationships, and no information on dose-response relationships. This study also documented evidence of tumor regression in some patients.

In a phase II trial of BCG immunotherapy by Guinan *et al.* [88], Tice BCG was administered by a single left deltoid region intradermal vaccination of 4.2×10^7 viable organisms in 0.5 ml every four months. The BCG treatment group consisted of 19 patients representing a variety of different stages of prostate cancer. The control and treatment groups were comparable in terms of age and tumor stage, but patients were not randomly assigned to the treatment groups, and the criteria for inclusion in the control group were not stated. In addition, seven patients in each group were also receiving concurrent endocrine therapy. The response to BCG therapy as assessed by mean survival time was reported to be 26.6 months in the BCG group as compared to 22.6 months for the untreated group. This survival difference was not statistically significant. Morbidity of the BCG vaccinations was described as minimal, but specific details were not given.

As a phase II trial, this study deals with a heterogeneous group of patients in terms of the extent of disease and other therapy received. Although the authors stated that survival was prolonged in BCG-treated patients the figures do not bear out a statistically significant benefit.

In summary, the available human studies on immunotherapy for prostatic carcinoma provide very limited, unconvincing evidence for a beneficial therapeutic effect arising from the agents and dose schedules reported. Moreover, the toxicity of nonspecific active immunotherapy with BCG is documented, and in some of these studies is substantial.

To our knowledge there have been no studies reported of passive immunotherapy for prostatic carcinoma. Much more work will need to be done to determine whether immunologic responses can be modified to the therapeutic benefit of prostate cancer patients.

We are aware of only two animal studies of immunotherapy for prostatic cancer. Pollard and coworkers [179] evaluated the effect of killed *C. parvum* administered in doses of 1.4 mg intravenously at weekly intervals on the development of metastases from the spontaneous adenocarcinoma of the prostate in germ-free Lobound-Wistar rats. *C. parvum* treated animals had significantly fewer pulmonary metastases (1.3 per lung) than controls (13 per lung). Pollard concluded that *C. parvum* protects against the development of metastatic lesions in this experimental tumor model.

The only other reported animal study of immunotherapy for prostatic carcinoma was reported by Weissman and coworkers [228]. This study used the R3327 AT prostatic cancer and F_1 hybrids of Copenhagen and Fischer rats. The investigators administered active specific immunotherapy with irradiated tumor cells and active nonspecific immunotherapy with injections of pyran copolymer. Neither pyran copolymer nor irradiated tumor cells protected against the outgrowth of a subcutaneous tumor cell inoculum or against local recurrences of surgically resected large tumors. However, pyran copolymer prevented recurrences of surgically excised small tumors.

3. CARCINOMA OF THE URINARY BLADDER

3.1. Evidence for tumor-associated antigens in bladder cancer

Several lines of evidence suggest that tumor-associated antigens are expressed on bladder cancer cells. In the early studies cell-mediated cytotoxicity assays were used to test lymphocyte-mediated cytotoxicity against bladder cancer cell lines. These studies were interpreted as showing a high degree of specificity in the cytotoxic activity of lymphocytes against bladder cancer target cells. Later studies showed less specificity, and it became apparent that the susceptibility of the target cells to cytolysis was an important consideration in interpreting cytotoxicity assay results. The latter studies further suggested that several cytotoxic mechanisms, including both tumor-specific and nonspecific reactions, occurred. Other lines of evidence including detection of humoral immune response and lymphokine production also suggested immune recognition of bladder cancer-associated antigens.

Bubenik and associates [30, 31] were the first to show that leukocytes from bladder cancer patients exhibited specific cytotoxic activity for bladder cancer target cells. These investigators used a microcytotoxicity assay in which leukocytes from patients with bladder cancer and from various control patients were cultured with bladder cancer target cells, non-bladder tumor cells or normal cells, and the number of target cells attaching to the growth surface was interpreted as a measure of the cytotoxic reactivity of the leukocytes. Using this assay, Bubenik and associates observed cytotoxicity only when leukocytes from bladder cancer patients were cultured with bladder cancer target cells. Cytotoxicity was observed with both autologous and allogeneic leukocytes. Control leukocytes, which included cells from patients with other malignancies, from patients with benign diseases and from normal control patients, were not cytotoxic to bladder cancer cells nor were leukocytes from bladder cancer patients cytotoxic to non-bladder cancer cell lines. These same investigators [31] examined the sera of bladder cancer patients for complement-mediated cytotoxicity against the same panel of bladder cancer and control target cells. Complement-fixing antibodies specific for bladder cancer cells were observed in sera from 8 of 13 bladder cancer patients. The conclusion was that leukocytes from bladder cancer patients recognized a cross-reactive tumor-specific antigen that was not expressed on normal bladder epithelium or other tumor cells.

The results of Bubenik and associates were confirmed by O'Toole and associates [170], who tested leukocytes from 54 bladder cancer patients and 32 control patients in a microcytotoxicity assay using autologous as well as long-term tissue culture cell lines, including the bladder cancer line designated T-24. These investigators also showed an inverse correlation between the degree of cytotoxic reactivity and the stage of the disease. Eighty-eight percent of the patients with local tumors showed specific cytotoxicity when assayed before treatment, while only 41% with advanced tumors showed specific cytotoxicity. Local radiotherapy (3500 to 8400 rads) decreased or eliminated cytotoxic activity, and the cytotoxicity remained depressed as long as radiation was being given. All patients with T-2 stage tumors redeveloped cytotoxicity within seven days after cessation of irradiation, while 80% of T-3 patients and 50% of the T-4 patients expressed cytotoxicity seven days after termination of treatment, suggesting that the effector cell that mediated the cytotoxicity was radiosensitive. Some patients with advanced tumors failed to redevelop cytotoxicity after radiation therapy, and these patients were found to develop distant metastases. O'Toole and associates [171] also reported that tumor resection resulted in the loss of cytotoxic activity while recurrence of tumor was associated with the return of cytotoxicity; they concluded that the presence of the tumor-associated antigen was required for the maintenance of cytotoxicity.

Contrasting results were reported by Troye and associates [217] using a ^{51}Cr release assay as a measure of cytotoxicity. These investigators studied seven bladder cancer patients whose tumors had been surgically excised before the time of assay. The patients as a group expressed greater cytotoxic activity against allogenic bladder cancer cell lines than to normal control patients.

Hakala and associates [95] tested 48 patients with histologically proven bladder cancer and 51 control patients for tumor-specific cytotoxicity in a microcytotoxicity assay. The bladder cancer target cells used were 253J and T-24 while the control cells included normal kidney and testis cell lines. The cytotoxic activity of bladder cancer patients was significantly ($p<0.001$) greater than control patients against the bladder cancer target cells, again suggesting tumor-specific cytotoxicity.

Bean and associates [12] measured the cytotoxicity of lymphocytes from 27 bladder cancer patients against T-24 target cells and other nonbladder cell lines in a ^{3}H-proline cytotoxicity assay. Specific cytotoxicity for T-24 cells was seen in lymphocytes from 10 of 27 bladder cancer patients, which was significantly greater than cytotoxicity in lymphocytes from normal patients (2 of 49). The specific cytotoxicity found in bladder cancer patients was predominantly in patients with superficial tumors (8 of 15 such patients displayed specific cytotoxicity). Nonspecific cytotoxicity occurred with equal frequency in bladder cancer and control patients.

O'Toole and associates [172] identified the effector cells mediating cytotoxicity by separating lymphocytes into those capable of forming spontaneous rosettes with sheep erythrocytes (E+), which are predominantly T-lymphocytes and those not capable of forming spontaneous rosettes (E−), which are predominantly B lymphocytes and null cells. O'Toole *et al.* showed that E− (no greater than 9% E+ contamination) cell populations mediated the tumor specific cytotoxicity, and antibody-dependent cell-mediated cytotoxicity (ADCC). The finding that tumor-specific cytotoxicity was mediated by E− lymphocytes was surprising since specific cytotoxicity is normally mediated by T lymphocytes.

Troye and associates [217, 218] suggested that the elevated specific cytotoxicity observed for bladder cancer patients may be attributed to antibody production, indicating that the specific cytotoxicity observed by O'Toole and associates [172] in the E− lymphoid fraction may be attributable principally to ADCC. In support of this hypothesis several other investigators [92, 93, 97, 176] have reported production of tumor-specific antibodies by bladder cancer patients (*vide infra*).

The questions surrounding the existence of tumor-specific cytotoxicity were amplified by Takasugi and associates [213] who reported that leukocytes from control as well as tumor-bearing patients mediated cytotoxicity against a variety of target cells. In a subsequent report [214] these investigators examined the cytotoxic activity of lymphocytes from patients with various cancers against 45 human tumor cell lines including the T-24 cell line. They observed a nonspecific pattern of cytotoxicity.

Bloom and associates [18] examined the cytotoxic activity of lymphocytes against T-24 target cells in patients with bladder, renal and prostatic carcinomas and nonmalignant genitourinary disorders. The lymphocytes from bladder cancer patients exhibited higher cytotoxic activity than the lymphocytes from normal donors against T-24 cells, but this level of activity was no different from that of patients with nonmalignant GU disorders. The investigators suggested that the specificity observed by other investigators resulted from varying susceptibility of target cells to lysis by lymphocytes.

In 1974, a workshop on cytotoxicity assays, sponsored by the National Cancer Institute and the American Cancer Society, was held at the Sloan-Kettering Institute in an effort to determine whether tumor-specific cytotoxicity was present in cancer patients [10]. Coded lymphocyte samples were supplied to the most prominent investigators in the field, but the results yielded no clear-cut findings on disease-related cytotoxicity.

Several investigators [19, 41, 98, 153] have been unable to detect tumor-specific cytotoxicity. Catalona and associates [41] performed a double-blind study in which 25 bladder cancer patients, 19 patients with non-transitional cell carcinoma and nine patients with the benign conditions were tested for tumor-specific cytotoxicity. Cytotoxicity of peripheral blood lymphocytes was measured in a ^{3}H proline-labeled tumor cell assay using T-24 and H-894 melanoma target cells. No significant differences with respect to patterns of cytotoxic reactivity among the various patient groups were observed.

Hakala and associates [98] developed an automated lymphocyte-mediated cytotoxicity assay in which cytotoxicity was expressed as the number of lymphocytes required to reduce target cell survival by 50%. These investigators observed a target cell specificity that did not appear to be related to tumor-associated antigens. Bolhuis [19] and Moore and Robinson [153] were also unable to detect tumor specific cytotoxicity by bladder cancer patients and suggested that the pattern of cytotoxicity often interpreted as tumor specific was related to the susceptibility of the target cell. In this regard, Catalona and associates [44] have shown that target cells vary in their susceptibility to lysis by various subpopulations of lymphoid cells, further emphasizing the importance of target cell selection.

Troye and associates [219] studied 54 patients with bladder cancer, 20 patients with other tumors and 24 healthy controls by menas of a ^{51}Cr-release assay using T-24 cells, normal bladder epithelial cells, colon cancer and malignant melanoma target cells. Bladder cancer lymphocytes exhibited cytotoxic activity against all the cell lines studied but their cytotoxicity was more elevated against T-24 target cells than against the others. These investigators concluded that *in vitro* cytotoxicity assays actually measure several different cytotoxic mechanisms simultaneously and that bladder cancer patients exhibit specific as well as nonspecific cytotoxicity. In subsequent studies Troye and associates [217, 218] suggested that antibody production against cross-reactive tumor-associated antigens mediated ADCC and therefore was responsible for the elevated cytotoxicity of bladder cancer cells against bladder cancer target cells.

Troye and associates [217, 218], using T-24 target cells, examined the effects of Fab fragments of IgG antibody directed against human immunoglobulin on the cytotoxic activity of lymphocytes from bladder cancer patients and control patients. Fab fragments were observed to significantly depress the cytotoxic activity of lymphocytes both from bladder cancer and control patients, suggeting a role for immunoglobulin in spontaneous cytotoxic activity [218]. Also, the effector cell responsible for the elevated cytotoxicity of lymphocytes from bladder cancer patients was identified as an E− lymphocyte that expressed receptors for Fc region of immunoglobulin.

Troye and associates [200] then obtained serum from bladder cancer patients and control patients and isolated immunoglobulin G, which was tested for its ability to mediate ADCC against T-24 and non-bladder cancer target cells. Significantly greater ADCC activity against T-24 target cells was observed with immunoglobulin G from bladder cancer patients than with immunoglobulin G from control patients.

Hakala and associates [93] also detected the presence of tumor-specific antibodies in serum from bladder cancer patients in studies performed to determine whether serum could mediate complement-dependent cytotoxicity with a specificity for bladder cancer cell lines. Serum from 6 of 7 patients with bladder cancer demonstrated significant ($p<0.05$) complement-mediated cytotoxicity against bladder cancer target cells. Only one of seven renal carcinoma patients and 2 of 6 patients without tumor demonstrated significant cytotoxicity against these target cells. The incidence of cytotoxicity of sera from the same patients was not significantly different when normal kidney cells were the target cells. Similar results were reported by Elhilali and associates [74].

Further studies by Hakala and associates [92, 97] showed that serum from bladder cancer patients was active in ADCC against bladder cancer target cells and that the active factor was immunoglobulin G. Immunoglobulin G from bladder cancer patients induced cytotoxicity in lymphocytes from normal as well as bladder cancer donors. The antibodies showed specificity for transitional cell carcinoma lines of the renal pelvis, ureter and bladder but not against normal adult or embryonic cells or against renal cell carcinomas.

Other methods were used to screen serum from bladder cancer patients for tumor specific antibodies. Phillips and Lewis [176] used the enzyme-linked immunoadsorbent assay (ELISA) to detect serum antibodies to tumor-associated antigens. The antigens were prepared by homogenizing tumor specimens at 4 °C followed by centrifugation to remove cellular debris. With this antigen preparation as the reactive agent, 43 of 53 (81 %) bladder carcinoma patients had detectable antibody in their serum, while no antibody was detected against prostate cancer antigen preparations. Eight of the 53 sera (15 %) also reacted with normal bladder antigen preparations. Twenty-four normal control sera were tested, none of which contained antibodies against bladder cancer, normal bladder or prostate cancer antigen preparations.

Sophen and O'Toole [207] used a quantitative membrane immunofluorescence assay to detect serum antibodies in patients with advanced squamous cell carcinoma of the bladder. Immunoglobulin M antibodies were found to react specifically with other squamous cell carcinoma cells but not with transitional cell carcinoma of the bladder, adenocarcinoma or melanoma cells.

Several investigators attempted to detect immune recognition of tumor-associated antigens by lymphokine production [17, 87, 199]. Guinan and coworkers [87] examined the responses of lymphocytes from 16 bladder cancer patients in a leukocyte adherence inhibition assay (LAI). In their system a potassium chloride extract of the tumor was used as the antigen and leukocytes were placed in test tubes containing either bladder cancer antigen, control renal cell carcinoma antigen or no antigen. Moreover, they evaluated LAI responses of age- and sex-matched control subjects as well as patients having urianry tract infections. They found that the mean percentage of nonadherent cells was significantly higher when lymphocytes from bladder cancer patients were incubated with the bladder cancer antigen than when they were incubated in the absence of antigen or with renal cancer antigen. In contrast, the mean percentage of nonadherent cells in control subjects was about the same whether cells were incubated in the absence of antigen or with bladder or renal cancer antigen. The percentage of individual patients having statistically positive LAI reactions was not stated in this study.

In contrast to the results of Guinan and coworkers [87], Bhatti and associates [17] observed no difference in the adherence of leukocytes from bladder cancer or control patients when treated with specific or nonspecific antigen. These investigators tested leukocytes from seven patients with bladder cancer and eight control patients using potassium chloride antigen extracts of bladder cancer and renal cell carcinoma in obtaining these results.

Schellhammer and associates [199] performed leukocyte migration inhibition (LMI) assays to detect tumor specific immune recognition. Leukocytes from 58 patients with bladder cancer, 16 patients with benign bladder disease, and 65 patients with other cancers or no disease were tested for the production of migration inhibition factor upon exposure to extracts from T-24 bladder cancer cells and extracts from renal and prostate cancer cell lines. There was a significant ($p<0.05$) increase in the frequency of migration inhibition in leukocytes from bladder cancer patients when exposed to T-24 extract as opposed to extracts from renal or prostatic carcinoma cell lines. Similarly, greater inhibition was observed in prostate and renal cancer patients when their leukocytes were exposed to the appropriate tumor antigen.

While no single line of evidence for tumor-associated antigens on bladder tumors can stand alone, taken together the data reported to date strongly suggest that the immune system recognizes antigenic determinants expressed on transformed bladder cells.

Animal model systems also have been examined for the presence of tumor-associated antigens. Daly and Prout [58] studied N-[4-(5-nitro-2-

furyl-2-thiazolyl] formamide (FANFT)-induced bladder tumors in rats. They demonstrated that lymphocytes from tumor-bearing rats expressed both specific cytotoxic activity and antibody production with specificities to the bladder tumor cells. Moreover, they showed that animals immunized with tumor cells rejected subsequent tumor challenge. These results have been confirmed for FANFT-induced bladder tumors in mice [53, 155].

Chapman and Taranger [47] showed that dogs immunized with methylcholanthrene-induced bladder papillomas developed fewer tumors when treated with methylcholanthrene than unimmunized controls. Also, specific cytotoxicity toward methylcholanthrene-induced bladder tumors was observed, further suggesting the presence of cross-reactive antigens on bladder tumors.

3.2. Impairment of Host Immune Mechanisms in Bladder Cancer

It is well established that immune responses of patients with bladder cancer are impaired and that the impairment correlates with progressive tumor growth. Early studies by O'Toole and coworkers [170] showed that the incidence of tumor-specific leukocyte-mediated cytotoxicity of bladder cancer patients decreased with progressive tumor growth. The impairment of the putative tumor-specific cytotoxicity was confirmed by others [17, 42, 43].

Ratliff and associates [186] extended these results by measuring two non-specific cytotoxic mechanisms, ADCC and spontaneous lymphocyte-mediated lympholysis, in bladder cancer patients. Both of these cytotoxic mechanisms were depressed in bladder cancer patients; however, no correlation with tumor stage was observed.

A general impairment of host cell-mediated immunity also occurs in association with bladder cancer, and this impairment also was shown to correlate with tumor stage. Olsson and associates [169] measured delayed cutaneous hypersensitivity responses to specific antigens in bladder cancer patietns. They examined 35 patients with biopsy-proven bladder cancer for their immunologic response to tuberculin purified protein derivative, streptokinase-streptodornase, mumps skin test antigen and keyhole-limpet hemocyanin. They observed an impaired response to the antigens in the bladder cancer patients compared to historical controls. These results were confirmed by others [38, 54, 112, 198]. Moreover, in the latter studies the incidence of the impaired response paralleled tumor stage and grade. Catalona and Chretien [38] studied the response of 25 bladder cancer patients to DNCB and observed an impaired response in 25% of the patients with noninvasive disease, 27% of the patients with T-1 and T-2 lesions, and 100% of those with T-3 and T-4 lesions. A similar correlation was observed with tumor grade.

McLaughlin and associates [140] showed that the nonspecific cellular response also was impaired in bladder cancer patients. They examined the proliferative response of lymphocytes to phytohemagglutinin (PHA) in 23 patients with bladder cancer and 63 control patients. They observed a significant ($p<0.01$) depression in the response of the patients compared to the response of control subjects. These results subsequently were confirmed by others [139, 164]. Moreover, Nishio and associates [164] observed an increase in the impairment of the proliferative response with increases in tumor stage and grade.

Herr and associates [111] showed that lymphocytes from bladder cancer patients expressed a decreased ability to function as stimulator cells in a one-way mixed lymphocyte culture (MLC). These investigators examined 55 unselected patients with bladder tumors for the lymphocytes ability to respond to and to stimulate activity in a one-way mixed leukocyte culture. The responses were compared to those of normal individuals. Lymphocytes from 31 of 55 (56%) patients with active disease exhibited decreased ability to stimulate in an MLC. In contrast, 26 of 31 patients (84%) expressed normal responsiveness to allogeneic lymphocytes. Surgical removal of the tumor restored the patients' ability to stimulate in 12 of 15 cases.

There is little information about the humoral response of bladder cancer patients. Merrin and Han [142] evaluated the humoral response in 10 patients with bladder cancer by serum protein electrophoresis and determining immunoglobulin levels in serum. By their criteria, all patients had normal humoral immunity. Other studies need to be performed to examine more specifically the humoral responses of bladder cancer patients.

The underlying reasons for the impairment of the immune response in bladder cancer patients are unclear although antigenic modulation of tumor-associated antigens, serum factors and suppressor cells have been implicated. Pizza and associates [128] examined the lymphocyte reactivity of two patients with transitional cell carcinoma of the bladder at various times during the course of their disease. Both had stage 2 disease at diagnosis. These patients showed a response to the primary tumor in both leukocyte migration and leukocyte proliferation, suggesting antigen recognition. However, in patient number 1, tumor from the fourth tumor recurrence, which appeared 24 months after the primary tumor, did not initiate a response in the leukocyte migration inhibition assay or leukocyte stimulation assay. The second patient showed a similar lack of reactivity to tumor cells at the third recurrence. The lack of response occurred in autologous as well as allogeneic AB serum eliminating possible serum blocking factors as a reason for the findings. The authors concluded that antigeneic modulation of tumor-associated antigens occurred, which allowed the tumor to escape immune recognition.

Early studies by Bubenik and associates [31] showed that the depression in cytotoxic reactivity was due in part to serum factors. Sera from four of nine bladder cancer patients were shown to block cytotoxicity. The factor responsible for blocking may have been immune complexes which have been shown to occur in a small percentage (13–15%) of bladder cancer patients [175].

Sera from bladder cancer patients also have been shown to impair the response of lymphocytes to mitogens. Nishio and associates [163] evaluated the effect of serum from normal patients, from tumor-bearing patients and fetal calf serum on the lymphocyte blastogenesis in response to PHA. The response of normal lymphocytes to PHA was significantly lower in the presence of bladder cancer patient serum than it was with autologous, fetal calf, or normal AB serum. There was a direct correlation of the lymphocyte response with stage and tumor grade. Others [139] also observed impaired lymphocyte proliferation in serum from bladder cancer patients. McLaughlin and Brooks [139] reported that the active factor in the suppressing sera migrated with the $alpha_2$ globulin fraction of the serum proteins. In contrast, Catalona and associates [42] detected serum-mediated impairment of lymphocyte proliferation in only 2 of 22 bladder cancer patients studied. These investigators suggested that the number of responding cells may be more important than serum factors in the impaired response of lymphocytes. They observed a significant decrease in the number of circulating T lymphocytes, which are the lymphocytes that respond to PHA, in bladder cancer patients.

Suppressor cells also have been shown to be important in the impairment of the immune response in bladder cancer patients. Herr [107, 108] studied lymphocytes from peripheral blood and draining lymph nodes from seven patients with locally advanced bladder carcinoma. All patients had received local radiation therapy (2000 rads) before a cystectomy. Lymph node lymphocytes from three patients showed a decreased ability to stimulate activity in a one-way mixed lymphocyte reaction. Moreover, the response of lymphocytes from normal patients was progressively impaired by increasing numbers of lymph node lymphocytes from these patients, suggesting that a suppressor cell was present. The suppressor cells observed in the three patients with disseminated disease were found only in the regional lymph nodes.

Catalona and associates reported the presence of suppressor cell precursors in the lymph nodes of bladder cancer patients [43]. The suppressor cells were activated by stimulation with the mitogen concanavalin A. Lymph node lymphocytes from four bladder cancer patients were studied; three of the patients had local disease. There was statistically significant suppression of the proliferative response of both syngeneic and allogeneic peripheral blood lymphocytes by lymph node lymphocytes from all bladder cancer patients.

Bean and associates [9, 11] observed a genetically restricted suppressor cell in the peripheral blood of a bladder cancer patient. Peripheral blood lymphocytes from this patient were unable to stimulate 3 of 27 responder lymphocyte preparations from normal individuals in a one-way mixed lymphocyte culture [11]. Depletion of T cells restored the ability of these cells to function as stimulator cells. Moreover, T-enriched preparations from this patient suppressed the responsiveness of the normal patients who had responded. These results suggest that immunologically depressed bladder cancer patients may possess genetically-restricted suppressor T cells. In a subsequent report, Bean and associates [9] studied in more detail the genetic restrictions associated with suppression by cells from this patient. Forty-three different normal individuals were tested for immunologic suppression by suppressor cells from this patients. Only those individuals bearing the antigen *HLA-B14* were immunologically suppressed. None of the individuals that responded normally in the presence of the suppressor cells expressed the *HLA-B14* antigen. Interestingly, the bladder cancer patient with the genetically restricted suppressor cells did not express the B14 antigen. No soluble suppressor factor has been detected.

3.3. Diagnostic and prognostic value of antigenic determinants on bladder tumors

Detecting the presence of bladder cancer antigens, including onconcofetal antigens, or the absence of normal antigens, including blood group antigens, has been examined as a possible means for detecting bladder tumors early in their development and predicting their clinical course. Monaco and associates [148] developed a rabbit antiserum to pooled bladder tumor extracts in efforts to develop a diagnostic test for bladder cancer. These investigators used a micro-complement fixation test to assay serum and a micro-Ouchterlony test to assay urine from 108 bladder cancer patients. Micro-complement fixation tests on serum were positive in 17 of 27 bladder cancer patients (62.9%) compared to only 1 of 29 normal patients (3.4%); however, 10 of 11 patients with urinary tract infections also had positive tests. Urine assays using the micro-Ouchterlony test yielded similar results when unadsorbed anti-serum was used. Adsorption of the serum with normal bladder mucosa membrane extracts reduced but did not eliminate the false-positive reactions. The Ouchterlony test with adsorbed serum detected 100% of grade 3 bladder tumors and 60% of all transitional cell papillomas; however, significant false-positive results remained in patients with urinary tract infections. The nature of the reactive material in the urine was unclear.

Colleen and coworkers [52] studied the concentration of CEA in the urine and serum of 213 patients with carcinoma of the bladder. The patients were followed for 1 year after diagnosis and CEA determinations were compared to grade, stage and recurrence of tumors. Neither serum nor urinary CEA levels correlated significantly with these parameters.

Hammarstrom and coworkers [99] used a heterologous antiserum to CEA in ADCC assay to detect CEA on T-24 target cells. No ADCC activity was observed, suggeting that CEA was not present on T-24 cells.

An area of more promising prognostic value is the study of the presence of ABO(H) blood group antigens on bladder tumors. Immune adherence tests for the expression of A, B or O(H) blood group isoantigens on tumor cells were evaluated as a means of predicting the malignant potential of bladder tumors. The basis for this test is that blood group antigens, normally expressed on epithelial cells, are not expressed on the cells of most bladder tumors that have a high malignant potential, even those that appear histologically well differentiated. Thus, this test detects ominous degrees of biochemical undifferentiation that may not be morphologically apparent. Because blood group antigens are composed largely of carbohydrate, they are stable to formalin fixation and thus formalin-fixed pathologic specimens can be examined retrospectively.

Clinical studies revealed that undifferentiated tumors (including *in situ* carcinoma [116, 227], invasive cancers [133], and metastatic lesions [77] generally do not express blood group antigens, while superficial, well differentiated tumors may or may not express these antigens [133]. The absence of antigens on a well-differentiated tumor indicates a high likelihood of the subsequent development of invasive cancer, usually within 10–30 months [116]. Approximately 80% of patients with antigen-negative tumors subsequently developed invasive lesions, while only about 10% with antigen-positive tumors did so [6, 54, 77, 116, 133, 136, 162, 189, 227, 237].

Falsely positive tests were encountered in patients having prior radiation therapy [6] and in some patients with invasive squamous cell carcinomas [190], and falsely negative tests occurred in patients with type O blood, presumably owing to the weakness of the H antigen expressed on the cells of individuals with type O blood [14], which results in negative immune adherence tests on normal urothelium in about one-third of cases [59].

There is conflicting evidence concerning the immune adherence test as a predictor of recurrence rates. Most evidence suggests that it is not, since many patients with antigen-positive tumors develop superficial recurrences [116, 133, 162]. In this regard, analyses of serial bladder tumor biopsies indicate that most patients retain their immune adherence characteristics on subsequent tumor recurrences [116, 133].

Johnson and Lamm [116] reported that normal-appearing epithelium adjacent to bladder tumors was antigen positive in all 155 specimens tested. In contrast, Weinstein and coworkers [227] reported that histologically normal-appearing adjacent epithelium was antigen-negative in five of nine bladders containing diffuse *in situ* carcinoma. Although Weinstein *et al.* [227] interpreted their results as suggesting that these antigen-negative areas may represent areas of low-grade carcinoma *in situ*, all five antigen-negative specimens were from patients with type A blood. Therefore, confirmation of Weinstein's results in patients with other than type O is needed.

Sadoughi and associates [196] examined bladder washing specimens from 12 patients who no history of bladder tumors and 20 patients with various stages and grades of transitional cell carcinoma of the bladder for the presence of blood group isoantigens. These results were compared with the results of tests for the presence of these antigens on the cell surfaces of original biopsy specimens. There was a high degree of correlation between amounts of antigen in the specimens from the bladder washings and on the biopsy specimens. These investigators suggested that the red cell adherence test on bladder washings also may provide a useful prognostic test.

Immune adherence tests have not been used as the sole indication for cystectomy, but may prove to be of value in identifying patients who need more careful clinical surveillance.

3.4. Immunotherapy of bladder cancer

Immunotherapy of bladder cancer has been extensively studied both in experimental animals and humans. It is beyond the scope of this chapter to review these studies in detail. The interested reader is referred to a recent review [40].

Studies of nonspecific active immunotherapy of transitional cell carcinoma in experimental animals have yielded conflicting results. de Kernion *et al.* [63] reported increased animal survival after injections of intramuscular Chicago BCG. Lamm *et al.* [128] reported delayed carcinogenesis and inhibition of tumor progression as a result of intravenous and intravesical as well as intralesional BCG. Adolphs and coworkers [4] reported reduction in tumor growth with use of Chicago BCG. Primm and Baldwin [179] reported elimination of human tumor outgrowth when tumor cells were mixed with Galaxo BCG and then transferred to nude mice. Negative results of BCG immunotherapy were reported by Adolphs and coworkers [4] using Chicago BCG intralesionally, Soloway [206] using Trudeau BCG intraperitoneally and Morales and coworkers [155] using Pasteur BCG intraperitoneally. The reasons for these discrepancies are not enterily clear, but differences in the type, routes of administration, and dose schedules of the BCG may be important factors. These studies also show that other agents, including *C. parvum* and levimosole [30] may be effective in treating experimental bladder cancer while intravesical DNCB [128] seems to be ineffective. Droller and Remington [69] demonstrated in a mouse system that growth of a transitional cell carcinoma was significantly less in Toxoplasma-infected animals. *In vitro* experiments showed that activated macrophages from Toxoplasma-infected mice killed tumor cells whereas control macrophages did not. Lymphocytes alone were not cytotoxic. In addition lymphocytes from Toxoplasma-infected mice did not convey cytotoxicity to control macrophages. Solid tumors appeared simultaneously in both toxoplasma-infected and control groups, and the survival period of both groups was also essentially the same.

Studies of specific active immunotherapy with either live or irradiated tumor cells or tumor membrane extracts [155] clearly indicate that chemical-induced bladder cancers are immunogenic in syngeneic hosts, and confer significant protection on the outgrowth of tumor cell inocula.

Human studies of immunotherapy for bladder cancer have yielded some of the most successful examples of immunotherapy reported to date in man. The studies of Morales [157], Lamm [129], and Camacho [35] using BCG intravesically and intradermally in patients with superficial bladder cancer demonstrated clearly that this form of immunotherapy significantly reduces the recurrence rate of superficial bladder cancer. Moreover, an uncontrolled study by Douville *et al.* [66] provided some evidence that intravesical BCG also caused the regression of established superficial tumors. A study by Kagawa [117] indicated that Streptococcal OK432 also produced a similar beneficial effect although the available data are too limited to permit the drawing of any definite conclusions. Studies by Purves and associates [183] using *C. parvum* in patients with more advanced bladder cancer indicate that this agent in the dose schedule used was not effective. Similarly a study by Herr [112] in patients with superficial bladder cancer seem to indicate that poly I:C is also ineffective. Studies by Symes and Feneley and their coworkers [80, 210–212] using specific passive immunotherapy with immune pig lymphocytes yielded some encouraging results, but need to be confirmed by other investigators before this form of therapy can be judged.

Droller and coworkers [67] examined the effect of human interferon *alpha* and *beta* on NK and ADCC activity against T-24 transitional cell carcinoma targets. Lymphocytes for these studies were obtained from normal volunteers. These investigators found that both *alpha* and *beta* human interferon augmented NK and ADCC activity. Clinical trials of interferons in the treatment of bladder cancer have not yet been initiated.

4. RENAL CELL CARCINOMA

Tumor-associated antigens expressed on human renal cancers have been evaluated with a variety of assays. Using microcytotoxicity assays, early investigators reported that leukocytes from renal cell carcinoma patients exhibited cytotoxicity against both autochthonous and allogeneic cultured renal cell carcinoma target cells, but that leukocytes from patients with nonrenal cancers and control subjects were not cytotoxic against renal cell carcinoma cell lines [29, 57, 73, 101]. The data suggested that renal cancers expressed cross-reactive tumor-associated antigens that were distinct from antigens expressed on normal kidney tissue or tumors of different histological types. Subsequent studies using similar assay systems revealed that leukocytes from normal individuals also often exhibited significant cytotoxicity against renal cell cancer target cells [32, 152].

Stjernsward and associates [209] reported that leukocytes from renal carcinoma patients could be stimulated in a mixed-lymphocyte tumor cell culture (MLTC) by autochthonous tumor cells but not by autochthonous normal kidney cells. Furthermore, Hemstreet and associates [104, 105] reported that autochthonous partially purified tumor plasma membranes induced significant proliferative responses (greater than responses to normal kidney extracts) in nylon wool-depleted lymphocytes from 75% of renal cancer patients. Allogeneic renal tumor extracts induced lymphocyte proliferation in only 14% of renal cancer patients, suggesting that lymphocyte-stimulating antigens expressed on renal cell carcinoma plasma membranes were not all cross-reactive.

Cell-mediated immune responses to renal cell carcinoma antigens also were evaluated by the leukocyte migration inhibition (LMI) test. Soluble extracts of renal cell carcinoma were shown by Wright and coworkers [235] to induce inhibition of leukocyte migration in 63% of renal cancer patients but in only 7% of normal subjects and 30% of patients with nonrenal cancers. Wright and coworkers [236] were able to induce specific LMI positive tests only in patients with renal cancer by fractionation of the tumor extract using preparative gradient polyacrylamide gel electrophoresis. Positive LMI assays were shown to correlate with the presence of active disease, and in this regard, 71% of patients clinically free of disease one year following nephrectomy lost their tumor-directed cell-mediated immune response. However, Kjaer and coworkers [119, 121] reported that patients with advanced metastatic disease also had low or absent responses as measured by the LMI test.

Shore and associates [202] were the first to show that sera from patients with renal cell carcinoma when added to renal cancer cells in tissue culture consistently inhibited the growth of renal cancer cells, as well as the growth of other cell types such as Chang and Hela. Serum toxicity did not correlate with extent of disease. Moreover, this serum factor was heat stable, sensitive to ultraviolet light and dialyzable. Antibodies in sera of renal cancer patients that direct complement-dependent cytotoxicity [94] and K-cell mediated ADCC [96, 127] against renal cancer targets also were described.

Hakala and coworkers [94] observed in certain patients with renal cell carcinoma humoral antibodies that effected tumor-specific, complement-dependent cytotoxicity against autochthonous and allogeneic renal cancer target cells. This humoral cytotoxicity was removed by adsorption of the serum with autochthonous tumor cells, but not by adsorption with autochthonous normal kidney cells. Similar findings were described by Elhilali and Nyack [73], suggesting that renal cancers express common cross-reacting tumor-associated antigens.

Interestingly, Ueda *et al.* [221] found natural antibodies to surface antigens of renal carcinoma cells in the sera of normal individuals; these could be removed by adsorption of the sera with renal cancer cells but not by absorption with normal kidney, fetal kidney or other nonmalignant and malignant cells.

Antigens expressed on renal cancer cells were reported to be restricted to the autologous tumor [185, 222], shared by allogeneic renal tumors of the same histological type [82], shared by allogeneic tumors of renal as well as nonrenal origin [222], or shared by malignant and normal cells. Numerous other serologic techniques, including immunofluorescence, mixed hemadsorption immune adherence, anti-C3 mixed hemadsorption, and *Staphylococcal* protein A binding, have been used to demonstrate the presence of antibodies directed against renal cell carcinoma-associated antigens [135, 187]. Ghose and associates [82], using autoradiography with ^{131}I-labeled xenogeneic antisera to human renal cell carcinoma, showed greater localization of radioactive antibody in renal cancer tissue sections than in tissue sections from normal kidney adjacent to cancerous tissue, suggesting a possible future diagnostic or therapeutic tool for radiolabelling in renal cancer.

Hakala and associates [96] also presented evidence for the existence of common tumor-associated antigens in patients with transitional cell carcinoma of the renal pelvis, ureter and bladder. Serum immunoglobulin G (IgG) from patients with transitional cell carcinoma induced lymphocyte (monocyte-depleted)-mediated antibody-dependent cell-mediated cytotoxicity against targets derived from transitional cell carcinoma of the renal pelvis, ureter and bladder but not against targets derived from normal kidney, testis, bladder, embryonic kidney, fibroblast or renal carcinoma cell lines.

Evidence for tumor-associated antigens in nephroblastoma (Wilms' tumor) was provided by cytotoxicity assays [64, 65, 126] and serologic studies [127]. Diehl and associates [64, 65] showed that lymphocytes from nephroblastoma patients had greater cytotoxicity for autochthonous, as well as allogeneic nephroblastoma target cells, than for nonmalignant cells, whereas lymphocytes from control subjects were cytotoxic to nephroblastoma and nonmalignant target cells to the same degree. Using membrane immunofluorescence, Kumar *et al.* [127] found tumor-specific antibodies against autochthonous and allogeneic Wilms' tumor cell surface antigens in sera of some patients with nephroblastoma. In addition, sera from some patients contained antibody that in the presence of killer (K) cells produced lysis of nephroblastoma targets. Interestingly, no serum from the nephroblastoma patients exhibited both membrane immunofluorescence and cooperation with K cells to elicit ADCC.

Various apparently distinct tumor-associated antigens of nephroblastomas were isolated and described, such as abnormal extracellular components [5], W-antigen [34], fetuin-like antigen [234], Wilms' tumor-associated antigen [223], and nephroblastoma-specific antigen [168].

Total levels of serum IgG, IgA and IgM were evaluated in renal cell carcinoma patients by immunodiffusion and IgG by radioimmunoassay and were shown not to correlate with the stage of disease or presence of malignancy in renal cancer [200].

Several investigators observed elevated (>2.5 ng/ml) serum levels of carcinoembryonic antigen (CEA) in patients with various types of urological malignancies, including renal cell carcinoma [49, 86, 137, 188]. Expression of elevated CEA levels occurred more often in patients with advanced disease than in patients with local or inactive disease [49, 188]. Lowered CEA levels were found in patients treated by nephrectomy for removal of the primary tumor by chemotherapy with 1-(2-chloroethyl)3-cyclohexyl-1-nitrosourea (CCNU) [49].

4.1. Immune Mechanisms Operative in Renal Cell Carcinoma

Indirect evidence suggests that host tumor immunity may be clinically manifest in renal cancer patients. Rarely, regression of metastases, almost always pulmonary, have been documented in the literature, indicating that renal cancer has relatively one of the highest rates of spontaneous regression among solid tumors [79, 81]. Spontaneous regressions are most apt to occur following ablation of the primary tumor. However, the rate of spontaneous regressions observed may be inflated [145].

Studies described above have shown that lymphocytes from both renal cancer patients and control patients often are cytotoxic to renal carcinoma targets. Hakala *et al.* [91] reported that lymphocytes from renal cancer patients induce more cytotoxicity than control lymphocytes against renal cancer targets, but not against melanoma target cells. This cytotoxicity was attributed to target-cell specificity, but not necessarily to tumor-cell specificity.

Lange [132] evaluated lymphocyte cytotoxicity in patients with advanced renal cell carcinoma who were receiving BCG therapy. Of the four patients who showed a rise in cytotoxicity concurrent with BCG therapy, one had complete regression of tumor, one was without recurrence, and the other two showed no evidence of tumor progression. Six patients with no cytotoxic response concurrent with BCG therapy showed continued progression of disease.

In vivo and *in vitro* exposure of lymphocytes of xenogeneic immune RNA isolated from sheep lymphoid cells immunized with human renal cancer cells increased cytotoxicity against renal cell cancer cells *in vitro* [28, 62, 208].

4.2. Impairment of Immune Mechanisms

Impaired host immune mechanisms in renal cancer patients have been documented. Immunological escape mechanisms operate in both humoral and cell-mediated immune responses.

In vitro proliferative responses of lymphocytes to the T lymphocyte mitogen phytohemagglutinin (PHA) were reported to be impaired in renal cancer patients [140, 156]. In addition, lymphocytes from renal cancer patients and normal control patients showed significantly lower proliferative responses to T-cell mitogens when cultured with serum from renal cancer patients [39, 139, 156, 181]. Suppression of T cell responses was found to correlate with increased levels of alpha-2 globulin serum proteins [139, 181] which previously were shown to contain immunosuppressive factors [56]. McLaughlin and associates [140] reported that impaired lymphocyte proliferation was a result of serum inhibitory factors and not caused by an intrinsic lymphocyte defect. Others have found both serum-mediated inhibition and T lymphocyte deficiencies operative in renal cancer patients [42].

Catalona, Chretien and Trahan [39] evaluated delayed cutaneous hypersensitivity reactions to dinitrochlorobenzene (DNCB) in renal cell cancer. They reported subnormal skin reactivity to DNCB in 50% of renal cancer patients and in only 4% of normal control patients. They noted that patients with metastatic disease had a higher, but not significantly so, incidence of impaired immunocompetence. deKernion and Ramming [62] reported that skin test responses seemed to bear no correlation with tumor burden or subsequent course of disease. Others have reported that delayed skin tests of renal cancer patients are normal to DNCB and several renal antigens [181].

Antibody-dependent cell-mediated cytotoxicity (ADCC) and natural killing (NK) were shown to be impaired in renal cancer [215]. These observations were supported by investigators studying these cytolytic effector cells in urologic cancers [44, 62, 186]. Mitogen-induced lymphocytotoxicity was also reported to be depressed in renal cancer patients [215]. It was shown, though, that ADCC, NK and mitogen-induced cytotoxicity return to normal levels following nephrectomy for removal of the primary tumor.

Monocyte chemotactic responses were reported to be depressed in renal cancer patients [24, 25, 106]. This may reflect on inability of the host to transport monocytes to the tumor focus. No correlation was observed between tumor stage and the degree of chemotactic defect [24], although depressed chemotactic levels returned to normal following radical nephrectomy [106]. In contrast to the depression of monocyte chemotaxis, *in vitro* macrophage-mediated cytotoxicity was reported enhanced in patients with urologic cancers [43].

Serum from renal cancer patients was shown to block cell-mediated cytotoxicity against both autochthonous and allogeneic renal carcinoma targets [51, 73, 102]. These serum blocking factors could be attributed to free circulating antigen, antigen-antibody complexes, blocking antibodies or a combination of these factors. Supportive evidence suggests a correlation between tumor growth *in vivo* and the presence of blocking serum *in vitro* [51, 102].

The number of T lymphocytes, as measured by spontaneous resetting with sheep erythrocytes, was significantly decreased in renal cancer patients [36, 37, 156]. However, Carmignani and associates [37] found that renal cancer patients had much lower numbers of sheep erythrocyte-rosetting lymphocytes in the neoplastic kidney renal vein than in their peripheral circulation, although there was no depression in total lymphocyte counts. They attributed this phenomenon to lymphocyte blocking activity produced by the tumor that was diluted in the peripheral circulation. These investigators reported that this impairment of E rosette levels was partially abrogated following nephrectomy, but not by angioinfarction [37].

Suppressor cells activated by concanavalin A (Con A) that suppress the proliferative response of autologous lymphocytes to Con A were demonstrated in regional lymph nodes of renal cancer patients [43], but spontaneous suppressor cells were not observed in the regional lymph nodes.

4.3. Immunotherapy

Results of immunotherapy trials for renal cancer have been discouraging although the various immunotherapeutic protocols used have not been adequately studied.

Passive immunotherapy using xenogeneic immune RNA, transfer factor and plasma transufisions has been attempted. Ramming and deKernion [185] and Skinner and associates [204] injected renal cell carcinoma patients with immune RNA. Only limited objective responses were observed, and significant improvement in survival as compared to historical controls was observed only in patients with metastases confined to the lungs. Richie and associates [190] exposed patient leukocytes *in vitro* to xenogeneic immune RNA and reinfused these cells. Of six patients treated, one showed complete remission of pulmonary metastases and two patients demonstrated partial response to therapy; however, five of six patients treated with this therapy died within 18 months.

Horn and Horn [113] transferred plasma from a donor with a history of renal cell carcinoma into one patient with metastatic renal cell carcinoma; there was no evidence of tumor recurrence following initiation of therapy.

The use of transfer factor in patients with disseminated renal cell carcinoma was examined by Montie and associates [151]. None of the patients with metastatic disease showed objective evidence of tumor remission.

Active nonspecific immunotherapy in renal cancer has been tried only with BCG. Lange [132], using Tice strain BCG to treat stage D renal cell carcinoma, observed complete regression of tumor in one patient, no tumor recurrence in one patient and no tumor progression in two patients. Six patients did not respond to therapy. Eidinger and Morales [71], using BCG (Institute Armand Fraipper) immunotherapy, demonstrated objective evidence of improvement in five of eight patients, although these favorable responses were transient. In a later study Morales and associates [158] observed partial and temporary evidence for tumor regression in 6 of 20 patients. In this study survival of treated patients did not significantly differ from that of concurrent control patients with renal cancer. Laucius and associates [134], using Galaxo BCG immunotherapy in conjunction with megestrol acetate, reported objective tumor regression of pulmonary metastases in only one of 16 patients with metastatic renal adenocarcinoma

Active specific immunotherapy has been attempted by either vaccination with autologous tumor or angioinfarction of the primary renal cell carcinoma prior to nephrectomy. Tykka and coworkers [221] vaccinated patients with advanced renal cell carcinoma with excised autologous primary and metastatic tumor polymerized with ethylchlorformide. The five-year survival rate was reported as 23.6% for the immunotherapy group as compared to 4.3% for control patients.

Angioinfarction of the primary tumor was performed by Bracken and associates [20] and Mohr and Whitesel [147]. Bracken and associates [20] reported only stabilization of metastases postinfarction in 3 of 17 patients with metastatic disease. Mohr and Whitesel [147] reported regression of pulmonary metastases in one patient treated following preoperative angioinfarction of the primary renal cell carcinoma.

5. FUTURE PROSPECTS

In speculating on the prospects for immunology as a useful tool in cancer, we are reminded of the historical vignette presented by Dr. Steven Rosenberg [195] concerning the early development of aviation. For centuries man had dreamed of flying and many abortive attempts to accomplish this were made. Naturally, there were both optimistic and pessimistic views regarding the possibilities of flight. There were even prophets. Jules Verne in the late 1800s predicted launching a rocketship to the moon from a site in Florida with a subsequent return landing in the Pacific.

Wilbur and Orville Wright, in their initial efforts to study aerodynamics, found may conflicting and confusing reports in the literature of the time. Orville Wright later wrote: 'truth and error were everywhere so intermingled and mixed as to be indistinguishable.' However, these brothers began their studies with investigations into basic mechanisms of aerodynamics and after several years of work designed their airplane. They deliberately chose Kitty Hawk as a testing ground because of the steady winds that prevailed there and because the sand dunes provided a safe landing spot. Then in 1903, Orville made the first manned flight, staying aloft for a grand total of 12 seconds. On the face of it is was not such an impressive feat, but the Wright brothers showed us that under a given set of circumstances, heavier than air flight was possible.

This is often the way of scientific discovery. There are always false leads, confusing data and unjustified optimism and pessimism. What is important is that fundamental studies need to be performed.

We believe that immunologic investigations will continue to make contributions to our understanding of cancer in the future.

REFERENCES

1. Ablin RJ, Bhatti RA, Guinan PD, Bruns GR: Evaluation of cellular immunologic responsiveness in the clinical management of patients with prostatic cancer. IV. Leukocyte adherence inhibition. Urol Int 31:459, 1976.
2. Ablin RJ, Gonder MJ, Soanes WA: Levels of immunoglobulins in the serum of patients with carcinoma of the prostate. Neoplasma 19:61, 1972.
3. Ablin RJ, Marrow C, Guinan PD, Bruns GR, Sadoughi N, John T, Bush IM: Evaluation of cellular immunologic responsiveness in the clinical management of patients with prostatic cancer. III. Inhibition of leukocyte migration. Urol Int 31:444, 1976.
4. Adolphs HD, Thiele J, Kiel H: Effect of intralesional and systemic BCG-application or a combined cyclophosphamide/BCG treatment on experimental bladder cancer. Urol Res 7:71, 1979.
5. Allerton SE, Beirle JW, Powars DR, Lucien A: Abnormal extracellular components in Wilms' tumor. Cancer Res 30:679, 1970.

6. Alroy J, Teramura K, Miller AW III, Pauli BU, Gottesman JE, Flanagan M, Davidsohn I, Weinstein RS: Isoantigens A, B and H in urinary bladder carcinomas following radiotherapy. Cancer 41:1739, 1978.
7. Avis F, Avis I, Cole AT, Freid F, Haughton G: Antigenic cross reactivity between benign prostatic hyperplasia and adenocarcinoma of the prostate. Urology 5:122, 1975.
8. Barzell W, Bean MA, Hilaris BS, Whitmore WF Jr: Prostatic adenocarcinoma: Relationship of grade and local extent tothe pattern of metastases. J Urol 118:278, 1977.
9. Bean MA, Akiyama M, Kodera Y, Dupont B, Hansen JA: Human blood T lymphocytes that suppress the mixed leukocyte culture reactivity of lymphocytes from HLA-B14 bearing individuals. J Immunol 123:1610, 1979.
10. Bean MA, Bloom BR, Herberman RB, Old LJ, Oettgen HF, Klein G, Terry WD: Cell-mediated cytotoxicity for bladder carcinoma: evaluation of a workshop. Cancer Res 35:2902, 1975.
11. Bran MA, Kodera Y, Cummings KB, Bloom BR: Occurrence of restricted suppressor T-cell activity in man. J Exp Med 146:1455, 1977.
12. Bean MA, Pees H, Fogh J, Grabstald H, Oettgen H: Cytotoxicity of lymphocytes from patients with cancer of the urinary bladder: detection by a 3-H prolene microcytotoxicity test. Int J Cancer 14:186–197, 1974.
13. Beierle JW, Wise KS, Trump GN, Allerton SE: Isolation of Wilm's tumor antigens by chelation. Clin Chim Acta 61:411, 1975.
14. Bergman S, Javadpour N: The cell surface antigen A, B or O (H) as an indicator of malignant potential in stage A bladder carcinoma: preliminary report. J Urol 119:49–51, 1978.
15. Bhatti RA, Ablin RJ, Guinan PD: Leucocyte adherence inhibition and immunoreactivity in prostatic cancer. II. Tissue and disease specificity of anti-tumor cell-mediated immunity. Eur J Cancer 15:133, 1979.
16. Bhatti RA, Ablin RJ, Guinan PD: Tumor-associated immunity in prostatic cancer as evaluated by tumor antigen induced leucocyte adherence inhibition: reactivity and specificity of responsiveness and relationship to stage, grade and therapy. J Reticuloendothel Soc 25:389, 1979.
17. Bhatti RA, McKiel CF, Flanagan MJ, Guinan PD, Rios EE, Ablin RJ: Antigen-induced leukocyte adherence inhibition. Evaluation of cellular immunity in patients with carcinoma of the urinary bladder. IRCS Medical Science 4:396, 1976.
18. Bloom ET, Ossorio RC, Brosman SA: Cell-mediated cytotoxicity against human bladder cancer. Int J Cancer 14:326, 1974.
19. Bolhuis RCH: Cellular microcytotoxicity in a human bladder cancer system; analysis of *in vitro* lymphocyte-mediated cytotoxicity against cultures target cells. Cancer Immunol immunother 2:245–256, 1977.
20. Bracken RB, Johnson DE, Goldstein HM, Wallace S, Ayala AG: Percutaneous transfemoral renal artery occlusion in patients with renal carcinoma. Urology 6:6, 1975.
21. Braf ZF, Gazit E, Many M: HLA-A and HLA-B antigens in transitional cell carcinoma of the bladder. J Urol 122:465, 1979.
22. Brannen GE, Gomolka DM, Coffey DS: Specificity of cell Membrane antigens in porstatic carcinoma. Cancer Chemother Rep 59:127, 1975.
23. Broder LE, Weintraub BD, Rosen SW, Cohen MH, Tejada F: Placental proteins and their subunits astumor markers in prostatic carcinoma. Cancer 40:211, 1977.
24. Brosman S, Hausman MS: Defective monocyte chemotactic response in genitourinary carcinoma. Urology 4:129, 1974.
25. Brosman S, Hausman M, Shacks SJ: Studies on the immune status of patients with renal adenocarcinoma. J Urol 114:375, 1975.

26. Brosman S, Hausman M, Shacks S: Immunologic alterations in patients with prostatic carcinoma. J Urol 113:841, 1975.
27. Brosman S, Hausman M, Shacks S: Immune response in bladder cancer patients. J Urol 121:162, 1979.
28. Brower PA, de Kernion JB, Ramming KP: Immune cytolysis of human renal carcinoma mediated by xenogeneic immune ribonucleic acid. J Urol 115:243, 1976.
29. Bubenik J, Jakoubková J, Krakora P, Baresová M, Helbich P, Viklický V, Malasková V: Cellular immunity to renal carcinomas in man. Int J Cancer 8:503, 1971.
30. Bubenik J, Perlmann P, Helmstein K, Moberger G: Immune response to urinary bladder tumors in man. Int J Cancer 5:39, 1870.
31. Bubenik J, Perlman P, Helmstein K, Moberger G: Cellular and humoral immune responses to human urinary bladder carcinomas. Int J Cancer 5:310, 1970.
32. Bukowski RM, Barna B, Deodhar SD, Hewlett JS: Nonspecific lymphocyte cytotoxicity in patients with malignant melanoma, renal cell carcinoma, and sarcomas,and in nontumor patients. Cancer 38:1962, 1976.
33. Burnet FM: The concept of immunological survaillance. Prog Exp Tumor Res 13:1, 1970.
34. Burtin P, Gendron MC: A tumor-associated antigen in human nephroblastomas. Proc Natl Acad Sci (Washington) 70:2051, 1973.
35. Camacho F, Pinsky C, Kerr D, Whitmore W, Oettgen H: Treatment of superficial bladder cancer with intravesical BCG. In: Immunotherapy of Cancer: Present Status of Trials in Man (abstract). National Cancer Institute, Bethesda, MD, April 28–30, 1980.
36. Carmignani G, Belgrano E, Puppo P, Cornaglia P: T and B lymphocyte levels in renal cancer patients: influence of preoperative transcatheter embolization and radical nephrectomy. J Urol 118:941, 1977.
37. Carmignani G, Belgrano E, Puppo P, Cornaglia P: T lymphocytes inhibiting factors in renal cancer: evaluation of differences between arterial and renal venous blood levels of E rosette forming cells. J Urol 120:673, 1978.
38. Catalona WJ, Chretien PB: Correlation among host immunocompetence and tumor stage, tumor grade and vascular permeation in transitional cell carcinoma. J Urol 110:526, 1973.
39. Catalona WJ, Chretien PB, Trahan EE: Abnormalities of cell-mediated immunocompetence in genitourinary cancer. J Urol 111:229, 1974.
40. Catalona WJ, McCool RE: Immunotherapy of genitourinary cancer. In: Recent Advances in Cancer Research. (Javadpour N, ed.) Baltimore: Williams & Wilkins, 1982, pp. 270–292.
41. Catalona WJ, Oldham RK, Herberman RB, Djeu JY, Cannon GB: Lack of specificity of lymphocyte mediated cytotoxicity against the bladder cancer lines T-24. JUrol 118:254, 1977.
42. Catalona WJ, Potvin C, Chretien PB: T lymphocytes in bladder and prostatic cancer patients. J Urol 112:378, 1974.
43. Catalona WJ, Ratliff TL, McCool RE: Concanavalin A-inducible suppressor cells in regional lymph nodes of cancer patients. Cancer Res 39:4372, 1979.
44. Catalona WJ, Ratliff TL, McCool RE: Discordance among cell-mediated cytolytic mechanisms in cancer patients: importance of the assay system. J Immunol 122:1009, 1979.
45. Catalona WJ, Smolev JK, Harty JI: Prognostic value of host immunocompetence in urologic cancer patients. J Uro 114:922, 1975.
46. Catalona WJ, Tarpley JL, Chretien PB, Castle JR: Lymphocyte stimulation in urologic cancer patients. J Urol 112:373, 1974.
47. Chapman WH, Taranger LA: Immunologic studies on urinary bladder tumors of rats and mice. Science 176:1337, 1972.

48. Chretien PB, Crowder WL, Gertner HR, Sample WF, Catalona WJ: Correlation of preoperative lymphocyte reactivity with the clinical course of cancer patients. Surg Gynecol Obstet 136:380, 1973.
49. Chu TM, Shukla SK, Mittleman AO, Murphy GP: Plasma carcinoembryonic antigen in renal cell carcinoma patients. J Urol 111:742, 1974.
50. Claflin J, McKinney EC, Fletcher Ma: The Dunning R3327 prostate adenocarcinoma in the Fischer-Copenhagen F_1 rat: a useful model for immunological studies. Oncology 34:105, 1977.
51. Cole AT, Avis I, Fried FA, Avis F: Call-mediated immunity in renal cell carcinoma-preliminary report. J Urol 115:234, 1976.
52. Colleen S, Ek A, Gullberg B, Johansson BG, Lindberg LG, Olsson AM: Carcinoembryonic antigen in urine in patients with urothelial carcinoma. An expression for the extent of inflammatory reaction of the urinary tract. Scand J Urol Nephrol 13:149, 1979.
53. Collste LG, Kostyrka-Claps ML, Darzynkiewicz Z, Devonec M, Traganos F, Whitmore WF, Melamed MR: Lymph node reactivity to experimental bladder tumor in preimmunized animals as measured by two parameter flow cytometry. Invest Urol 17:191, 1979.
54. Coon JS, Weinstein RS: Variability in the expression of the O(H) antigen in human transitional epithelium. J Urol 125:301, 1981.
55. Cooper SM, Hirsen DJ, Freou CJ: Spontaneous cell-mediated cytotoxicity against Chang cells by nonadherent, non-thymus-derived, Fc receptor-bearing lymphocytes. Cell Immunol 32:135, 1977.
56. Cooperband SR, Badger AM, Davis RC, Schmid K, Mannick JA: The effect of immunoregulatory α globulin (IRA) upon lymphocytes *in vitro.* J Immunol 109:154, 1972.
57. Cummings KB, Peter JB, Kaufman JJ: Cell-mediated immunity to tumor antigens in patients with renal cell carcinoma. J Urol 110:31, 1973.
58. Daly JJ, Praut GR Jr, Ahl CA: Demonstration of specific antigen in N-[4-(5-Nitro-2-Furyl-2-Thiazolyl] Formamide induced rat bladder tumor. J Urol 109:253, 1973.
59. Daly JJ, Prout GR, Ahl CA, Lin JC: Specificity of cellular immunity to renal cell carcinoma. J Urol 111:448, 1974.
60. Davidsohn I, Ni LY: Loss of isoantigens A, B, and H in carcinoma of the lung. Am J Pathol 57:307, 1969.
61. Decenzo JM, Allison R, Leadbetter GW Jr: Skin testing in genitourinary carcinoma: 2-year follow-up. J Urol 114:271, 1975.
62. de Kernion JB, Ramming KP: Treatment of hypernephroma with xenogeneic immune RNA. Natl Cancer Inst Monogr 49:347, 1978.
63. de Kernion JB, Ramming KP, Fraser K: A bladder tumor model response to immunotherapy. Natl Cancer Inst Monogr 49:333, 1978.
64. Diehl V: Microcytotoxicity test for detection of cellular immunity to nephroblastoma in man. In: Applied Tumour Immunology. (Götz H, Bücher ES, eds.) Berlin: Walter de Gruyter, 1975, p. 86.
65. Diehl V, Jereb B, Stjernswärd J, O'Tolle C, Ahström, L: Cellular immunity to nephroblastoma. Int J Cancer 7:277, 1971.
66. Douville Y, Pelouze G, Roy R, Charrois R, Kibrite A, Martin M, Dionne L, Coulonval L, Robinson J: Recourrent bladder papillomata treated with bacillus Calmette-Guerin: a preliminary report (phase I trial). Cancer Treat Rep 62:551, 1978.
67. Droller MJ, Borg H, Perlman P: *in vitro* enhancement of natural and antibody-dependent lymphocyte mediated cytotoxicity against tumor target cells by interferon. Cell Immunol 47:248, 1979.
68. Droller MJ, O'Toole C: The cellular immune response to carcinoma of the urinary bladder: correlation to clinical stage and treatment. Br J Cancer 28 (Suppl 1):266, 1973.

69. Droller MJ, Remmington JS: A role for macrophage *in vivo* and *in vitro* resistance to murine bladder tumor cell growth. Cancer Res 35:49, 1975.
70. Ehrlich P: Ned Erst Helf, No. 5. Tijdschr Geneeskd, 1909.
71. Eidinger D, Morales A: BCG immunotherapy of metastatic adenocarcinoma of the kidney. Natl Cancer Inst Monogr 49:339, 1979.
72. Elhilali MM, Brosman SA, Vescera C, Paul JG, Fahey JL: The effects of treatment on delayed cutaneous hypersenitivity responses (DNCB, Croton oil, and recall antigen) in patients with genitourinary cancer. Cancer 41:1765, 1978.
73. Elhilali MM, Nayak SK: Immunologic evaluation of human renal cell carcinoma. *in vitro* studies. Invest urol 13:60, 1975.
74. Elhilali MM, Nayak SK: Immunologic evaluation of human bladder cancer: in vitro studies. Cancer 35:419, 1975.
75. Elhilali MM, Nayak SK: In vitro cytotoxicity studies in bladder and renal cell cancer. Urology 7:488, 1976.
76. Elliott AY, Fraley EE, Cleveland P, Castro AE, Stein N: Isolation of RNA virus from papillary tumors of the human renal pelvis. Science 179:393, 1973.
77. Emmott RC, Javadpour N, Bergman SM, Soares T: Correlation of cell surface antigens with stage and grade in cancer of the bladder. J Utol 121:37, 1979.
78. Evans CM, Bowen JG: Immunological tests in carcinoma of the prostate. Proc R Soc Med 70:417, 1977.
79. Everson TC: Spontaneous regression of cancer. Ann NY Acad Sci 114:721, 1964.
80. Fenely RCL, Eckert H, Riddell AG, Symes MO, Tribe CR: The treatment of advanced bladder cancer with sensitized pig lymphocytes. Br J Surg 61:825, 1974.
81. Garfield DH, Kennedy BJ: Regression of metastatic renal cell carcinoma following nephrectomy. Cancer 30:190, 1972.
82. Ghose T, Belitsky P, Tal J, Janigan DT: Production and characterization of xenogeneic antisera to a human renal cell carcinoma-associated antigen. J Natl Canc Inst 63:301, 1979.
83. Green MI, Dorf ME, Pierres M, Benacerrof B: Reduction of syngeneic tumor growth by anti-I-J-alloantiserum. Proc Natl Acad Sci USA 74:5118, 1977.
84. Gross L: Intradermal immunization of C3H mice against a sarcoma that originated in an animal of the same line. Cancer Res 3:326, 1933.
85. Guinan PD: Cited as personal communication in Grayhack JT, Lee C, Kolbusz W, Oliver L, Lee C: Detection of carcinoma of the prostate utilizing biochemical observations. Cancer 45:1896, 1980.
86. Guinan P, Ablin RJ, Barakat H, John T, Sadoughi, Bush IM: Carsinoembryonic antigen in patients with urologic cancer. Urol Res 1:101, 1973.
87. Guinan P, McKiel C, Flanigan M, Bhatti R, Pessis D, Ablin RJ: Cellular immunity in bladder cancer patients. J Urol 119:747, 1978.
88. Guinan PD, John T, Sahadevan V, Crispen R, Nagale V, McKiel C, Ablin RJ: Prostate carcinoma: immunostaging and adjuvant immunotherapy with BCG. Natl Cancer Inst Monogr 49:355, 1978.
89. Gursel EO, Megalli MR, Veenema RJ: Serum immunoglobulins in patients with prostate cancer. Urol Res 1:145, 1973.
90. Gursel EO, Roberts M, Veenema RJ: Regression of prostatic cancer following sequential cryotherapy in the prostate. J Urol 108:928, 1972.
91. Hakala TR: Transitional cell and renal carcinoma: cell-mediated immunity as determined by the lymphocyte titration technique. Natl Canc Inst Monogr 49:151, 1978.
92. Hakala TR, Lange PH, Castro A, Elliot A, Fraley E: Antibody induction of lymphocyte mediated cytotoxicity against human transitional cell carcinomas of the urinary tract. N Engl J Med 291:638, 1974.

93. Hakala TR, Castro A, Elliott A, Fraley R: Humoral cytotoxicity in human transitional cell carcinoma. J Urol 111:382, 1974.
94. Hakala TR, Castro AE, Elliott AY, Fraley EE: Humoral cytotoxicity in human renal cell carcinoma. Invest Urol 11:405, 1974.
95. Hakala TR, Lange PH, Castro A, Elliott A, Fraley EE: Cell mediated cytotoxicity against human transitional cell carcinomas ofthe urinary tract. Cancer 34:1929, 1974.
96. Hakala TR, Lange PH, Castro AE, Elliott AY, Fraley EE: Lymphocyte antibody interaction in cytotoxicity against human transitional cell carcinoma. J Urol 113:663, 1975.
97. Hakala TR, Lange TH: Serum-induced lymphoid cell-mediated cytotoxicity to human transitional cell carcinoma of the genitourinary tract. Science 184:795,1974.
98. Hakala TR, Lange PH, Fraley E: Human cell mediated cytotoxicity estimated by lymphocyte titration. Cancer Res 36:2915, 1976.
99. Hammarstrom S, Troye M, Wahlund G, Svenberg T, Perlmann P: K cell-mediated lysis of cultured colon carcinoma and urinary bladder carcinoma cells induced by nonspacific antisera against carcinoembryonic antigen (CEA) and two CEA-related normal glycoproteins. Int J Cancer 19:756, 1977.
100. Hausman J, Brosman S, Fahey JL, Snyderman R: Defective mononuclear leukocyte chemotactic activity in patients with genitourinary carcinoma. Clin Res 21:646, 1973.
101. Hellström I, Hellström KE, Sjögren HO, Warner GA: demonstration of cell-mediated immunity to human neoplasms of various histological types. Int J Cancer 7:1, 1971.
102. Hellström I, Sjögren HO, Warner GA, Hellström KE: Blocking of cell-mediated tumor immunity by sera from patients with growing neoplasms. Int J Cancer 7:226, 1971.
103. Hellström KE, Hellström I: Immunological enhancement as studied by cell culture techniques. Ann Rev Microbiol 24:373, 1970.
104. Hemstreet GP: Renal cell carcinoma: tumor membrane lymphocyte stimulation assay. Natl Canc Inst Monogr 49:165, 1978.
105. Hemstreet GP, Dawson JR, Seigler HF: Tumor-membrane lymphocyte stimulation assay in patients with renal cell carcinoma. Cancer Res 38:1447, 1978.
106. Hemstreet GP, Snyderman R: Monocyte chemotactic mechanisms in patients with hypernephroma. Natl Cancer Inst Monogr 49:115, 1978.
107. Herr HW: Suppressor cell activity in lymph nodes regional to bladder carcinoma. Surg Forum 28:546, 1977.
108. Herr HW: Suppressor cells in pelvic lymph nodes regional to bladder cancer. J Surg Oncol 11:289, 1979.
109. Herr HW: Immune reactivity of lymph nodes regional to prostatic cancer. J Surg Res 24:409, 1978.
110. Herr HW: Suppressor cells in immunodepressed bladder and prostate cancer patients. J Urol 123:635, 1980.
111. Herr HW, Bean MA, Whitmore WF: Decreased ability of blood leukocytes from patients with tumors of the urinary bladder to act as stimulator cells in mixed leukocyte culture. Cancer Res 36:2754, 1976.
112. Herr HW, Kemery N, Yagoda A, Whitmore WF: Poly I: C immunotherapy in patients with papillomas or superficial carcinomas ofthe bladder.Natl Canc Inst Monogr 49:325, 1978.
113. Horn L, Horn HL: An Immunological approach to the therapy of cancer? Lancet 2:466, 1971.
114. Huus JC, Kursh ED, Poor P, Persky L: Delayed cutaneous hypersensitivity in patients with prostate adenocarcinoma. J Urol 114:86, 1975.
115. Jereb B, Diehl V, Ahström L, Juhlin I: Relation between cellular immunity to nephroblastoma and the phase of the disease. Acta Paediat Scand 61:709, 1972.

116. Johnson JD, Lamm DL: Prediction of bladder tumor invasion with the mixed all agglutination test. J Urol 123:25, 1980.
117. Kagawa S, Ogura K, Kurokawa K, Uyama K: Immunological evaluation of a streptococcal preparation (OK-432) in treatment of bladder carcinoma. J Urol 122:467, 1979.
118. Kaneti J, Thomson DMP, Reid EC: Prostaglandin E_2 affects the tumor immune response in prostatic carcinoma. J Urol 126:65, 1981.
119. Kjaer M: In vitro demonstration of cellular hypersensitivity to tumor antigens by means of the leukocyte migration technique in patients with renal carcinoma. Eur J Cancer 10:523, 1974.
120. Kjaer M: The dose-related effect of tumor extract on the *in vitro* migration of leukocytes from patients with renal carcinoma. Eur J Cancer 11:281, 1975.
121. Kjaer M, Christensen N: Ability of renal carcinoma tissue extract to induce leukocyte migration inhibition in patients with nonmetastatic renal carcinoma: correlation with clinical and histopathological findings. Cancer Immunol Immunother 2:41, 1977.
122. Klein G: Tmor antigens. Ann Rev Microbiol 20:223, 1966.
123. Klein G, Sjögren HO, Klein E, Hellstrom KE: Demonstration of resistance against methylcholanthrene-induced sarcomas in the primary autochthonous host. Cancer Res 20:1561, 1960.
124. Krutchik AN, Sullivan C, Sinkovics JG, Ayala A: Chemoimmunotherapy of sarcomatoid renal cell carcinoma. Med Pediatr Oncol 5:9, 1978.
125. Kumar S, Taylor G: Non-organ-specific and tumor-specific antibodies in children with Wilms' tumor. Int J Cancer 16:448, 1975.
126. Kumar S, Taylor G, Steward JK, Waghe MA, Pearson D: Cellular immunity in Wilms' tumor and neuroblastoma. Int J Cancer 10:36, 1972.
127. Kumar S, Waghe M, Taylor G: Tumor specific antibodies reactive with cell-surface antigens in children with Wilms' tumor. Int J Cancer 19:351, 1977.
128. Lamm DL, Harris SC, Gittes RF: Bacillus Calmette-Guerin and dinitrochlorobenzene immunotherapy of chemically induced bladder tumors. Invest Urol 14:369, 1977.
129. Lamm DL, Thor DE, Harris SC, Stogdill VD, Radwin HW: Intravesical and percutaneous BCG immunotherapy of recurrent superficial bladder cancer. In: Immunotherapy of Cancer: Present Status of Trialsin Man (abstract). National cancer Institute, Bethesda, MD, April 28–30, 1980.
130. Lamm DL, Yee GN, Reichert DF, Radwin HM: Levamisole immunotherapy of experimental transitional cell carcinoma. Invest urol 16:286, 1979.
131. Lang W, Zobl H, Georgii A: The effect of neonatal thymectomy on the growth kinetics of a virus-induced renal sarcoma of the rat. Eur J Cancer 14:431, 1978.
132. Lange PH: Lymphocyte-mediated cytotoxicity in patients with renal and transitional call carcinoma receiving BCG. Natl Cancer Inst Monogr 49:343, 1978.
133. Lange PH,Limas C, Fraley EE: Tissue blood-group antigens and prognosis in low stage transitional cell carcinoma of the bladder. J Urol 119:52, 1978.
134. Laucius JF, Patel YA, Lusch CJ, Koons LS, Bellet RE, Mastrangelo MJ: A phase II evaluation of Bacillus Calmette-Guerin plus megestrol acetate in patients with metastatic renal adenocarcinoma. Med Pediatr Oncol 3:237, 1977.
135. Leblanc PA, Taffet SM, Fried FA, Avis FP: Staphylocaccal protein A assay for detection of antibody directed at renal cancer cells. J Urol 121:724, 1979.
136. Limas C, Lange P, Fraley EE, Vessela RL: A, B, H antigens in transitional cell tumors of the urinary bladder. Cancer 44:2099, 1979.
137. Lo Gerfo P, Krupey J, Hansen HJ: Demonstration of an antigen common to several varieties of neoplasia: assay using zirconyl phosphate gel. N Engl J Med 285:138, 1971.
138. Lopez DM, Voigt W: Adenocarcinoma R3327 of the Copenhagen rat as a suitable model for immunological studies of prostate cancer. Cancer Res 37:2057, 1977,

139. McLeughlin AP, Brooks JD: A plasma factor inhibiting lymphocyte reactivity in urologic cancer patients. J Urol 112:366, 1974.
140. McLaughlin ap, Kessler WO, Triman K, Gittes RF: Immunologic competence in patients with urologic cancer. J Urol 111:233, 1974.
141. Menon M, Stefani SS: Search For blocking factors in sera of patients with prostatic cancer. J Urol 122:503, 1979.
142. Merrin C, Han T: Immune response in bladder cancer. J Urol 111:170, 1974.
143. Merrin C, Han T, Klein E, Wajsman Z, Murphy GP: Immunotherapy of prostatic carcinoma with Bacillus Calmette-Guerin. Cancer Chemother Rep 59:157, 1975.
144. Mickey DD, Seal E, Paulson DF: Detection of oncornavirus antigenic activity in human urothelial tissues. J Urol 113:658, 1975.
145. Middleton RG: Surgery for metastatic renal carcinoma. J Urol 97:973, 1967.
146. Mikulski Sm, Billing R, Terasaki PI: Inhibition of effector cell function in human antibody-dependent cellular cytotoxicity by sera from cancer patients. J Natl Cancer Inst 58:1485, 1977.
147. Mohr SJ, Whitesel JA: Spontaneous regression of renal cell carcinoma metastases after preoperative embolization of primary tumor and subsequent nephrectomy. Urology 14:5, 1979.
148. Monaco AP, Gozzo JJ, Schlesinger RM, Codish SD: Immunological detection of human bladder carcinoma. Ann Surg 182:325, 1975.
149. Moncure CW, Johnson CL Jr, Koontz WW Jr, Smith MV: Investigation of specific antigens in prostatic cancer. Cancer Chemother Rep:105, 1975.
150. Mondal S, Iype PT, Griesbach LM, Heidelberger C: Antigenicity of cells derived from mouse prostate cells after malignant transformation in vitro by carcinogenic hydrocarbons. Cancer Res 30:1593, 1970.
151. Montie JE, Bukowski RM, Deodhar SD, Hewlett JS, Stewart BH, Straffon RA: Immunotherapy of disseminated renal cell carcinoma with transfer factor. J Urol 117:553, 1977.
152. Montie JE, Stratton RA, Deodhar SD, Barma B: In Vitro Assessment of cell-mediated immunity in patients with renal cell carcinoma. J Urol 115:239, 1976.
153. Moore M, Robinson A: Cell-mediated cytotoxicity in carcinoma of the human urinary bladder. Cancer Immunol Immunother 2:233, 1977.
154. Morales A: Adjuvant immunotherapy in superficial bladder cancer. Natl Cancer Inst Monogr 49:315, 1978.
155. Morales A, Djeu J, Herberman RB: Immunization by irradiated whole cells or cell extracts against an experimental bladder tumor. Invest Urol 17:310, 1980.
156. Morales A, Eidinger D: Immune reactivity in renal cancer: a sequential study. J Urol 115:510, 1976.
157. Morales A, Eidinger D, Bruce AW: Intracavitary Bacillus Calmette-Guerin in the treatment of superficial bladder tumors. J Urol 116:180, 1976.
158. Morales A, Wilson JL, Pater JL, Loeb M: cytoreductive surgery and systemic BCG therapy in meatastatic renal cancer. J Urol (in press).
159. Nadler SH, Moore GE: Immunotherapy of malignant disease. Arch Surg 99:376, 1969.
160. Nairn RC, Philip J, Ghose T, Porteous IB, Fothergill JE: Production of a precipitin against renal cancer. Br Med J 1:1702, 1963.
161. Nelson DL, Bundy BA, Pitchon HE, Blaese RM, Strober W: The effector cell in human peripheral blood mediating mitogen-induced cellular cytotoxicity and antibody-dependent cellular cytotoxicity. J Immunol 117:1472, 1976.
162. Newman AJ Jr, CarltonCE Jr, Johnson S: Cell surface A, B or O(H) blood group antigens as an indicator of malignant potential in stage A bladder carcinoma. J Urol 124:27, 1980.

163. Nishio S, Horii A, Morikawa Y, Kawakita J, Nishijima T, Kishimoto T, Maekawa M: Studies of the nonspecific cellular immune response in patients with urinary bladder carcinoma. II. Immunodepressive effect of sera from bladder carcinoma. Invest Urol 16:342–345, 1979.
164. Nishio S, Horii A, Morikawa Y, Kawakita J, Nishijima T, Kishimoto T, Maekawa M: Studies of the nonspecific cellular immune response in patients with urinary bladder carcinoma. I. PHA-induced lymphocyte transformation. Invest Urol 16:336, 1979.
165. O'Boyle PJ, Cooper EH, Williams RE: Evaluation of immunologic reactivity in bladder cancer. Br J Urol 46:303, 1974.
166. Ohtsuki Y, Seman G, Dmochowski L, Bowen J, Johnson D: Virus-like particles in a case of human prostatic carcinoma. J Natl Cancer Inst 58:1493, 1977.
167. Okabe T, Ackermann R, Wirth M, Frohmuller HGW: Cell-mediated cytotoxicity in patients with cancer of the prostate. J Urol 122:628, 1979.
168. Okada S, Itaya K, Kurata Y: Identification of a tumor-specific antigen in the insoluble fraction of human nephroblastoma (preliminary communication). Eur J Cancer 15:1085, 1979.
169. Olsson CA, Rao CN, Menzoian OJ, Byrd WE: Immunologic unreactivity in bladder cancer patients. J Urol 107:607, 1972.
170. O'Toole C, Perlmann P, Unsgaard B, Moberger G, Edsmyr F: Cellular immunity to human urinary bladder carcinoma. I. Correlation to clinical stage and radiotherapy. Int J Cancer 10:77, 1972.
171. O'Toole C, Perlman P, Unsgaard B, Almgard LE, Johansson B, Moberger G, Edsmyr F: Cellular immunity to human urinary bladder carcinoma. II. Effect of surgery and preoperative irradiation. Int J Cancer 10:92, 1972.
172. O'Toole C, Stejskal V, Perlmann P, Karlsson M. Lymphoid cells mediating tumor specific cytotoxicity to carcinoma of the urinary bladder. Separation of the effector population using a surface marker. J Exp Med 139:457, 1974.
173. Papsidero LD, Wang MC, Valenzuela LK, Murphy GP, Chu TM: A prostate antigen in sera of prostatic cancer patients. Cancer Res 40:2428, 1980.
174. Paulson DF, Robson A, Fraley EE: Viral neoplastic transformation of hamster prostatic tissue *in vitro*. Science 159:200, 1968.
175. Pesce AJ, Phillips TM, Ooi BS, Evans A, Shenk RA Ill, Lewis MG: Immune complexes in transitional cell carcinoma. J Urol 123:486, 1980.
176. Philips TM, Lewis MG: Immune reactions in patients with bladder and prostate cancer. Aust NZ J Surg 48:545, 1978.
177. Pimm MV, Baldwin RW: BCG treatment of human tumor xenograftsin athymic nude mice. Br J Cancer 38:699, 1978.
178. Pizza G, Viza D, Fini M, Cuzzocrea D, Meaniti DE, Corrado F: Transitional cell carcinoma of the bladder. Differences between primary tumor and following relapses. Eur Urol 6:45, 1980.
179. Pollard M, Chang CF, Burleson GR: Investigations on prostate adenocarcinoma in rats. Cancer Treat Rep 61:153, 1977.
180. Pontes JE, Choe B, Rose N, Pierce JM Jr: Indirect immunofluorescence for identification of prostatic epithelial cells.J Urol 117:459, 1977.
181. Prager MD, Gregg DE, Walter MC: Effect of sera of patients with genitourinary tract cancers on transformation of lymphocytes stimulated with anti-thymocyte globulin. Natl Cancer Inst Monogr 49:127, 1978.
182. Prahn RT, Main JM: Immunity to methylcholanthrene-induced sarcomas. J Natl Cancer Inst 18:769, 1957.
183. Purves EC, Snell M, Cope WA, Addison JE, Copland RFP, Berenbaum MC: Subcutaneous Corynebacterium parvum in bladder cancer. Br J Urol 51:278, 1979.

184. Pyrhönen S, Mäntyjärvi R, Tykkä H, Sarna S, Tallberg T: Bk and Herpes Simplex virus antibodies in renal cell carcinoma. Med Biol 56:194, 1978.
185. Ramming KP, de Kernion JB: Immune RNA therapy for renal cell carcinoma: survical and immunologic monitoring. Ann Surg 186:459, 1977.
186. Rattliff TL, McCool RE, Catalona WJ: Antibody-dependent and spontaneous lympholysis in urologic cancer patients. Br J Cancer 39:667, 1979.
187. Ravitz G, Watne AL, Milan DF: Autoantibodies to human renal cell carcinoma. J Urol 107:26, 1972.
188. Reynoso G, Chu TM, Guinan P, Murphy GP: Carcinoembryonic antigen in patients with tumors of the urogenital tract. Cancer 30:1, 1972.
189. Richie JP,Blute RD Jr, Waisman J: Immunologic indicators of prognosis in bladder cancer: the importance of cell surface antigens. J Urol 123:22, 1980.
190. Richie JP, Wang BS, Steele GD, Wilson RE, Mannick JA: *In vivo* and *in vitro* effects of xenogeneic immune RNA in patients with advanced renal cell carcinoma: a phase I study. J Urol (Submitted).
191. Robinson MRG, Nakhala LS, Whitaker RH: Lymphocyte transformation in carcinoma of the prostate. Br J Urol 43:480, 1971.
192. Robinson MRG, Rigby CC, Pugh RCB, Dumonde DC: Adjuvant immunotherapy with BCG in carcinoma of the prostate. Br J Urol 49:221, 1977.
193. Robinson MRG, Rigby CC, Pugh RCB, Dumonde DC: Prostate carcinoma: intratumor BCG immunotherapy. Natl Cancer Inst Monogr 49:35, 1976.
194. Rosenberg EB, Herberman RB: Serum factors in renal carcinoma, Lancet 2:1153, 1971.
195. Rosenberg SA: Prospects for immunotherapy. Cancer 36:821, 1975.
196. Sadoughi N, Rubenstone A, Mlsna J, Davidsohn I: The cell surface antigens of bladder washing specimens in patients with bladder tumors, a new approach. J Urol 123:19, 1980.
197. Sanford EJ, Dagen JE, Geder L, Rohner TJ, Rapp F: Lymphocyte reactivity against virally transformed cells in patients with urologic cancer. J Urol 118:809, 1977.
198. Schellhammer PF, Bracken RB, Bean MA, Pinsky CM, whitmore WF Jr: Immune evaluation with skin testing. A study of testicular, prostatic and bladder neoplasms. Cancer 38:149, 1976.
199. Schellhammer PF, Wright GL Jr Rosato FE, Faulconer RJ: Leukocyte migration inhibition assay in patients with bladder cancer. J Urol 122:746, 1979.
200. Schmidt JD, Feldbrush TL, Weinstein SH, Bonney WW: Serum immunoglobulins in genitourinary malignancies. J Urol 115:293, 1976.
201. Schwarze G, Dietz R, Pappas A: Studies on cellular immunity in patients with renal carcinoma: radiation-induced inhibition of leukocytemigration. Eur J Cancer 15:205, 1979.
202. Shore B, Wise GJ, McBride RA, Brendler H: Tissue culture of human renal cell carcinoma: effect of serumon monolayer growth. J Urol 103:554, 1970.
203. Sjögren HO, Hellström I, Klein G: Resistance of polyoma virus immunized mice to transplantation of established polyoma tumors. Exp Cell Res 23:204, 1961.
204. Skinner DG, de Kernion JB, Brower PA, Ramming KP, Pilch YH: Advanced renal cell carcinoma: treatment with xenogeneic immune ribonucleic acid and appropriate surgical resection. J Urol 115:146, 1976.
205. Soanes WA, Ablin RJ Gonder MJ: Remission of metastatic lesions following cryosurgery in prostate cancer. J Urol 104:154, 1970.
206. Soloway MS: Effectiveness of long-term chemotherapy and/or BCG on murine bladder cancer. Natl Canc Inst Monogr 49:327, 1978.
207. Sophen H, O'Toole C: Anti-squamous tumor antibodies in patients with squamous cell carcinoma. Cancer Res 38:199, 1978.

208. Steele G Jr, Wang BS, Richie J, Wilson RE, Ervin T, Yankee R, Fallon M, Mannick JA: In vivo effect and parallel in vitro lymphocyte-mediated tumor cytolysis after phase I xenogeneic immune RNA treatment of patients with widespread melanoma or metastatic renal cell carcinoma. Cancer Res 40:2377, 1980.
209. Stjernsward J, Almgard LE, Franzen S, von Schreeb T, Wadstrom LB: Tumor-distinctive cellular immunity to renal carcinoma. Clin Exp Immunol 6:963, 1970.
210. Symes MO, Riddell AG: The use of immunized pig lymph node cells in the treatment of patients with advanced malignant disease. Br J Surg 60:176, 1973.
211. Symes MO, Riddell AG, Feneley RCL, Tribe CR: The treatment of advanced bladder cancer with sensitized pig lymphocytes. Br J Cancer 28 (Suppl. I):276, 1973.
212. Symes MO, Eckert H, Feneley RCL, Lai T, Mitchell JP, Roberts JBM, Tribe CR: Adoptive immunotherapy and radiotherapy in the treatment of urinary bladder cancer. Br J Urol 50:328, 1978.
213. Takasugi M, Mickey MR, Terasaki PI: Reactivity of lymphocytes from normal persons on cultured tumor cells. Cancer Res 33:2898, 1973.
214. Takasugi M, Mickey MR, Terasaki PI: Studies on specificity of cell-mediated immunity to human tumors. J Natl Cancer Inst 53:1527, 1974.
215. Thatcher N, Barnard RJ, Gasiunas N, Crowther D: Changes in cellular immunity following nephrectomy for localized and metastatic hypernephroma. Eur J cancer 13:951, 1977.
216. Thomas L: In: Cellular and Humoral Aspects of the Hypersensitive State. (Lawrence HS, ed.) New York: Hoeber-Harper, 1961, p. 529.
217. Troye M, Vilien M, Pape GR, Perlmann P: Cytotoxicity *in vitro* of blood lymphocytes from bladder cancer patients and controls to allogeneic or autologous tumor cells derived from established cell lines or short-term cultures. Int J Cancer 25:33, 1980.
218. Troye M, Perlmann P, Pape GR, Spiegelberg HL, Noslund I, Gidlof A: The use of Fab fragments of anti-human immunoglobulin as analytic for establishing the involvement of immunoglobulin in the spontaneous cytotoxicity to culture tumor cells by lymphocytes from patients with bladder carcinoma and from healthy donors. J Immunol 119:1061, 1977.
219. Troye M, Perlmann P, Larsson A, Blomgren H, Johansson B: Cellular cytotoxicity *in vitro* in transitional cell carcinoma of the human urinary bladder: ^{51} Cr release assay. Int J Cancer 20:188, 1977.
220. Troye M, Hansson Y, Paulie S, Perlmann P, Blomgren H, Johansson B: Lymphocyte-mediated lysis of tumor cells *in vitro* (ADCC), induced by serum antibodies from patients with urinary bladder carcinoma or from controls. Int J Cancer 25:45, 1980.
221. Tykkä H, Oravisto KJ, Lehtonen T, Sarna S, Tallberg T: Active specific immunotherapy of advanced renal cell carcinoma. Eur Urol 4:250, 1978.
222. Ueda R, Shiku H, Pfreundschuh M, Takahashi T, Li LTC, Whitmore WF, Oettgen HF, Old LJ: Cell surface antigens of human renal cencer defined by autologous typing. J Exp Med 150:564, 1979.
223. Waghe M, Kumar S: Demonstration of a Wilm's tumor associated antigen using xenogeneic antiserum. Eur J Cancer 13:993, 1977.
224. Wallace AC, nairm RC: Renal tubular antigens in kidney tumors. Cancer 29:977, 1972.
225. Wang MC, Valenguela LA, Murphy GP, Chu TM: Purification of human prostate specific antigen. Invest Urol 17:159, 1980.
226. Wechsler M, Lo Gerto P, Feminella J, Lattimer JK: The cancer associated antigen test as an index to failure of complete removal of urological cancer. J Urol 109:699, 1973.
227. Weinstein RS, Alroy J, Farrow GM, Miller AW Ill, Davidsohn I: Blood group isoantigen deletion in carcinoma *in situ* of the urinary bladder. Cancer 43:661, 1979.
228. Weissman RM, Coffey DS, Scott WW: Cell Kinetic studies of prostatic canner: adjuvant therapy in animal models. Oncology 34:133, 1977.

229. White TG, Mebust WK, Mirikitani FK: Induction of canine autoantibody to prostatic neoantigen. Clin Exp Immunol 33:174, 1978.
230. Whitmore WF, Gittes RF: Studies on prostate and testis as immunologically privileged sites. Cancer Treat Rep 61:217, 1977.
231. Williams RD, Bronson DL, Elliott AY, Gehrke CW, Kuo K, Fraley EE: Biochemical markers of cultured human prostatic epithelium. J Urol 119:768, 1978.
232. Williams RD, Bronson DL, Elliott AY, Fraley EE: Production of carcinoembryonic antigen by human prostate epithelial cells *in vitro*. J Natl Cancer Inst 58:115, 1977.
233. Williams G, Castro JE: The diagnostic and prognostic significance of delayed hypersensitivity skin testing in patients with urological cancer.Br J Urol 47:97, 1975.
234. Wise KS, Allerton SE, Trump G, Powars D, Beierle JW: A fetuin-like antigen from human nephroblastoma. Int J Cancer 16:199, 1975.
235. Wright GL, Schellhammer PF, Rosato FE, Faulconer RL: Cell mediated immunity in patients with renal cell carcinoma as measured by leukocyte migration inhibition test. Urology 12:525, 1978.
236. Wright GL, Schellhammer PF, Faulconer RL: Isolation of a soluble tumor-associated antigen from human renal cell carcinoma by gradient acrylamide gel electrophoresis. Cancer Res 37:4228, 1977.
237. Young AK, Hammond E, Middleton AW Jr: The prognostic value of cell surface antigens in low grade, non-invasive, Transitional cell carcinoma o of the bladder. J Urol 122:462, 1979.

8. Does Radiotherapy Alter the Course of Genitourinary Cancer?

MILJENKO V. PILEPICH and CARLOS A. PEREZ

1. INTRODUCTION

In order to assess accurately the impact of a treatment modality on the course of a disease (malignancy) one would ideally need to compare a group of untreated patients with a group of patients with comparable stage malignancy receiving the treatment in question. Understandably, this task is rarely feasible in current medical practice. The use of 'historical controls' as an alternative is associated with numerous pitfalls. An 'improvement' in the treatment results can simply be an expression of refinement of the general medical care or a selection of patients with particular prognostic factors rather than the application of a specific treatment. In addition, it is recognized that the natural course of a disease can change with time. Comparability of patient populations (in terms of staging, histological subtype of the malignancy, associated medical conditions, etc.) is always questionable when using historical series as a baseline.

Similar problems are encountered when comparing the impact of different treatment modalities. Unless comparison is done in the form of a controlled, prospective randomized trial, the problem of comparability of patient populations will arise. Selection criteria usually favor one modality over the other in the sense that patients with certain tumor stages or more favorable general condition are more likely to be accepted for treatment by one of the modalities.

We will try to review the available data in order to assess the effects of radiotherapy on local control, disease-free survival and survival in genitourinary malignancies and try to compare these with the results obtained by other modalities.

We will confine our discussion to radiotherapy used in curative (definitive) mode, in patients with localized or regional malignancies. In that context several general comments should be made. The probability of eradica-

D.F. Paulson (ed.), Genitourinary Cancer 1, 215-238.

tion of a tumor by radiotherapy in a given anatomical region depends on several factors:

a) Size of tumor. Smaller tumors have a greater probability of tumor control than larger lesions.
b) 'Radiosensitivity' of the tumor. While radiobiologists have no difficulties in defining radiosensitivity of a certain cell line *in vitro* (as defined by the shape of the cell survival curve), it is much more difficult to define radiosensitivity in a clinical set-up and the term is best avoided in clinical practice. While seminomas are no doubt quite radiosensitive tumors, epithelial tumors (squamous cell carcinomas, transitional cell carcinomas, and adenocarcinomas) share similar radiosensitivity in cell culture. The radioresponsiveness (this term simply refers to the rate of regression) can differ remarkably, however, from one tumor to the other. The rate of regression does not however necessarily have a significant bearing on the final results of treatment. An example of this is carcinoma of the prostate which may take up to two years or even longer to regress but it is still quite controllable locally. It is generally agreed that epithelial tumors require similar doses of radiation regardless of cell type.
c) Adequate coverage of all tumor and its regional extensions by the treatment fields.
d) Total tumor dose delivered. For a similar tumor size there is a greater probability of tumor control with higher doses of irradiation. The doses that can be administered safely are usually limited by the tolerance of the normal tissues.

The primary factor in determining the doses required to eradicate a tumor, in the majority of clinical situations, would therefore be the tumor size (initial number of tumor cells). Subclinical, microscopic tumor extensions can be controlled with a high degree of consistency with doses in the order of 4500–5000 rad given in four and one half to five weeks. Doses of this magnitude are commonly used in combination with surgery to eliminate microscopic extensions either before or after the removal of the gross tumor.

Doses of 2000 rad or even less are sometimes given preoperatively. These doses are not sufficient to eradicate even micrometastases. Potential benefit from this type, low dose, preoperative radiation lies in devitalization of the tumor and prevention of seeding of the wound and dissemination of viable tumor cells through the systemic circulation during surgical manipulation.

If radiotherapy is to be used as the only modality of treatment and if it has to deal with gross (macroscopic) disease, doses of at least 6000 rad or more given in six weeks will generally be needed to achieve permanent local control.

2. RENAL CELL CARCINOMA

The doses of radiation that can be safely delivered to the renal area are limited by the tolerance of the surrounding structures (primarily the GI tract). Although renal cell carcinoma can be expected to exhibit radiosensitivity similar to that in other epithelial tumors, limitations in total doses that can be safely delivered to the kidneys and surrounding areas make renal cell carcinoma a primarily surgical disease with radiotherapy being used only as a adjuvant either preoperatively or postoperatively.

Preoperative irradiation could theoretically, as in other tumors, convert unresectable lesions into resectable ones and reduce incidence of dissemination and local seeding during surgical manipulation. Both pre- and postoperative radiotherapy should eliminate microextensions of the tumor and reduce the incidence of local and/or regional recurrence.

As early as 1935, Waters [1] reported on the conversion of inoperable renal cell carcinomas into operable. Riches [2, 3] made similar observation in his own series. Initially, he applied preoperative radiotherapy only to advanced tumors but later expanded its use to all patients. In his experience, and also in that of Flock and Kadesky [4], preoperative radiation appeared beneficial in terms of improving resectability, reducing the rate of local recurrence and improving survival.

A prospective trial of preoperative radiotherapy was started in 1965 by the Rotterdam urologists and the Rotterdam Radiotherapy Institute [5]. Operable patients were randomized to either simple nephrectomy or preoperative radiotherapy followed by simple nephrectomy. Radiation consisted of 3000 rad in three to four weeks. Of 174 eligible patients, 89 received preoperative radiation while 85 underwent immediate simple nephrectomy. In patients with locally extensive tumors invading the perinephric fat or renal hilum, 35% of those who had surgery only showed positive resection margins while only 11% of those that had preoperative radiotherapy showed tumor in the plane of resection. There was however no difference in survival in the two groups.

A randomized trial of preoperative radiotherapy was instituted in 1970 by the Genitourinary Oncology Group. The results of the study which tested 4500 rad in four to six weeks preoperative radiotherapy against nephrectomy alone have not been published yet.

The results of postoperative radiotherapy in renal carcinoma are also controversial. Rafla [6] analyzed a series of 244 patients of whom 96 were treated with nephrectomy alone, and 94 received postoperative radiotherapy. Thirty-seven percent of the first and 56% of the second group survived five years. The 10 year survival figures were 19% for the first and 34% for the second group. The difference between the groups was most prominent in patients with the tumor involving capsulary tissues and renal pelvis. The five-year survival in the subgroup of patients with capsule involvement was 29.8% in the surgery alone group and 57% in the surgery plus radiotherapy group. In the British Association of Urological surgeons series as reported by Riches [3] the five- and ten-year survival of patients undergoing nephrectomy only was 30% and 17% while in those that received postoperative radiotherapy the survival was 49% and 27% respectively. The positive effect of postoperative radiotherapy was most noticeable in patients with renal vein involvement. Riches [2] in his personal series observed an improvement in survival with postoperative radiotherapy in patients with evidence of perinephric spread or involvement of lymph nodes. Peeling [7] in a retrospective analysis of cases seen at London Hospital between 1940 and 1965 could not substantiate an improvement of survival in patients receiving postoperative radiotherapy. The doses given and the technique employed were not specified. It should be noted that the patients with more advanced disease were more likely to receive radiotherapy. Finney [8] conducted a controlled trial of postoperative radiotherapy. The patients were randomized by the date of birth into no postoperative radiotherapy or 5500 rad in 27 treatments given in five and one half weeks. There were four instances of liver failure in patients with right-sided tumors who received radiotherapy. The trial showed no advantage in patients receiving postoperative radiotherapy. The criticism of the trial is primarily in the small number of patients available, diluted even further by the inclusion of early stage tumor (43 patients with Stage I tumors that would not ordinarily be considered for postoperative radiotherapy) and also randomization by the date of birth which can introduce a bias since the referring surgeon could be influenced by his advance knowledge of whether the patient would receive postoperative radiotherapy.

In summary, the available data cannot support routine preoperative radiotherapy in all patients planned for radical nephrectomy. However, radiotherapy appears effective in converting locally advanced unresectable renal carcinomas into resectable and also reduce the incidence of positive resection margins and local recurrence. With the modern radiographic methods it is possible to select locally advanced tumors prior to exploration and apply radiotherapy preoperatively. Postoperative irradiation is likely to benefit patients with residual tumor, positive margins and those with documented invasion of the perinephric fat and/or regional lymph nodes.

3. CARCINOMA OF THE RENAL PELVIS AND URETER

It is generally recognized that carcinomas arising in the renal pelvis and ureter manifest not only histological features, but also patterns of spread and biological behavior in general similar to much more common bladder cancer. Primary treatment is surgical. Although several authors have suggested the potential for the use of radiotherapy in this tumor the data is quite scarce.

Brady *et al.* [9] reported on six patients with carcinoma of the ureter treated with radiotherapy. Two were treated for recurrent tumor and four for either unresectable or residual disease. Three of five patients available for follow-up survived five years.

Administration of preoperative radiotherapy had been suggested by Almgard *et al.* [10] who is conducting a study investigating this approach. Preoperative radiotherapy might be impractical due to difficulties in diagnosis and assessment of tumor extend. These difficulties are lessened by the availability of the modern radiographic procedures.

Postoperative radiotherapy as suggested by Batata *et al.* [11] and employed by Babaian and Johnson [12] appears likely to improve surgical results in high stage tumors but the data to support this approach are still lacking.

4. CARCINOMA OF BLADDER

Radiotherapy is employed in bladder carcinoma either as the sole modality of treatment or in combination with surgery (preoperatively or postoperatively). Although considerable experience has accumulated with its use, the guidelines for its optimal application in either definitive form or as an adjuvant to surgery have not been completely defined for the various presentations of this exceedingly heterogeneous type of tumor.

4.1. Definitive Radiotherapy

Patients with bladder carcinoma who are referred to definitive radiotherapy are usually those with residual or recurrent tumor post-transurethral resection who for various reasons are not candidates for definitive surgery (cystectomy).

In the M.D. Anderson Hospital series of 533 patients treated with radiotherapy alone [13], most were in advanced stage (79 % of patients were clinically staged as B_2, C or D). Local (pelvic) recurrences were observed in 44 % of the patients. The incidence of local recurrence was remarkably constant in all the stages (48 % in Stage A and 45 % in Stage D_1, for example). Survival, on the other hand, decreased with more advanced stages and histological grade reflecting higher incidence of distant metastases.

At Stanford University [14], 384 patients were treated with definitive radiotherapy and 176 (50%) failed in the bladder. It is of interest that 48% of the 44 patients who underwent cystectomy after failure of radiotherapy remained disease-free at various intervals. Similar salvage rates have been reported by Wallace and Bloom [15], Galleher *et al.* [16] and Johnson *et al.* [17].

The value of definitive radiotherapy relative to surgery alone has not been evaluated adequately on a large scale, randomized trial. Radiotherapy had proven inferior to a combination of radiotherapy and surgical resection in several trials [13, 15, 18].

It is clear that patients treated with definitive radiotherapy show a substantial rate of local recurrence and that surgical salvage of these recurrences is quite successful. By applying definitive radiotherapy first and using salvage cystectomy in recurrent tumors, one can achieve satisfactory results and, at the same time, save a substantial number of bladders.

4.2. Preoperative Irradiation

Results of surgical management in bladder carcinoma are far from satisfactory, particularly in invasive high-grade tumors where five-year survival in most reports varies between 10 and 30% [19]. Cystectomy is associated with a substantial incidence of local recurrences. At Memorial Hospital [20] 37% of patients undergoing radical cystectomy with lymph node dissection developed pelvic recurrences.

Pelvic recurrences are attributed to either incomplete resection usually due to microscopic extensions into the perivesical fat or lymphatics, or intraoperative seeding (implantation). The role of lymphatic and hematogeneous dissemination due to tumor manipulation during surgical procedure may conceivably play an important role in the development of treatment failures, but is difficult to assess quantitatively.

The value of adjuvant, preoperative radiotherapy in improving results of surgical resection has been evaluated in several major trials.

At Memorial Hospital, preoperative radiotherapy has been systematically applied since the late 1950's [20–22]. It initially consisted of 4000 rad in twenty fractions to the true pelvis, followed by radical cystectomy with lymph node dissection within four to twelve weeks. This approach was used between 1959 and 1965. Between 1966 and 1970, the treatment policies changed to 2000 rad in one week to the true pelvis, followed by radical cystectomy with lymph node dissection within one week. Since 1971, the field of radiation was increased to cover the whole pelvis to the same dose, followed by the same type of surgery. The results of these consecutive series

Table 1. Site of first recurrence

	Group 1	Group 2	Group 3	Group 4
	No radiation	4000 rad	200 rad true pelvis	2000 rad whole pelvis
Recurrence				
Pelvic only	38 (28%)	19 (16%)	12 (14%)	9 (9%)
Distant only	10 (7%)	21 (18%)	17 (20%)	25 (25%)
Both	12 (9%)	10 (8%)	5 (6%)	8 (8%)
Undetermined	7 (5%)	3 (3%)	2 (2%)	4 (4%)
Total	67 (49%)	53 (45%)	36 (42%)	46 (46%)

Smith *et al.*: Cancer (in press). By courtesy of Lippincott Publishing Company.

of patients have been correlated with a group of patients treated with radical surgery alone prior to 1959. When comparing the results in the four consecutive groups of patients, the contention is made that the groups were comparable and that the surgical technique has not changed significantly during the period in question. A reduction in the incidence of pelvic recurrences has been observed in all groups that received preoperative radiotherapy. The incidence of pelvic recurrences is lowest in the group treated to whole pelvis (Table 1). An improvement in survival at five years is twice as high as in the group treated with surgery alone (Table 2).

Downstaging was most frequent in the group receiving 4000 rad in four weeks. This is to be expected since not only was the dose higher, but the tumor was allowed enough time to respond.

At M.D. Anderson Hospital preoperative radiotherapy in bladder carci-

Table 2. Five-year survival according to clinical stage *

Stage	Group 1	Group 2	Group 3	Group 4
	No radiation	4000 rad	2000 rad true pelvis	2000 rad whole pelvis
Superficial				
CIS	5/7 (71%)	8/9 (89%)	1/1 (100%)	2/2 (100%)
T_1	11/17 (65%)	8/13 (62%)	4/6 (67%)	5/7 (71%)
T_2	19/42 (45%)	18/36 (50%)	10/22 (45%)	7/17 (41%)
Deep				
T_3	10/64 (16%)	17/50 (34%)	21/52 (40%)	21/52 (40%)
T_4	0/6 (0%)	0/11 (0)	0/5 (0%)	4/20 (20%)

* From Smith *et al.*: Cancer (In Press). By courtesy of Lippincott Publishing Company.

noma consists of 5000 rad in twenty-five fractions over five weeks, followed within six weeks by total cystectomy without lymph node dissection. In a group of 125 patients, 35% survived five years and 29% showed no residual tumor at the time of surgery [23]. Fifty-four percent of patients with no residual tumor who had cystectomy (these were clinical Stage B_2 and C) survived five years while only 25% of patients with residual tumors survived five years. These findings are in agreement with those of van der Werf-Messing [24]. Preoperative radiotherapy in her series consisted of 4000 rad in twenty fractions in four weeks followed by cystectomy in one to two weeks without lymphadenectomy. Of 35 patients with deeply invasive tumors (Stage T_3) who showed downstaging postradiotherapy, approximately 80% survived five years while none of the 19 patients whose tumor failed to respond to radiotherapy survived five years.

In the Urological Cancer Research Group Study [25, 26], 35% of the patients (clinical Stage B_2 or higher) receiving 4500 rad in four and one-half weeks and undergoing cystectomy four to eight weeks later had no residual tumor in the specimen. A statistically significant difference in survival between irradiated and unirradiated groups was noted in the clinical stage B_2 and C provided there was no tumor in the cystectomy specimen. A decreased incidence of lymph node involvement was noted in patients who received preoperative radiotherapy versus those who underwent surgical resection only.

Bloom [18] reported on the Institute of Urology controlled trial that involved patients with T_3 tumors who received 4000 rad in four weeks and four weeks later, radical cystectomy with lymph node dissection. Another group of patients received radiotherapy alone. Forty-seven percent of the patients were downstaged and of these, 51% were alive at five years versus 23% of those who were not downstaged.

In summary, it would appear that preoperative radiotherapy does produce significant impact on bladder carcinoma. With moderately high doses (4000–5000 rad), downstaging is observed in two-thirds of the patients and no residual tumors in one-third of the patients. The incidence of detectable lymph node involvement in the lymphadenectomy specimen is also reduced. Incidence of pelvic recurrences is reduced remarkably, even with the relatively low dose of 2000 rad in one week.

An improvement in survival and disease-free survival is, however, more difficult to document. It is demonstrable in deeply-invasive tumors, particularly those that were downstaged following irradiation or which have regressed completely. The possible reasons for modest improvement in survival with preoperative radiotherapy may lie in the fact that a large proportion of patients with bladder carcinoma fail with distant metastases. Another proportion of patients, probably in the vicinity of 15–25% can be controlled with resection alone. There is, therefore, only a limited population of patients who can be significantly helped with adjuvant radiotherapy. These appear to be primarily those with deeply invasive tumors, particularly those that respond morphologically to preoperative radiotherapy. Slack and Prout [26] suggested that the group of patients with invasive papillary tumors might be the ones who are likely to benefit from preoperative radiation.

4.3. Postoperative Radiotherapy

Experience with postoperative radiotherapy in bladder carcinoma is quite limited. In clinical practice, patients referred for radiotherapy postoperatively are those with known or suspected residual tumor post-resection. Miller and Johnson [13] reported on a group of 62 patients who received postoperative radiotherapy at M.D. Anderson Hospital to a maximum of 6000 rad in six weeks. Over 40% survived five years. This was a highly selected population with a substantial number of patients with early stage tumors. It is, therefore, difficult to make any conclusion from their report.

In 1978, RTOG (Radiation Therapy Oncology Group) undertook a pilot study of 'sandwich' adjuvant radiotherapy [27]. The pre-op dose was quite low, consisting of only 500 rad given immediately prior to cystectomy. The purpose of this low dose was prevention of seeding and dissemination at surgery. Post-cystectomy the patients received 4500 rad in four and a half to five weeks if the pathological stages were B_2, C or high grade B_1. The actuarial survival at two years was 82% and no local failures have been recorded. Only 6% major complication rate has been observed. The approach allows for accurate staging and optimal selection of patients prior to postoperative radiation. The very promising results need to be confirmed in a larger group of patients. In 1980, RTOG started a randomized study comparing the 'sandwich' postoperative radiation therapy with the 2000 rad in one week preoperative radiotherapy regimen.

There is no doubt a pressing need to further define various subgroups of patients and establish criteria for selection for preoperative and postoperative irradiation.

It is quite likely that if and when the means of controlling systemic micrometastatic (subclinical) disease become available, local control will be a more important determinant for cure in a larger percentage of patients and radiotherapy might play an increasingly important role in the future treatment of bladder carcinoma.

5. CARCINOMA OF THE PROSTATE

Radiotherapy has been an increasingly important treatment modality in the definitive (curative) management of carcinoma of the prostate. Although various forms of radiation sources had been applied with variable degrees of success since the early part of the century, the real impetus began with the technological advances of the last two decades which made possible safe and precise delivery of adequate doses to the tumor bearing area and surrounding pelvic structures using external beam. At the same time, a new form of isotope (I-125) for interstitial implants became available. At present there are two main curative radiotherapeutic approaches to carcinoma of the prostate: external beam radiotherapy and interstitial implant.

Definitive external beam radiotherapy is applicable to all stages of potentially curable tumor, confined to the pelvis. The primary tumor, prostate and the periprostatic tissues are treated with a dose of 6500–7000 rad, 175-200 rad per day. In patients with high risk of lymph node involvement (high grade, high stage) or documented lymph node involvement (either radiographically or at staging laparotomy) regional lymphatics are treated with a dose of 4500-5000 rad, 175-200 rad per day.

Interstitial implants either in the form of Iodine (I-125), gold (Au 198) or Radon (Rn 222) are usually applied to Stage B lesions, less often to early C_1 lesions [28–30]. Following an exploratory laparotomy with pelvic lymphadenectomy the gland is exposed and permanently implanted with radioactive 'seeds'. Iodine 125 has a long half-life of 60 days. The tumoricidal dose which is usually defined as 15 000 rad or more is delivered over approximately one year. The energy of the Gamma radiation is quite low, with rapid fall-off resulting in very little exposure outside the implanted volume. Due to the long half-life the exposure rate is quite low allowing for improved tolerance of tissues.

Radioactive gold (Au 198), has a half-life of 2.7 days so that most of the effective dosage is delivered within several weeks. Full tumoricidal doses cannot therefore be delivered with implant only due to the severe local reactions that would result from such an exposure. The implants with short-lived isotopes are limited to approximately 3000–3500 rad and supplemented by external beam usually to the whole pelvis to a dose of 4000–4500 rad [28]. Energy of emitted radiation is higher (0.42 Mev for Au 198) and the tissues around the implanted volume receive a considerably higher dose. There is also an increased exposure of the hospital personnel.

The natural course of carcinoma of the prostate is exceedingly variable. While some patients can live with tumor for a number of years without being significantly affected and ultimately die of other causes, others die of widely disseminated rapidly growing tumors [31]. Most patients are elderly and survival is often affected by unrelated medical problems. These factors make an accurate assessment of the effect of any treatment on the course of disease quite difficult. Since late relapses occurring ten years or later after the completion of treatment are not unusual, the term 'cure' is seldom applied to prostatic carcinoma. We will however try to compare the end results of different modalities in terms of local control, disease-free survival, and absolute survival.

Assessment of local tumor control following external radiotherapy is a somewhat controversial issue. It is well recognized that in the majority of patients prostatic carcinoma regresses at a very slow rate. Although time to complete regression appears to be inversely related to probability of local control [32] some tumors may persist several years before complete regression is recorded. Biopsies of the prostate at various intervals following radiotherapy have shown a high 'positivity' rate during the first several months. Cox and Stoffel [33] conducted a prospective study in 38 patients who received radical radiotherapy to a dose of 7000 rad to the prostate. A total of 139 biopsies were done serially. At six months 60% (Fig. 1) of

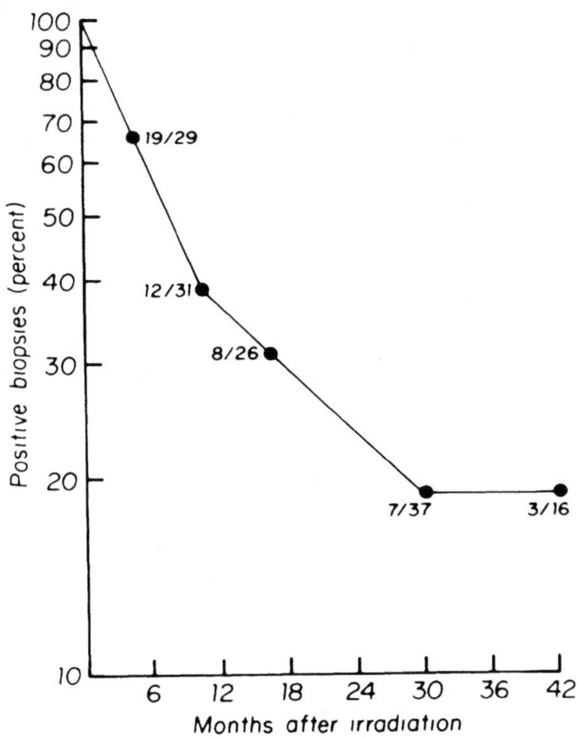

Figure 1. Correlation of biopsy results with postirradiation interval. From Cox and Stoffel, Cancer 40: 158; by courtesy of Lippincott Publishing Company.

biopsies were histologically positive, at 12 months 37%, at 18 months 30% and two and one-half years 19%. Hill [34] reported on biopsy results in 21 patients obtained from six months to seven years post-treatment. Seventy-six percent of biopsies were negative one year after completion of treatment. Although conversion from positive to negative was observed even two years after the treatment, clinical (rectal) examination correlated quite well with biopsy results one year or more after the treatment. Sixteen of seventeen clinically negative prostates had negative biopsies and four of four prostates with palpable residual tumor showed positive biopsies. Presence of histologically identifiable carcinoma cells in the specimen does not necessarily imply reproductive capability of the cells. The cells may be active metabolically and appear normal under the microscope, but the damage to cell's reproductive material may prevent it from dividing and sustaining further tumor growth. The only unequivocal evidence of local failure is tumor progression.

Local control with external radiotherapy is dependent primarily on tumor stage, to a certain degree on tumor size, and on the dose of radiotherapy [35]. At Washington University only three of 45 patients (6.6%) with stage B tumor failed in the pelvis while 25 of 155 patients (16.1%) with stage C tumors failed locally. All tumors smaller than 2 cm regardless of stage were controlled locally. Increase in doses of radiation improved local control rate. Most publications, however, do not analyze the local control by stage. Overall local control rates reported by Ray [36] is 87%, McGowen [37] 90%, and Cox [33] 93%.

Local recurrences following radical prostatectomy are not uncommon. In Jewett's classical series [38], 16% of patients with early stage B nodule developed local recurrence. In Belt's series [39], 22.2% of patients with pathological stage C (this group of patients included those staged as B clinically) developed clinically manifest local recurrence. Survival and disease-free survival are listed in Table 3 for several radiotherapy and surgical series. It is apparent that both modalities achieve similar survival rates ranging from 75 and 95% to stage A and B at five years, and from 40 to 55% for stage C at five years. The disease-free survival is somewhat lower.

Similarity of survival with radiotherapy and radical prostatectomy is quite remarkable in view of the fact that selection criteria, if anything, would be likely to favor surgical series. Patients with smaller tumors and better general condition are more likely to be approached surgically. Other selection processes can sometimes apply. In the series by Veenema *et al.* [40] tumor was of well-differentiated histology in 146 or 159 patients. Survival rates in the series by Belt and Schroeder [39] refer to pathological (not clinical) stages and should be interpreted in view of frequent clinical understaging in prostate carcinoma.

Table 3. Survival following definitive radiotherapy and radical prostatectomy

	No. of patients	Stage	5 Year		10 Year	
			% Sur-vival	% Disease-free	% Sur-vival	% Disease-free
Radiotherapy						
Pistenma *et al.* [44]	230	B	71*	70^{+}	45*	42^{+}
	200	C	41*	37^{+}	31*	29^{+}
Harisiadis *et al.* [45]	13	A	88.2*			
	21	B	86.8*			
	112	C	58*		35*	
Hill *et al.* [34]	19	A & B	80	70		
	49	C	42	31		
Lipsett *et al.* [46]	23	A & B	95*			
	56	C	55*			
McGowan [47]	21	A	88*	84*		
	43	B_1	90*	61*		
	30	B_2	66*	43*		
	13	C	39*	37*		
Perez *et al.* [32]	42	B	80*			
	141	C	56*			
Surgery						
Veenema *et al.* [40]	159	A & B	84		52	
Belt and Shroeder [39]	185	path B	78.3		55.2	
	267	path C	63.3		37.3	
Vickery and Kerr [48]	196	B	70.6		39.2	
Williams *et al.* [49]	52	B	75		35	

* Actuarial survival
$^{+}$ Direct survival

The local control rate and survival with Iodine-125 implants appear comparable [29, 30, 41] with those reported using external beam radiotherapy or surgery but larger numbers of patients and longer follow-up periods are needed.

While the effect of each of the modalities on the natural course of prostatic cancer is difficult to ascertain in the absence of a comparable population of patients observed untreated, it is apparent that if the measurable endpoint, i.e. survival, appears similar then, the choice of treatment should probably be based on the type and incidence of complications. The choice between beam and radioactive implant, for example, is often based on the patient's potency and his wish to retain it. Treatment with Iodine-125 implant has a 95% rate of preservation of potency [42, 43] in comparison with 70% reported incidence of potency following external beam treatment [36].

6. CARCINOMA OF THE URETHRA

Treatment and prognosis in carcinoma of the urethra varies considerably in tumors arising at the different anatomical divisions of the organ in both the male and the female.

6.1. Male Urethra

Carcinoma of the male urethra is quite uncommon and accumulated experience with its treatment is limited. Carcinomas of the distal (penile) urethra are curable in a high percentage of patients by either resection [50, 51] (usually penectomy) or irradiation [52]. Results of treatment in lesions arising in the bulbomembranous urethra are dismal with either modality [50, 51]. Lesions of the prostatic urethra show an intermittent overall prognosis [50, 51]. The role of radiotherapy in lesions arising at this location has not been defined yet.

6.2. Female Urethra

Carcinoma of the anterior urethra can be approached with partial urethrectomy but this results in a high local recurrence rate [53]. Radiotherapy in the form of interstitial implant either alone or in combination with external radiotherapy seems to be the treatment of choice in lesions of the anterior urethra resulting in satisfactory control rates and preservation of function [54–58]. Lesions of the proximal urethra and those involving the whole urethra have poor prognosis due to difficulties in achieving adequate local control and also due to tendency of the tumor to involve pelvic lymph nodes and also to produce distal metastases. A combination of several modalities including external beam, implant and resection has been advocated by several authors [50, 53, 54, 59].

7. CARCINOMA OF THE PENIS

Therapeutic considerations in carcinoma of the penis are usually discussed in two separate phases – the one dealing with management of primary tumor, and the one dealing with the regional lymphatics.

Surgical approach to the primary lesions in carcinoma of the penis consists of local excision only on rare occasions. Early lesions of the prepuce are amenable to local excision with acceptable results [60, 61]. A majority of patients, however, require partial or total penectomy with the associated functional and psychological mutilation. Although local control with penectomy is good, conservative treatment in the form of radiotherapy offers the obvious advantage of organ preservation.

Numerous radiotherapeutic approaches have been utilized in the treatment of the primary penile lesion. One of the earliest methods was application of mould to the surface of the organ [62, 63]. Interstitial implants, contact therapy, electron beam and megavoltage radiation have all been utilized in the treatment of this disease. Analysis of results is tempered by innumerable variations in the techniques, dosage and fractionation patterns quite often unacceptable by today's standards. In the series by Almgard [64] for example, patients were treated during the period from 1920 to 1955 with daily doses ranging from 500 to 900 rad to a total dose of 4000–6100 rad.

Local control rate in the treatment of the primary lesion in several representative series of patients treated with radiotherapy is listed in Table 4. Local control varies between 50 and 100%, depending on the type of method used and patient selection. Adequate dosage delivered by external beam results in excellent local control clearly superior to historical series in which other methods of treatment and inadequate doses were employed. It should be stressed that local recurrences can be salvaged surgically further improving the control rates. In the classical series by Engelstad [65] for example,

Table 4. Radiotherapy in carcinoma of the penis and control of primary lesion with radiotherapy

Author	No. of patients	Treatment method	Dosage	Local control (%)
Engelstad [65]	72	Mould Teleradium	3500–3700 rtg 500–700 rtg/day	50
Jackson [63]	39	Mould (most cases) External beam (some cases)	?	49
Murrell [72] and Williams	108	External beam	3000–6700 rad 200 rad/day	52
Kelley *et al.* [73]	10*	External beam (electrons)	5100–5400 rad 300/day	100
Haile [74] and Delclos	20	Mould Implant External beam	?	90
Pointon [75]	32	External beam	5250–5500 rad in 16 Rx/22 days	84.4

* All tumors except one were 3 cm or less in size.

although only 50% of lesions were controlled locally with radiotherapy, 24 of 27 locally persistent or recurrent lesions could be controlled by surgical resection.

Management of regional lymph nodes in penile carcinoma remains a controversial issue. Although approximately 30 to 55% of patients present with palpable inguinal lymph nodes at the time of diagnosis only 40–60% of palpable lymph nodes show histological evidence of tumor involvement, while 10–20% of clinically negative nodes contain tumor [60, 61, 66–68]. Surgical resection of the involved regional nodes can salvage approximately 30–40% of patients [61, 68, 66]. Prophylactic dissection of clinically negative inguinal lymph nodes is generally not considered advisable due to high morbidity associated with groin dissection and at the same time high salvage rate in patients undergoing dissection at the time the lymph nodes become clinically positive [69].

Radiotherapy in adequate doses can be an effective means of control of the tumor involving lymph nodes. In the report by Staubitz [70], 5 of 13 patients with biopsy proven nodal involvement survived five years in comparison to a group of patients with positive lymph node biopsies who underwent radical lymph node dissection and of whom 8 of 18 survived five years.

There is limited information on the value of prophylactic inguinal irradiation in patients with penile carcinoma with clinically negative groins. However, one would need to note the excellent survival rates in the two series in which prophylactic lymphatic irradiation was employed. Survival rates at five years in most series range from 40–60% [61, 67, 68, 71, 72], while 69% of patients reported by Ekstrom and Edsmyr [66] and 66.7% of those in Engelstad's [65] series survived five years.

In summary, radiotherapy can be applied successfully in the treatment of both the primary lesion and lymph node metastases. Of particular interest is the use of radiotherapy in early lesions in younger patients who wish to retain a functional organ. Excellent control rates and preservation of sexual function can be achieved.

8. TESTICULAR TUMORS

8.1. Seminoma

Seminoma is one of the most radioresponsive tumors. This property, along with its orderly spread through the lymphatic system and late occurrence of hematogenous metastases accounts for the excellent treatment results with radiotherapy.

The staging following orchiectomy should include lymphangiogram and determination of tumor markers (beta chain HCG and AFP). Patients with negative lymphangiogram (Stage I) receive prophylactic radiotherapy to the ipsilateral pelvic lymph nodes and para-aortic and renal hilum lymph nodes (2500 rad, usually given in three weeks).

Patients with positive lymphangiograms (Stage II) receive a somewhat higher dose, 3000–3500 rad in three and one-half to four weeks to regional lymphatics followed by prophylactic mediastinal irradiation to a dose of 2500 rad in three weeks. Patients with massive retroperitoneal tumor deposits receive whole abdominal irradiation to approximately 1500–2000 rad followed by a boost to the detectable tumor masses to a total of 3500–4000 rad.

In Stage III (supradiaphragmatic lymphatic involvement), the policies of treatment are not uniformly defined due to the rarity of this presentation. In the past, patients were treated with mediastinal and whole lung irradiation in addition to subdiaphragmatic irradiation. At present, most institutions employ radiotherapy to bulky disease and proceed with adjuvant chemotherapy.

In clinical Stage I, it is highly unusual to see a failure following the treatment described. In several series [76, 77] no failures were reported in Stage I seminomas and in the majority of reports, the cure rates approach or exceed 95% [78–80]. In Stage II, cure rates are about 90% [2, 8, 13, 16].

Treatment results in Stage III and IV are difficult to interpret due to rarity of patients in this stage and the variety of treatment methods applied. Three of five patients (60%) with Stage III seminomas survived thirty-six months with no evidence of disease in the M.D. Anderson Hospital series [81]. In Stanford series [76], three or four patients remained disease-free. Long-term control (cure) with radiotherapy had been reported in a proportion of patients presenting with recurrent and/or disseminated seminoma [82].

Stage III and IV patients are currently approached in most institutions with a combination of radiotherapy and cytotoxic agents.

Anaplastic seminoma is a histological variety of the tumor, the treatment of which is somewhat controversial [83]. Kademian suggested that anaplastic seminoma had a poor prognosis in comparison with the same stage typical (classical) seminoma. Maier [84] and Johnson [85] on the other hand, found no difference in prognosis stage per stage. It is clear that the patients with anaplastic seminoma present in more advanced stages. It is not completely established, however, whether the doses or fields should be any different from those routinely employed in typical seminoma with the same stage tumor.

With refinement of the staging methods (lymphangiogram and CT scan) and with wide use of marker determination (beta chain HCG and AFP) it is likely that the already excellent results in radiotherapy of seminoma would improve further and that it will become highly unusual to see a patient fail on treatment.

8.2. Testicular Carcinomas

Management of testicular carcinomas (embryonal carcinoma and teratocarcinoma) has undergone considerable changes in the recent years, primarily due to the appearance of effective chemotherapy.

Although testicular carcinomas do not respond to radiotherapy as promptly as seminoma, radiotherapy in moderately high doses can control lymph node metastases in a substantial percentage of cases. At the M.D. Anderson Hospital [86, 87], thirty-four patients received 2500 rad in three weeks to the para-aortic and the ipsilateral lymph nodes followed one to two weeks later by lymphadenectomy. The lymphadenectomy findings were compared with those patients who did not receive preoperative radiotherapy. Both groups were staged clinically by lymphangiogram prior to treatment. Although the irradiated patients presented with more advanced disease than those who did not receive preoperative radiotherapy, the incidence of histologically positive lymph nodes in the lymphadenectomy specimens was much lower in the preoperative radiotherapy group! Zero vs. 17% in clinical Stage I, 32% vs. 90% in clinical Stage II-A and 80% vs. 100% in clinical Stage II-B had histologically positive lymph nodes. Stage II-B in the M.D. Anderson Hospital series is defined as disease presenting with massive retroperitoneal lymph nodes.

At a number of institutions in Europe, radiotherapy is used routinely instead of lymphadenectomy in testicular carcinomas. In the series from Royal Marsden Hospital in London [88], 95% of cases with clinical Stage I disease were controlled in the retroperitoneum with 4000 rad in four to five weeks. In clinical Stage II, following 4500 rad in five to six weeks to the retroperitoneal lymph nodes, 86% of patients remained disease-free if the metastatic deposits were 2.0 cm in diameter or less as measured on lymphangiogram. If the deposits measured more than 2.0 cm in diameter, only 33% of patients remained disease-free.

It is apparent that irradiation to moderately high doses can consistently erradicate microscopic (sub-clinical) lymph node disease in testicular carcinomas and that it is quite effective even in macroscopic (radiographically detectable) disease, provided that metastatic deposits are of limited size. Lymphadenectomy is needed as a debulking procedure in patients with massive retroperitoneal disease.

Results of radiotherapy as the only therapeutic modality following orchiectomy, directed to the retroperitoneal lymph nodes are quite satisfactory in patients with clinical Stage I testicular carcinomas. Several reported series [77, 79, 80] cite long term survival in 85–90% of patients. The results in clinical Stage II with minimal or moderate amount of tumor burden are also satisfactory. Eighty-two percent of patients in the Walter Reed Hospital experience [79] survived three years with no evidence of disease. As mentioned previously, 86% of patients at Royal Marsden Hospital remained NED provided the metastatic deposits measured 2.0 cm or less.

Radiotherapy is a viable alternative to lymphadenectomy in clinical Stage I and early Stage II. This would particularly apply to younger patients who are interested in retaining fertility. While an overwhelming majority of patients who undergo bilateral retroperitoneal lymphadenectomy develop ejaculatory impotence, most patients who receive radiotherapy to the retroperitoneum remain fertile [89, 90].

A high percentage of patients with advanced Stage II and Stage III patients fail with disseminated metastases and therefore need adjuvant systemic chemotherapy. Prophylactic (in advanced Stage II) and therapeutic in Stage III, supradiaphragmatic irradiation is rarely employed in testicular carcinomas. It is not only of limited value but would also compromise tolerance to systemic chemotherapy.

Lymphadenectomy and retroperitoneal irradiation have often been combined. Hussey [86, 87] found a remarkably decreased incidence of retroperitoneal recurrences in patients with advanced Stage II disease who received preoperative irradiation. There was also a suggestion of an improvement in survival in patients who were treated preoperatively.

Combination of radiotherapy and lymphadenectomy in the form of a so-called 'sandwich technique' has been used widely. Patients receive approximately 2500 rad in three weeks to the retroperitoneal lymph nodes followed by lymphadenectomy and (usually if the nodes were found positive) postoperative irradiation to a dose of about 2000 rad. A randomized trial has been carried out at Walter Reed Hospital [79] comparing this method with radiotherapy only in Stage I and II. The results in both groups were comparable, showing no definite advantage of 'sandwich technique' over radiotherapy alone.

REFERENCES

1. Waters CA: Preoperative irradiation of cortical renal tumors. Am J Roentgenol 33:149, 1935.
2. Riches E: The place of irradiation. JAMA 204:230–233, 1968.
3. Riches EW, Griffiths IH, Thackray AC: New Growths of the kidney and ureter. Br J Urol 23:297–339, 1951.
4. Flocks RH, Kadesky MC: Malignant neoplasms of the kidney: An analysis of 353 patients followed five years or more. J Urol 79:196–201, 1958.

5. Van der Werf-Messing B: Carcinoma of the kidney. Cancer 32:1056–1061, 1973.
6. Rafla S: Renal cell carcinoma. Cancer 25:26–40, 1970.
7. Peeling WB, Mantel BS, Shepheard BGF: Post-operative irradiation in the treatment of renal cell carcinoma. Br J Urol 23–31, 1978.
8. Finney R: An evaluation of postoperative radiotherapy in hypernephroma treatment – a clinical trial. Cancer 32:1332–1340, 1973.
9. Brady LW, Gislason GJ, Faust DS, Kazem I, Antoniades J, Davis JA: Radiation therapy – a valuable adjunct in the management of carcinoma of the ureter. JAMA 206:2871–2874, 1968.
10. Almgard LE, Freedman D, Ljungqvist A: Carcinoma of the ureter. Scand J Urol Nephrol 7:165–167, 1973.
11. Batata MA, Whitmore WF, Hilaris BS, Tokita N, Grabstald H: Primary carcinoma of the ureter: A prognostic study. Cancer 35:1626–1632, 1975.
12. Babaian RJ, Johnson DE: Primary carcinoma of the ureter. J Urol 123:357–359, 1980.
13. Miller LS, Johnson DE: Megavoltage irradiation for bladder cancer: Alone, postoperative, or preoperative. Seventh Natl. Cancer Conf Proc 1973, pp. 771–782.
14. Goffinet DR, Schneider MJ, Glatstein EJ, Ludwig H, Ray GR, Dunnick NR, Bagshaw MA: Bladder Cancer: Results of radiation therapy in 384 patients. Radiology 117:149–153, 1975.
15. Wallace DM, Bloom HJG: The management of deeply infiltrating (T3) bladder carcinoma: Controlled trial of radical radiotherapy versus preoperative radiotherapy and radical cystectomy (First Report). Br J Urol 48:587–594, 1976.
16. Galleher EP, Young JD, Campbell EW: Wizenberg MJ, Jacobs JA, Millstein DI: Pre-cystectomy irradiation for carcinoma of the bladder: 17 year experience. J urol 118:179–183, 1977.
17. Johnson DE, Lamy S, Bracken RB: Salvage cystectomy after radiation failure in patients with bladder carcinoma. South Med J 70:1279–1281, 1977.
18. Bloom HJG: Multi-modal treatment of deep infiltrating (T3) Bladder cancer. In: Hazra TA, ed., Progress in Clinical and Biological Research. Vol. 25. New York: M.C. Beachley, 1978, pp. 117–134.
19. Prout GR: The role of surgery in the potentially curative treatment of bladder carcinoma. Cancer Research 37:2764–2770, 1977.
20. Smith JA, Batata M, Grabstald H, Sogani PC, Herr H, Whitmore WF: Preoperative irradiation and cystectomy for bladder cancer. Cancer (In press).
21. Whitmore WF, Batata MA, Hilaris BS, Reddy GN, Unal A, Ghoneim MA, Grabstald H, Chu F: A comparative study of two preoperative radiation regimens with cystectomy for bladder cancer. Cancer 40:1077–1086, 1977.
22. Whitmore WF, Batata MA, Ghoneim MA, Grabstald H, Unal A: Radical cystectomy with or without prior irradiation in the treatment of bladder cancer. J Urol 118:184–187, 1977.
23. Miller LS: Bladder Cancer. Superiority of preoperative irradiation and cystectomy in clinical stages B2 and C. Cancer 39:973–980, 1977.
24. Van der Werf-Messing B: Carcinoma of the bladder treated by preoperative irradiation followed by cystectomy. Cancer 32:1084–1088, 1973.
25. Prout GR, Slack NH, Bross IDJ: Preoperative irradiation and cystectomy for bladder carcinoma, IV: Results in a selected population. 7th Natl Cancer Conf Proc 1973, pp 783–791.
26. Slack NH, Prout GR: The heterogeneity of invasive bladder carcinoma and different responses to treatment. J Urol 123:644–652, 1979.
27. Mohiuddin M, Kramer S, Newell J, Parson J, Willey A: Combined pre- and postoperative adjuvant radiotherapy in bladder cancer. Cancer (In press).

28. Carlton CE, Hudgins PT, Guerrieo WG, Scott R: Radiotherapy in the management of stage C carcinoma of the prostate. J Urol 116:206–210, 1976.
29. Hilaris BS, Whitmore WF, Batata MA, Barzell W: Behavioral patterns of prostate adenocarcinoma following an I-125 Implant and pelvic node dissection. Int J Radiat Oncol Biol Phys 2:631–637, 1977.
30. Hilaris BS, Whitmore WF, Batata MA, Barzell W, Takita N: I-125 implant of the prostate: Dose-response considerations. Front Radiat Ther 12:82–90, 1978.
31. Hanash KA, Utz DC, Cook EN, Taylor WF, Titus JL: Carcinoma of the prostate: A 15-year follow-up. J Urol 107:450–453, 1972.
32. Perez CA, Walz, BJ, Zivnuska FR, Pilepich MV, Prasad K, Bauer W: Irradiation of carcinoma of the prostate localized to the pelvis: Analysis of tumor response and prognosis. Int J Radiat Oncol Biol Phys 6:555–563, 1980.
33. Cox JD, Stoffel TJ: The significance of needle biopsy after irradiation for stage C adenocarcinoma of the prostate. Cancer 40: 156–160, 1977.
34. Hill DR, Crews QE, Walsh PC: Prostate carcinoma: Radiation treatment of the primary and regional lymphatics. Cancer 34:156–160, 1970.
35. Pilepich MV, Perez CA, Bauer W: Prognostic parameters in radiotherapeutic management of localized carcinoma of the prostate. J Urol 124:485–487, 1980.
36. Ray GR, Cassady JR, Bagshaw MA: Definitive radiation therapy of carcinoma of the prostate. Radiology 106:407–418, 1973.
37. Neglia WJ, Hussey DH, Johnson DE: Megavoltage radiation therapy for carcinoma of the prostate. Int J Radiat Oncol Biol Phys 2:873–882, 1977.
38. Jewett HJ, Eggleston JC Yawn DH: Radical prostatectomy in the management of carcinoma of the prostate: Probable cause of some therapeutic failures. J Urol 107:1034–1040, 1972.
39. Belt E, Schroeder FH: Total perineal prostatectomy for carcinoma of the prostate. J Urol 107:91–96, 1972.
40. Veenema RJ, Gursel EO, Lattimer JK: Radical retropubic prostatectomy for cancer: A 20-year experience. J Urol 117:330–331, 1977.
41. Barzell W, Bean MA, Hilaris BS, Whitmore WF: Prostatic adenocarcinoma: Relationship of grade and local extent to the pattern of metastases. J Urol 118:278–282, 1977.
42. Fowler JE, Barzell W, Hilaris BS, Whitmore WF: Complications of I-125 implantation and pelvic lymphadenectomy in the treatment of prostatic cancer. J Urol 121:447–451, 1979.
43. Herr HW: Preservation of sexual potency in prostatic cancer patients after pelvic lymphadenectomy and retropubic I-125 implantation. J Urol 121:621–623, 1979.
44. Pistenma DA, Ray GR, Bagshaw MA: The role of megavoltage radiation therapy in the treatment of prostatic carcinoma. Seminars in Oncology 3:115–122, 1976.
45. Harisiadis L, Veenema RJ, Senyszyn JJ, Punchner PJ, Tretter P, Romas NA, Chang CH, Lattimer JK, Tannenbaum M: Carcinoma of the prostate: Treatment with external radiotherapy. Cancer 41:2131–2142, 1978.
46. Lipsett JA, Cosgrove MD, Green N, Casagrande JT, Melbye RW, George FW: Factors influencing prognosis in the radiotherapeutic management of carcinoma of the prostate. Int J Radiat Oncol Biol Phys 1:1049–1058, 1976.
47. McGowan DG: Radiation therapy in the management of localized carcinoma of the prostate. Cancer 39:98–103, 1977.
48. Vickery AL, Kerr WS: Carcinoma of the prostate treated by radical prostatectomy. Cancer 16:1598–1608, 1963.
49. Williams J, Marshall VF, Gray GF: Radical perineal prostatectomy with bilateral orchiectomy for carcinoma of the prostate. J Urol 113:380–384, 1975.
50. Grabstald H: Tumors of the urethra in men and women. Cancer 32:1236–1255, 1973.
51. Mandler JI, Pool TL: Primary Carcinoma of the male urethra. J Urol 96:67–72, 1966.

52. Raghavaiah NV: Radiotherapy in the treatment of carcinoma of the male urethra. Cancer 41:1313–1316, 1978.
53. Bracken RB, Johnson DE, Miller LS, Ayala AG, Gomez JJ, Ruthledge E: Primary carcinoma of the female urethra. J Urol 116:188–192, 1976.
54. Antoniades J: Radiation therapy in carcinoma of the female urethra. Cancer 24:70–76, 1969.
55. Chu AM: Female urethral carcinoma. Radiology 107:627–630, 1973.
56. Prempree T, Wizenberg MJ, Scott RM: Radiation treatment of primary carcinoma of the female urethra. Cancer 42:1177–1184, 1978.
57. Staubitz WJ, Carden LM Oberkircher OJ, Lent MH, Murphy WT: Management of urethral carcinoma in the female. J Urol 73:1045–1053, 1955.
58. Taggart CG, Castro JR, Rutledge FN: Carcinoma of the female urethra. Am J Roentgenol 114:145–151, 1972.
59. Grabstald H, Hilaris B, Henschke U, Whitmore WF: Cancer of the female urethra. JAMA 197:835–842, 1966.
60. DeKernion JB, Tynberg P, Persky L, Fegen JP: Carcinoma of the Penis. Cancer 32:1256–1262, 1973.
61. Skinner DG, Leadbetter WF, Kelley SB: The surgical management of squamous cell carcinoma of the penis. J Urol 107:273–277, 1972.
62. Hope-Stone H: Carcinoma of the penis. Proc Royal Soc Med 68:777–779, 1975.
63. Jackson SM: The treatment of carcinoma of the penis. Br J Surg 53:33–35, 1966.
64. Almgard LE, Edsmyr F: Radiotherapy in treatment of patients with carcinoma of the penis. Scand J Urol Nephrol 7:1–5, 1973.
65. Engelstad RB: Treatment of cancer of the penis at the Norwegian Radium Hospital. Radiology 60:801–806, 1948.
66. Ekstrom T, Edsmyr F: Cancer of the penis. Acta Chir Scand 115:23–45, 1958.
67. Gursel EO, Georgountzos C, Uson AC, Melicow MD, Veenema RJ: Urology 1:569–578, 1973.
68. Hardner GJ, Bhanalaph T, Murphy GP, Albert DJ, Moore RH: Carcinoma of the penis. Analysis of therapy in 100 consecutive cases. J Urol 108:428–430, 1972.
69. Baker BH, Spratt JS, Perez-Mesa C, Watson FR, Leduc RJ: Carcinoma of the Penis. J Urol 116:458–461, 1976.
70. Staubitz WJ, Lent MH, Oberkircher OJ: Carcinoma of the penis. Cancer 8:371–378, 1955.
71. Marcial VA, Figueroa-Colon J, Marcial-Rojas RA: Carcinoma of the penis. Radiology 79:209–220, 1962.
72. Murrell DS, Williams JL: Radiotherapy in the treatment of carcinoma of the penis. Br J Urol 37:211–222, 1965.
73. Kelley CD, Arthur K, Rogoff E, Grabstald H: Radiation therapy of penile cancer. Urology 4:571–573, 1974.
74. Haile K, Delclos L: The place of radiation therapy in the treatment of carcinoma of the distal end of the penis. Cancer 45:1980–1984, 1980.
75. Pointon RCS: External beam therapy. Proc Royal Soc Med 68:779–781, 1975.
76. Earle JD, Bagshaw MA, Kaplan HS: Supervoltage radiation therapy of the texticular tumors. Am J Roentgenol 117:653–661, 1973.
77. Van der Werf-Messing B: Radiotherapeutic treatment of testicular tumors. Int J Radiat Oncol Biol Phys 1:235–248, 1976.
78. Lee F, Perez CA: Radiation Therapy in the management of testicular tumors. J Urol 111:201–204, 1974.
79. Maier JG, Mittemeyer B: Carcinoma of the Testis, Cancer 39:981–986, 1977.

80. Peckham MJ, McElwain TJ: Radiotherapy of testicular tumors. Proc Royal Soc Med 67:14–17, 1974.
81. Doornbos JF, Hussey DH, Johnson DE: Radiotherapy for pure seminoma of the testis, Radiology 116:401–404, 1975.
82. Friedman M, Purkayastha MC: Recurrent seminoma: The management of late metastasis, recurrence, or a second primary tumor. Amer J Roentgenol 83:25–42, 1960.
83. Kademian M, Bosch A, Caldwell WL, Jaeschke W: Anaplastic seminoma. Cancer 40:3082–3086, 1977.
84. Maier JG, Sulak MH, Mittemeyer BT: Seminoma of the testis: Analysis of treatment success and failure, Amer J Roentgenol 120:596–602, 1968.
85. Johnson DE, Gomez JJ, Ayala, AG: Anaplastic seminoma, J Urol 114:80–82, 1975.
86. Hussey DH: Experience with preoperative radiotherapy and lymphadenectomy for germinal cell tumors of the testis other than pure seminoma. In: Johnson DE, Samuels ML, eds.: Cancer of the genitourinary tract, New York, Raven Press 1979, pp. 149–158.
87. Hussey DH, Luk KH, Johnson DE: The role of radiation therapy in the treatment of germinal cell tumors of the testis other than pure seminoma. Radiology 123:175–180, 1977.
88. Tyrrell CJ, Peckham MJ: The response of lymph node metastases of testicular teratoma to radiation therapy. Br J Urol 48:363–370, 1976.
89. Orecklin JR, Kaufman JJ, Thompson RW: Fertility in patients treated for malignant testicular tumors. J Urol 109:293–295, 1973.
90. Smithers DW, Wallace DM, Ausin DE: Fertility after unilateral orchidectomy and radiotherapy for patients with malignant tumors of the testis. Br Med J 4:77–79, 1973.

9. Current Status of Androgen Receptor Measurements in Prostatic Cancer

JOHN TRACHTENBERG

1. INTRODUCTION

Prostatic cancer is the second most common malignancy in American males and the majority of patients are found to have advanced stages of the disease at the time of its discovery [1, 2]. Since the discovery by Huggins and Hodges that prostatic cancer is an androgen-dependent tumor the treatment of advanced prostatic cancer has centered on methods designed to decrease circulating levels of androgen [3]. The majority of patients so treated, either by castration or by the administration of pharmacologic doses of estrogens, display both subjective and objective evidence of tumor regression, but the duration of response to these modes of therapy is variable [4]. Ten percent of patients with metastatic prostatic cancer treated by hormonal manipulations survive less than one year, 50% survive less than three years, and 10% survive more than ten years [5]. Alternative methods of treatment such as chemotherapy are usually reserved for patients who fail to respond to a trial of hormonal therapy [6]. Thus, if one could identify those patients unlikely to obtain a prolonged response to hormonal manipulation they could be spared the side-effects of an unsuccessful course of hormonal therapy and instead be started earlier on alternate modes of therapy at a time when they are most likely to tolerate and thus possibly more likely to respond to these treatment. While a variety of clinical, histological, and biochemical parameters have been studied to predict the biological response of prostatic cancer none have proven completely satisfactory [7–9].

Current concepts of steroid hormone action dictate the presence of specific intracellular proteins – receptors – for hormonally mediated events to occur. Steroid, not bound to serum protein, passively diffuses across the cell membrane and in the cytoplasm of target cells binds to receptor proteins of high affinity, narrow specificity and limited capacity. The steroid receptor

D.F. Paulson (ed.), Genitourinary Cancer 1, 239-250. All rights reserved.

complex then undergoes a conformational change termed activation, translocates into the nucleus and binds to an acceptor site in the chromatin. It is there that transcription occurs with the initiation of protein synthesis and tissue growth [10, 11].

In certain experimental models of endocrine responsive tissue such as rat uterus, vagina and chemically induced mammary tumors, the presence of specific hormone receptors strongly correlates with hormonal responsiveness [12, 13]. Conversely, in the absence of functioning receptor proteins target cells are insensitive. This has been demonstrated in the kidney of the tfm/y mouse and the preputial gland of the tfm/y rat where androgen receptors are absent and in rat mammary cancer where estrogen receptors are absent and the tissues are thus insensitive to regulation by effector steroid [14, 15]. These observations have been successfully translated into clinical practice for the treatment of advanced human mammary cancer. Estrogen receptor content of breast carcinoma has been found not only to identify the hormonal dependence of that tumor, but also to provide a useful prognostic index in selected groups of patients [16].

Because prostatic cancer is an androgen-dependent tumor, a vigorous investigative effort has thus been expended to determine if, as in breast cancer, the prostatic content of steroid receptors would correlate with the hormonal dependence and duration of response to hormonal therapy of this tumor.

2. BASIC PRINCIPLES

Testosterone, the principal circulating androgen, enters the prostatic cell through nonenergy dependent processes and is then irreversibly reduced to dihydrotestosterone (DHT) by membrane-bound NADPH-dependent Δ4-3-ketosteroid 5 oxidoreductase (5 ∝ reductase) [17, 18]. DHT may be further metabolized into other 5 ∝ reduced products whose exact function and fate are less well defined [19]. In the cytoplasm dihydrotestosterone encounters macromolecular binding proteins (receptors) of high affinity (Kd of approximately 10^{-9} molar) and narrow specificity. On sucrose density gradient centrifugation this receptor protein sediments in a heterogeneous aggragated form in low salt solutions not containing glycerol; in the presence of glycerol it sediments at 8S [20]. The receptor can be converted to a 3-4S form by heating briefly to 30 °C or by increasing the ionic concentration of the containing buffer to 0.4–0.6 molar KCl [20]. The receptor precipates in the 0–30% ammonium sulfate fraction, has an acidic isoelectric point (pI 5.8), is precipated by protamine sulfate and when complexed to DHT binds to DNA cellulose [21]. The DHT-receptor complex then undergoes a temperature dependent translocation to the nucleus. It has been demonstrated that following brief warming of the cytosolic androgen-receptor complex to 37 °C *in vitro* there is a physical alteration in structure with a reduction in its sedimentation coefficient from 8 to 3–4S and an alteration in its isoelectric point [22]. Because the physical properties of the activated cytoplasmic receptor are identical to the sedimentation coefficient and isoelectric point of the nuclear receptor it is assumed that the cytoplasmic receptor is transferred to the nucleus.

Once in the nucleus, the dihydrotestosterone-receptor complex can be demonstrated to be both tightly bound (salt resistant) and loosely bound (salt extractable) to chromatin [23]. The biological significance of this partition of nuclear steroid receptor complex content is as yet unclear but the dihydrotestosterone receptor complex is felt to exert its major influence at this stage with the initiation of transcription, the formation of messenger RNA, the increase in protein synthesis and tissue growth [10, 11].

Although the quantitation of androgen receptor content in prostatic tissue has proven attractive to many investigators as a means to better understand the hormonal regulation of this tissue, many obstacles have hampered the development of reliable assay techniques for the measurement of prostatic androgen receptor content. One problem has been the contamination of tissue preparations with Testosterone-Estradiol Binding Globulin (TeBG), a serum carrier protein that binds to dihydrotestosterone with an affinity similar to that of the intracellular androgen receptor. TeBG is a 4–5S protein that has a neutral isoelectric point and is not precipitated by protamine sulphate, but is precipitated by 50% ammonium sulfate [21].

Because contamination of prostatic tissue with as little as 4% serum may add as much as 2000 femtomoles of high affinity androgen binding per gram of tissue, it became essential to develop techniques to distinguish between binding to the androgen receptor from binding to TeBG. Therefore, in order to separate these two proteins many methods were devised to exploit the physical chemical differences between TeBG and the androgen receptor. These methods include gel electrophoresis, ammonium sulfate or protamine sulfate precipitation, density gradient centrifugation, ion exchange techniques and gel filtration [24–28]. Although all of these methods have certain merits, none have proven totally acceptable [29].

Other complicating factors in the development of an acceptable assay include the high endogenous content of dihydrotestosterone in prostatic tissue necessitating the development of exchange type assays and the abundant quantity of enzymes within the prostate capable of degrading both steroid and receptor.

The introduction and subsequent popularization by Bonne and Raynaud of a radio-labelled potent synthetic androgen of high specific activity (6-

7-^{3}H) methyltrienolone (R 1881) has largely eliminated the need for the above separation techniques [30]. R 1881 binds with high affinity to the androgen receptor but does not bind to TeBG. Furthermore, because (^{3}H) R 1881 is not significantly metabolized in prostatic tissue it serves both as a stable source of steroid to bind the receptor and as a known source of radioactivity, not an unknown metabolic product, in assays that depend on measured radioactivity to quantitate binding [31]. Thus, utilizating R 1881 in an exchange assay under conditions that minimized degradation of the receptor it has been possible to characterize the androgen receptor in human prostatic tissue.

3. DEVELOPMENT OF A RELIABLE MEASURE OF ANDROGEN RECEPTOR CONTENT IN PROSTATIC TISSUE

Minimal criteria for the demonstration of a steroid receptor are high affinity and limited capacity binding and steroid specificity. Utilizing the cytostolic and 0.6M KCl nuclear extracts of benign prostatic hyperplasia tissue (BPH) as a source of androgen receptor Walsh and colleagues demonstrated high affinity and limited capacity specific binding of R 1881 by Scatchard analysis [32–34]. In ten determinations the number of apparent binding sites in cytostol was found to be 48 ± 7 (mean $\pm$ S.E.M.) femtomoles/mg protein and in nuclear extract 104 ± 10 femtomoles/mg protein. The equilibrium dissociation constant for cytosol was 1.3 ± 0.2 nM and for nuclear extract was 2.8 ± 0.3 nM. The steroid specificity of R 1881 binding was examined utilizing dihydrotestosterone and progestrone as competitors. Cytosol and nuclear extract were incubated with 10 nM (^{3}H) R 1881 alone or in the presence of 10-, 25-, or 50-fold excess nonradioactive steroid. Nonspecific binding, defined as binding not displaced by the addition of 50-fold excess of nonradioactive R 1881 was subtracted in all instances. A concentration of R 1881 required to displace 50% of specific binding was determined and assigned a relative binding affinity of 100. The concentration of other competing steroids causing 50% displacement was compared to this and constituted their relative binding affinity. By this technique high affinity binding of (^{3}H) R 1881 in nuclear extract was shown to possess the steroid specificity of an androgen receptor whereas the binding in cytosol demonstrated the primary characteristics of a progesterone receptor. The apparent binding of R 1881 to both progesterone- and androgen-binding proteins in prostatic tissue thus further complicated the measurement of androgen receptor content in human BPH cytosol and emphasized the need for careful steroid specificity studies when utilizing R 1881. Attempts to improve the androgen specificity of R 1881 binding by masking the progesterone receptor with high concentrations of progestins proved unsuccessful, however, because the majority of progestins evaluated also demonstrated binding to the androgen receptor. Triamcinolone acetonide, a synthetic glucocorticoid, binds to both the progesterone and glucocorticoid receptor but does not bind to the androgen receptor. In molar concentrations of 500–1000 times that of R 1881, triamcinolone acetonide effectively inhibits the binding of R 1881 to the progesterone receptor without interfering with its binding to the androgen receptor [33, 35]. Steroid specificity studies repeated in the cytostol of prostatic tissue in the presence of 10 micromolar triamcinolone acetonide clearly demonstrated the androgen-like characteristics of R 1881 binding.

In paired experiments in which R 1881 binding was measured in cytostol in the presence or absence of triamcinolone acetonide, the number of binding sites was reduced 60% by the addition of triamcinolone acetonide. Similar experiments conducted with nuclear extract did not show any decrease in R 1881 binding. The binding of R 1881 to human prostatic cytostol in the presence of 1000-fold molar excess of triamcinolone acetonide relative to R 1881 is of high affinity, limited capacity and specific for androgen binding and thus is an appropriate ligand system to measure androgen receptor content in human prostatic cytostol.

The human prostate possesses an high endogenous content of androgens. Thus, the majority of prostatic androgen receptor sites are thought to be occupied by androgen. In order to quantitate receptor content, unoccupied receptor sites and those sites already occupied by native androgen must therefore be measured. Exchange assays have thus been developed to measure both these sites. To determine the optimal conditions under which total receptor sites could be quantitated, a time/temperature evaluation of both association and dissociation of (^{3}H) R 1881 binding was carried out. When cytosol containing a 1000-fold excess of triamcinolone acetonide or nuclear extract was incubated at 4 °C with 10 nM (^{3}H) R 1881, maximal specific binding was achieved at 20–24 h. When incubations were performed at 15 °C for 24 h the number of specific binding sites in cytosol was less than the binding site number measured at 4 °C; in nuclear extract the content was similar at both temperatures. To determine the stability of the receptor, incubations were performed for an additional 20 h. Although this resulted in a small reduction in the cytosolic receptor (11% at 4 °C and 9% at 15 °C), there was no decrease in the nuclear receptor. To evaluate the dissociation of bound androgen, 100-fold nonradioactive R 1881 was added to cytosol that had been previously incubated for 24 h with 10 nM (^{3}H) R 1881 in the presence of 10 micromolar triamcinolone acetonide. At 4 °C, by 20 h, 85% of the radiolabelled androgen had been displaced by R 1881; similar findings were noted at 15 °C. In nuclear extract, complete dissociation occurred at both temperatures by 20 h. Thus, total androgen receptor content of prostatic cytosol in nuclear extract can be determined utilizing assay conditions of 4 °C for 20 h.

4. DEVELOPMENT OF MICROASSAY

The majority of patients who will be candicates for the clinical quantitation of prostatic androgen receptor are likely to suffer from metastatic prostatic cancer and, thus, would not be amenable to surgical procedures that would allow for the collection of large quantities of tissue. Consequently, an assay was developed that would yield accurate estimates of androgen receptor content from as little as 200 mg of tissue [33]. This amount of tissue can be readily obtained at the time of needly biopsy for diagnostic purposes. As previously demonstrated in detail, a single saturating dose technique was developed utilizing incubations of 10 nM (^{3}H) R 1881 for nuclear extract and 5 nM (^{3}H) R 1881 plus 5 micromollar triamcinolone acetonide for cytosol at 4 °C for 20 h. Briefly, tissue frozen in liquid nitrogen was pulverized with a tissue pulverizer (Thermovac Industries Corporation, Copiague, NY). The powdered tissue was added to ten volumes of TEDG buffer (10 mM Tris, 1.5 mM EDTA, 1 mM dithiothreitol, 10% (weight/volume) glycerol, pH 7.4, 22 °C) and homogenized in an all-glass Duall homogenizer (Kontes Company, Vineland, N.J.) for three periods of 5–10 s (pestle speed 1350 rpm) with a cooling-off period of 60 s at 4 °C between. An aliquot (0.5 ml) was saved for DNA determination. The homogenate was then centrifuged at 800 g for 20 min (4 °C). The resulting supernatant was decanted and then centrifuged at 104 000 **g** for 1 h at 4 °C to yield a supernant cytosol fraction. The nuclear myofibrillar pellet obtained from the 800 **g** centrifugation was washed twice in two volumes of TEDG buffer (800 **g**, 15 min) and resuspended in ten volumes of TEDK buffer (10 mM Tris, 1.5 mM EDTA, 1 mM dithiothreitol, 0.6 M KCl, pH 7.4 at 22 °C). This suspension was homogenized with a Polytron PT-10-35 (5 s, setting 5) (Brinkman Instrument Inc., Westbury, NY) and centrifuged for 1 hour at 4 °C at 104 000 **g** to yield a supernatant nuclear extract.

Protein concentration was determined rapidly by measuring absorbance at 230 nm and 260 nm and correcting the values to mg/ml: $(A230 \times 184) - (A260 \times 76.1) = $ mg protein/ml [36]. An appropriate quantity of buffer was added to give a protein concentration of 1–2 mg/ml for nuclear extract and 2–3 mg/ml for cytosol. DNA was measured by the method of Burton using calf thymus DNA as standard [37].

Two hundred µl of cytosol or nuclear extract was incubated in triplicate with (^{3}H) R 1881 (5 nM for cytosol, 10 nM for nuclear extract) with and without a 50-fold excess of R 1881. All cytosol incubations were performed in the presence of 1000-fold molar excess triamcinolone acetonide. After an incubation period of 20 h at 4 °C, 500 μl of a 0.25 % dextran-coated charcoal suspension (0.25 % acid washed activated charcoal, 0.0025 % dextran in TED buffer) were added to each assay tube. The tubes were shaken for 15 min at 4 °C, followed by centrifugation for 20 min at 5000 **g**. The entire supernatant was transferred to a liquid scintillation vial and the radioactivity counted in 10 ml of ACS^R (Amersham/Searle Corporation, Arlington Heights, IL). The data were expressed as fmol/mg DNA.

When this assay was applied to needle biopsy specimens, the estimates of androgen receptor content correlated well with matched evaluations of bulk tissue performed by saturation analysis studied by Scatchard plots. The number of cytosolic androgen receptor sites estimated by the single saturating dose determination averaged 75% ($\pm$20 S.D.: range 51–101; r = 0.82) of the number estimated from Scatchard plots. In nuclear extracts, the binding sites estimated from a single saturating dose determination averaged 80 % ($\pm$19 S.D.; range 72–117; r = 0.91). Although these data indicate that assays performed on needle biopsy specimens provide a modest underestimation of the actual number of binding sites, in relative terms, this technique provides representive information for clinical comparisons.

5. APPLICATION OF MICROASSAY TO HUMAN PROSTATIC ADENO CARCINOMA

Using the above microassay for the measurement of prostatic androgen receptor content a prospective trial was initiated to determine the correlation between pretreatment tumor androgen receptor content and duration of response to hormonal therapy of patients with metastatic prostatic cancer [38]. Twenty-three patients were thus submitted to percutaneous biopsy of their primary prostatic tumor prior to initiation of hormonal therapy for symptomatic disease. No patient had received anti-androgen therapy before. The patients were followed for 6–40 months until relapse or death. Every patient demonstrated an initial objective response to treatment. The duration of this response, however, was variable. Because all tumors contained androgen receptors and because all patients responded to treatment, an attempt was made to establish the relationship between the duration of response and androgen receptor content. The correlation coefficient comparing cytosolic or nuclear androgen receptor content and duration of response was −0.096 and 0.370 respectively. While these values demonstrate a weak negative correlation between cytosolic androgen receptor content and a weak positive correlation between nuclear receptor content and duration of response, neither was statistically significant. No significant correlation existed between histological grade as scored by the Gleason System and duration of response; similar results have been reported by others [39].

In this study cytosolic androgen receptor content did not correlate with the duration of response to hormonal therapy. These results are in accord with the report of Wagner and Schulze, and DeVogt and Dingjan who, using agar gel electrophoretic methods, failed to demonstrate a relationship between cytosolic androgen receptor content and qualitative response to hormonal therapy [40, 41]. However, Ekman *et al.* demonstrated that cytostolic methyltrienolone binding did correlate with a response to hormonal treatment [42]. Methyltrienolone binds to both the androgen and progesterone receptor in human prostatic cytostol. Therefore, it is possible that this correlation resulted from the measurement of the cytostol progesterone receptor, implying that progesterone receptor content may represent a biochemical discriminant of androgen sensitivity.

In early studies attempting to establish the relationship between estrogen receptor content and the estrogen dependence of human breast cancer it was recognized that these tumors segregated into receptor-rich and receptor-poor populations [43]. Using empirically derived criteria to define receptor-rich and receptor-poor tumors estrogen receptor assays were then demonstrated to predict correctly a clinical response to hormonal therapy in approximately two thirds of patients with receptor rich tumors and essentially all those of the receptor-poor group [44]. Those patients with receptor-rich tumors tended to respond to hormonal manipulation while those with receptor-poor cancers were found to derive little benefit from endocrine manipulation and were felt to be better treated directly with cytotoxic chemotherapy [45].

Using a similar rationale the above patients with prostatic cancer were empirically divided into receptor-rich and receptor-poor groups on the basis of nuclear androgen receptor content. The 'critical level' assigned to this tumor system was 110 femtomoles/mg DNA. All patients with prostatic nuclear androgen receptor content of less than 110 femtomoles/mg DNA were thus termed receptor-poor and they all relapsed from hormonal treatment within one year. Conversely, 60% of patients with receptor-rich tumors (>110 femtomoles/mg DNA) responded for more than 12 months. The mean duration of response of patients with receptor-poor tumors was 6.9 months which was significantly less than the 15.5 month duration of response of the group of patients with receptor-rich tumors.

These data bear a strong similarity to the large body of knowledge already accumulated relating estrogen receptor content of breast cancer and response to hormonal manipulation [44]. In this study of patients with metastatic prostatic cancer, low nuclear androgen receptor content identified a population of patients who responded poorly to hormonal therapy. At present, when a diagnosis of metatastic carcinoma of the prostate is made, hormonal theapy is withheld until the patient develops symptoms and alternate forms of treatment, such as chemotherapy are reserved until patients fail to respond to endocrine treatment. At this point these patients are usually weak and quite ill and often are unable to tolerate chemotherapy. These data suggest that patients with receptor poor tumors might be candidates for early treatment with chemotherapy as they are unlikely to derive significant benefit from endocrine manipulation.

If future studies involving larger groups of patients confirm the above hypothesis, then a significant change in the treatment of patients with metastatic prostatic cancer could be initiated. Symptomatic patients with low prostatic nuclear androgen receptor content would be started immediately on chemotherapy, whereas patients with high levels of nuclear androgen receptor content would be managed by conventional endocrine manipulation. This change in patient management combined with the utilization of effective chemotherapeutic agents would hopefully improve the survival of patients with prostatic cancer.

6. FUTURE TRENDS

Efforts are being directed at improving the sensitivity and reliability of assays of prostatic androgen receptor content. Techniques to enhance conventional radioreceptor assays have centered about methods to prevent receptor losses during homogenization and further processing of prostatic tissue. Recent reports suggest that molybdate containing buffers and the use of proteolytic inhibitors as well as the use of hydroxylapatite adsorption techniques to separate free and bound steroid may be of use in this regard [46]. Novel techniques to quantitate receptor content are also under development. Jensen has described several monoclonal antibodies directed against the human cytosolic estrogen receptor and has suggested various techniques (immunoradiometric or enzyme-linked immunosorbent) whereby these antibodies could be used to quantitate receptor content [45]. Similar efforts are being made to develop immunoassays of the androgen receptor.

7. SUMMARY

Prostatic cancer is a major cause of death due to malignancy in the ageing male population. Although hormonal manipulation appears effective in the treatment of advanced stages of this disease a significant proportion of patients with this disease derive little benefit while sustaining all the side-effects associated with hormonal therapy. Androgen receptor assays have been developed, verified and are now under clinical trial to assess the correlation between androgen receptor content and response to hormonal therapy. Present studies indicate that low nuclear androgen receptor content identifies a population of patients unlikely to benefit from hormonal therapy. If further trials using either conventional assays or more refined techniques confirm the above, then those patients identified as unlikely to enjoy a prolonged response to hormonal therapy might be commenced on alternate modes of therapy at a time when they are more likely to respond to this therapy. This basic change in the treatment of advanced prostatic cancer will hopefully improve the survival of patients so affected.

ACKNOWLEDGEMENTS

Much of the data presented in this article originated in the laboratories of Dr. Patrick Walsh at Johns Hopkins Hospital, Baltimore, MD. It is through his courtesy that this information is presented.

REFERENCES

1. American Cancer Society: Cancer Statistics. Cancer 30:24, 1980.
2. Klein LA: Prostatic Carcinoma: N Engl J Med 300:824, 1979.
3. Huggins C, Hodges CV: Studies on prostatic cancer. I. The effect of castration, of estrogen and of androgen injection on serum phosphates in metastatic carcinoma of the prostate. Cancer Res 1:293, 1941.
4. Scott WW, Menon M, Walsh PC: Hormonal Therapy of prostatic cancer. Cancer 45:1929, 1980.
5. Blackard CE, Byar DP, Jordan WP: Orchiectomy for advanced prostatic carcinoma. A re-evaluation. Urology 1:553, 1973.
6. Resnick MI, Grayhack JT: Treatment of stage IV carcinoma of the prostate. Urol Clin North Am 2:141, 1975.
7. Ray Gr, Pistenma DA, Castellino RA, Kepson RL, Bagshow MA: Operative staging of apparently localized adenocardinoma of the prostate. Cancer 38:73, 1976.
8. Seal US, Doe RP, Byar DP, Corle MS: Response of plasma fibrinogen and plasminogen to hormone treatment and the relation of pre-treatment value to mortality in patients with prostatic cancer. Cancer 38:1108, 1976.
9. Bailer JC, Mellinger GT, Gleason DF: Survival rates of patients with prostatic cancer, tumor stage, and differentiation: preliminary report. Cancer Chemother Rep 50:129, 1966.
10. Baxter JD, Funder JW: Hormone receptors. N Engl J Med 301:1149, 1979.
11. Gorski J, Gannon F: Current models of steroid hormone action: A critique. Ann Rev Physiol 38:425, 1976.

12. Jensen EV, Block GE, Smith S, Kyser K, De Sombre ER: In: estrogen target tissues and (Dao TL, ed.) Chicago: University of Chicago Press, 1972, pp. 23–57.
13. McGuire WL, Huff K, Jennings A, Chamness GC: Mammary carcinoma: a specific biochemical defect in autonomous tumors. Science 173:335, 1971.
14. Bullock LP, Bardin CW: Androgen receptors in mouse kidney: a study of male, female and androgen-insensitive (tfm/y) mice. Endocrinology 94:746, 1974.
15. Bullock L, Bardin CW: Decreased dihydrotestosterone retention by preputial gland nuclei from the androgen insensitive pseudohermaphrodite rat. J Clin Endrocrinol Metab 31:113, 1970.
16. De Sombre ER, Carbone PP, Jensen EV, MvGuire WL, Wells SA, Jr: Wittliff JL, Lipsett MB: Steroid receptors in breast cancer. N Engl J Med 301:1011, 1979.
17. Bruchovsky M, Wilson JD: The conversion of testoterone to 5a-androstan-17B-ol-3one by rat prostate in vivo and in vitro. J Biol Chem 243:2012, 1968.
18. Bruchovsky M, Wilson JD: The intranuclear binding to testosterone and 5a-adrostan-17B-ol-3-one by rat prostate. J Biol Chem 243:5953, 1968.
19. Isaacs JT, McDermott IR, Coffey DS: Characterization of two new enzymatic activities of the rat ventral prostate: 5a-androstane-3B-, 17B-Diol 6a-Hydrozylase and 5a-androstane-3B, 17B-diol 7a-Hydroxylase. Steroids 33:6:675, 1979.
20. Hoisaeter PA: The androgen cytosol receptor in the ventral prostate of the rat. Biochim Biophy Acta 317:492, 1973.
21. Menon M, Tananis CE, McLoughlin MG, Walsh PC: Androgen receptors in human prostatic tissue. Cancer Treat Rep 61:265, 1977.
22. Mainwaring WIP, Mangan FR, Wilce PA, Milroy EJG: Androgens 1. Review of current research on the binding and mechanism of action of androgenic steroids notably 5α dihydrotestosterone. In: Receptors for Reproductive Homones. O'Malley BW, Means AR, eds.) New York: Plenum, 1973, pp. 197–231.
23. Barrak ER, Coffey DS: The specific binding of estrogen and androgens to the nuclear matrix of sex hormone responsive tissues. J Biol Chem 255(15):7265, 1980.
24. Wagner RK, Schulze KH, Jungblut PW: Estrogen and androgen receptor in human prostate and prostatic tumor tissue. Acta Endocrinol (Suppl.) (Kbh) 193:52, 1975.
25. Fang S, Jsu RS: Characterization of androgen binding components in human prostate cytosol. Fed Proc 34:279, 1975.
26. Menon M, Tananis CE, McLoughlin MG *et al.*: The measurement of androgen receptors in human prostatic tissue utilizing sucrose density gradient centrifugation and a protamine precipitation assay. J Urol 117:392, 1977.
27. Hsu RS, Middleton RC, Fang S: Androgen receptors in human prostates. In: Normal and Abnormal Growth of the Prostate. (Goland M, ed) Springfield: Charles C Thomas, 1975, pp.663–675.
28. Geller J, Cantor T, Albert J: Evidence for a specific dihydrotestosterone-binding cytosol receptor in human prostate. J Clin Endocrinol Metab 41:854, 1975.
29. Menon M, Tananis C, McLoughlin MG, Walsh PC: Androgen receptors in human prostatic tissue: a review. Cancer Treat Rep 61:265, 1977.
30. Bonne C, Raynaud JP: Assay of androgen binding sites by exchange with methyltrienolone (R 1881). Steroids 27:497, 1976.
31. Snochowski M, Pousette A, Ekman P, Bression D, Anderson L, Hagberg B, Sustafsson JA: Characterization and measurement of the androgen receptor in human benign prostatic hyperplasia and prostatic cancer. J Clin Endocrinol Metab 45:720, 1977.
32. Menon M, Tananis CE, Hicks LL, Hawkins EF, McLoughlin MG, Walsh PC: Characterization of the binding of a potent synthetic androgen, methyltrienolone (R 1881) to human tissues. J Clin Invest 61:150, 1978.

33. Hicks LL, Walsh PC: A microassay for the measurement of androgen receptors in human prostatic tissue. Steroids 33:389, 1979.
34. Walsh PC, Hicks LL: Prostate cancer and hormone receptors. In: Characterization and measurement of androgen receptors in human prostatic tissue. Murphy GP, Sandberg AA, eds.) New York: Alan R Liss, 1979, p. 51.
35. Zava DT, Landrum B, Horwitz KB, McGuire WL: Androgen receptor assay with (^{3}H) methyltrienolone (R 1881) in the presence of progesterone receptors. Endocrinology 104(4):1007, 1979.
36. Kalk VF, Bernlohr RW: A 260/230 method for the determination of protein concentration in the presence of nucleic acids. Fed Proc 34:546, 1975.
37. Burton K: A study of the conditions and mechanism of the diphenylamine reaction for the colorometric estimation of deoxyribunucleic acid. Biochem J 62:315, 1956.
38. Trachtenberg J, Walsh PC: Androgen receptors and response to hormonal therapy in advanced prostatic cancer. J Urol 1981. (In press.)
39. Hovespian JA, Byar DP: The Veterans Administration Cooperative Research Group: Quantitative radiology for staging and proganosis of patients with advanced prostatic carcinoma. Urology 14:145, 1979.
40. Wagner RK, Schulze KH: Clinical relevance of androgen receptor content in human prostatic carcinoma. Acta Endocrinol 215 (Suppl.): 139, 1978.
41. De Voogt HJ, Dingjan P: Steroid receptors in human prostatic cancer. A preliminary evaluation. Urol Res 6:151, 1978.
42. Ekman P, Snochowski M, Zetterberg A, Hogberg B, Gustafsson JA: Steroid receptor content in human prostatic carcinoma and response to endocrine therapy. Cancer 44:1173, 1979.
43. Jensen EV, Smith S, DeSombre ER: Hormone dependency in breast cancer. J Steroid Biochem 7:911, 1876.
44. DeSombre ER, Greene GL, Jensen EV: Estrophilin and endocrine responsiveness of breast cancer. In: Homones, receptors and breast cancer. (McGuire WL,ed.) New York: Raven Press, 1978, pp. 1–14.
45. Jensen EV: Hormone dependency of breast cancer. Cancer 47:2318, 1981.
46. Trachtenberg J, Hicks LL, Walsh PC: Methods for the determination of androgen receptor content in human prostatic tissue. Invest Urol 18:349.

SUBJECT INDEX

2-Acetylaminofluorene, 10
Acid phosphatase, prostatic (PAP), 47, 49, 61, 127, 176
  counterimmunoelectrophoresis for, 127-28
  immunofluorescent assay for, 128
  radioimmunoassay for, 62, 127, 128
Adenocarcinoma of the prostate, *see* Prostatic cancer
Aflatoxin Bl, 15, 30
Alkaline phosphatase, 57, 78
Alpha-fetoprotein (AFP), 47, 64, 65, 95, 172
Alpha-2-globulin, 57, 178, 199
Anaplastic seminoma, 92
Adrogen receptor measurement, 240-44
  future trends in, 247
  microassay for, 244-47
Angioinfarction, in renal cell carcinoma, 201
Aniline dyes, 6
Antibodies, monoclonal, 67
Antigen(s)
  blood-group, 54, 57-59, 85, 193-94
  glycoprotein, 53-54, 85
  major histocompatability complex, 50
  oncodevelopmental, 48-49, *see also* Carcinoembryonic antigen
  tumor-associated, 169-70, 172
    in bladder cader, 183-89
    in nephroblastomas, 198
    in prostatic cancer, 61-64, 174-79
    in renal cell carcinoma, 55-57, 78, 196-98
    in testicular cancer, 64-67
    in transitional cell carcinoma, 57-61
  tumor-specific transplantation, 47-48, 169
  viral, 176
Asbestos, 14
Avian leukosis viruses, 16-17

Bacillus Calmette-Guérin (BCG), 173
  for bladder cancer, 163, 194-95
  for prostatic cancer, 180-82
  for renal cell carcinoma, 201
Balkan endemic neprhopathy, 11
B cells, 170
Benign prostatic hyperlasia, *see* Prostatic cancer
Benzo (a)pyrene, 22
Beta-aminoisobutyrate (BAIB), 52, 60
Beta-glucuronidase, 60
Biologic markers, *see* Tumor markers
Bladder cancer
  benign paillomas, 82
  etiologic factors in, 5, 6, 8-11
  and herpes virus, 6
  immunotherapy in, 194-95
  impairment of host immune mechanism in, 189-92
  prognostic indicators in, 81-86
  radiotherapy in, 219-23
  role of chemical agents in, 6-8
  tumor-associated antigents in, 183-89, 192-94
Bladder cancer, superficial
  characteristics of, 143
  immunotherapy in, 162-63
  intravesical chemotherapy in, 147-61
  radiotherapy in, 162
  recurrent tumors in, 143-46
Blood-group antigents, 54, 57-59, 85, 193-94

Cadmium, 14, 21-22
Carcinogenesis, 3-5
  viral, 6, 16
Carcinoma of the renal pelvis and ureter, 5, 11, 219
Carcinoembryonic antigen (CEA), 48-49, 56, 59, 53, 127, 175, 192-93, 198

Carcinogenic agents, 1-3, *see also* names of specific agents
Cervical cancer, relation of, to circumcision, 33
Chemicals, as potential carcinogens, 2-3, *see also* specific chemical names
Chemotherapy, *see also* names of specific agents
in renal cell carcinoma, 198
in superficial bladder cancer, 147-61
1-(2-chloroethyl)3-cyclohexyl-1-nitrosourea (CENU), 198
Cholesterol, as tumor marker
in prostatic cancer, 63
in renal cell carcinoma, 56
Choriocarcinoma, 93
Chorionic gonadotropin, *see* Human chorionic gonadotropin
Chromatin, 241
Chromosome pattern, as prognostic indicator in bladder cancer, 83
Chromosome translocations, 13
Cigarette smoking, role of
in bladder cancer, 8-9, 12
in lung cancer, 2
in renal cell carcinoma, 13-14
Circumcision
and penile cancer, 31-32
and relation to carcinoma of uterine cervix, 33
13-*Cis*-retinoic acid, 163
Citrulline, 17
Coffee, and bladder cancer, 10
Coley's toxin, 180
Comparability of patient populations, problems in, 215
Computed tomography, 45
Concanavalin A (Con A), 200
Corynebacterium parvum (*C. parvum*), 173, 182, 194, 195
Counterimmunoelectrophoresis, 127-28
Creatine kinase-BB, 63, 127
Croton oil, 4
Cryotherapy, in prostatic cancer, 180
Cryptorchidism, 28, 30
Cycasin, 15
Cystectomy, 220, 222, 223
Cytomegalovirus (CMV), 25
Cytotoxicity
antibody-dependent cell-mediated, 179, 185, 186, 187, 199-200
assay, 171-72
in bladder cancer, 183-87
in prostatic cancer, 174
in renal cell carcinoma, 196-98

Diabetes, 9, 13
Dicarboxydine, 23
Diet, role of
in bladder cancer, 9, 10, 11
in prostatic cancer, 26-27
in renal cell carcinoma, 14
Dihydrolestosterone (DHT), 240, 241
7,12-dimethylbenz(a)anthracene, 32
N,N-dimethylguanosine, 52
Dimethylnitrosamine (DMN), 16
Dinitrochlorobenzene reactivity, 177, 179-80, 194, 199
DNA, effects of chemical carcinogens on, 4-5
Doxorubicin, 158-59
Dysuria, 152

Embryonal carcinoma, 93
Endocrine therapy, in prostatic cancer, 180, 181
Environment, role of, in carcinogenesis, 1-2, 3
Environmental Protection Agency (EPA), 2
Enzymes, as tumor markers, 49, 78
Epodyl, 159
Erythrocytosis, 78
Erythropoietin, 55
Ethylnitrosourea, 17

Familial susceptibility to cancer, *see* Heredity
Fibrin degradation products, 53, 57, 59
Fibronectin, 53, 64
Flocks and Kadeskey staging system for renal cell carcinoma, 75-76
N-[4-[5-nitro-2-furyl-2-thiazolyl] Formamide FANFT), 189
Fuchsin, 6

Gamma glutamyltranspeptidase (GGT), 56
Genes, immune response, 170
Genetics, role of, in carcinogenesis, *see* Heredity
Gleason histologic grading system for prostatic cancer, 86, 87, 88, 125-26
Glycoproteins, 53-54, 85
Glycosphingolipids, 53, 54
Gold, use of, in interstitial irradiation, 131-32, 224
Gonorrhea, 24

Haptoglobin, 57
Hemorrhage, treatment of, in renal cell carcinoma, 113-14
Hepatosplenomegaly, 78
Heredity, role of
in bladder cancer, 7

in carcinogenesis, 2, 3
in renal cancer, 13
in testicular cancer, 30
in nephroblastoma, 17
Herpes virus, role of
in bladder cancer, 6
in prostatic cancer, 25
in renal cancer, 16
Hormones, *see also* Androgen receptor mesurement
role of, in prostatic cancer, 23
role of, in testicular cancer, 31
steroid, 239-40
Hormone therapy, in treatment of renal cell carcinoma, 116-17
Host immunocompetence, in prostatic cancer, 179-80
Human chorionic gonadotrpin (HCG), 45, 47, 172
in prostatic cancer, 175
in renal cell carcinoma, 57, 78
in testicular cancer, 64, 65, 66, 95
in transitional cell carcinoma, 61
Hybridomas, 67
Hydroxyproline, 53, 63
Hygiene, role of, in penile cancer, 32-33
Hypercalcemia, 56, 114
Hypertension, 78

Immune complexes, 54
Immune response, 170, *see also* Tumor immunology
Immunofluorescent assay for prostatic acid phosphatase, 128
Immunoglobulin A, 198
Immunoglobulin G, 187, 197, 198
Immunoglobulin M, 187, 198
Immunotherapy, 173
in bladder cancer, 162-63, 194-95
in prostatic cancer, 180-83
in renal cell carcinoma, 200-01
Implantation, as cause of recurrent bladder tumors, 146
Impotence, 132, 136, 233
Incontinence, 131, 136
Infarction, percutaneous, in renal cell carcinoma, 113, 116-17
Inguinal hernia, 28
Interferon, 195
Iodine, use of, in interstitial irradiation, 131-32, 224, 227
Irradiation, interstitial, *see* Radiotherapy
Isoenzymes, as tumor markers, 49

Juvenile embryonal cell carcinoma, *see* Yolk sac tumor

Keyhole-limpet hemocyanin, 189
Kidney tumors, *see* Renal cell carcinoma
Killer cells, 170

Lactate dehydrogenase (LDH), 57, 66, 67
Lead, 15
Leukocyte adherence inhibition (LAI), 175, 179, 188
Leukocyte migration inhibition (LMI), 188, 196
Leukopenia, 152
Life-style, and incidence of cancer, 3
Lung cancer, 2
Lymphadenectomy
in prostatic cancer, 123-24, 132
in renal cell carcinoma, 106-09
in testicular cancer, 232, 233
Lymphangiography, 123

Macrophages, 170
Marker proteins, *see* Tumor markers
Megestrol acetate, 201,
Metastatic disease
in prostatic cancer, 124
in renal cell carcinoma, 80, 101-02, 106
Methylcholanthrene, 22, 176, 189
1-Methylinosine, 52
N-methyl-N^1-nitro-N-nitrosoguanidine (MNNG), 22
Methylnitrosourea (MNU), 146
(6-7-^{3}H) methyltrionolone (R 1881), 242, 246
Microassay of prostatic androgen receptor, 244-47
Mitomycin C, 160-61
Mormons, incidence of cancer among, 20
Mutation, 17
Mycotoxins, 3, 15

2-Naphthylamine, 6, 7, 8
Nephrectomy
adjunctive, 114-16
palliative, 113-14, 115
with percutaneous infarction, 116-18
radical, 102-06
Nephroblastoma, 12, 17, 197-98
Nitrosamine carcinogenesis, 15-16
N-nitroso compounds, 8
Nucleosides, methylated, 52

Occupation, and carcinogenic exposure, 3, 608
Oncodevelopmental antigents, 48-49

Oncofetal antigens, *see* Oncodevelopmental antigens
Oncornaviruses, 8
Opium, 9

Pancytopenia, 152
Penectomy, 229
Penile cancer, 31-33, 228-30
Penile implantation, 131
Phenacetin, 11
Phimosis, 32
Phytothemagglutinin (PHA), 177, 178, 190, 191, 199
Placental alkaline phosphatase (PIAP), 66, 67
Polyamines, as tumor markers, 52-53, 57, 59
Polycyclic aromatic hydrocarbon, 4
Polyoma virus, 171
Potassium chloride extracts, cutaneous hypersensitivity reactions to, 174-75
Potency, preservation of, in radiotherapy, 227-28
Proctitis, 132
Prolactin, 57
Prophylaxis
- in bladder cancer, 152-59
- in penile cancer, 230

Prostaglandin E_2, 175
Prostatic cancer
- androgen dependence of, 239, 240
- adrogen receptor measurement in, 240-47
- benign prostatic hyperplasia, 25-26, 174
- clinical staging system for, 121-23,
  - stage A, 133-36
  - stage B, 136-39
- cryotherapy for, 180
- demographic incidence of, 19-21
- etiologic factors in, 23-27
- geographic incidence of, 2, 18
- Gleason histologic grading system for, 86, 87, 88, 125-26
- immunotherapy for, 180-83
- impairment of host immune mechanism in, 26, 177-80
- latent, 18-19
- occupational incidence of, 21-22
- prognostic indicators in, 87-90
- radical prostatectomy for, 130-31, 135, 136, 138, 139, 226
- radiotherapy in, 224-27
- screening methods for, 126-29
- spontaneous, 23
- tumor markers in, 61-64, 174-76

Prostatectomy, radical, 130-31, 135, 136, 138, 139, 226
Proteins
- marker, *see* Tumor markers
- oncodevelopmental, 61
- serum, 50-51, 60

Pseudouridine, 52
Pulmonary metastases, in renal cell carcinoma, 114-15, 117
Pyran copolymer, 182, 183

Radiation, as carcinogenic agent, 1
Radiation therapy, *see* Radiotherapy
Radioimmunoassay (RIA), 46, 62, 127
Radioimmunodetection, 65-66
Radiotherapy
- in bladder cancer, 162, 219-23
- factors determining probability of tumor eradication, 216
- in carcinoma of the renal pelvis and ureter, 219
- in carcinoma of the urethra, 228
- interstitial irradiation, 112-13, 131-32, 162, 224
- in penile cancer, 228-30
- in prostatic cancer, 131-33, 136, 137, 224-27
- in renal cell carcinoma, 111-13, 114, 217-18
- in testicular cancer, 230-33

Radon, use of, in interstitial irradiation, 112-13, 224
Regan isoenzyme, *see* Placental alkaline phosphatase
Renal adenocarcinomas, 73, 78
Renal cell carcinoma
- age-specific and geographic incidence of, 12-13
- etiologic factors in, 13-17
- immunotherapy for, 200-01
- impairment of host immune mechanism in, 199-200
- prognostic indicators in, 74-80, 102-03
- radiotherapy for, 111-13, 114, 217-18
- spontaneous regression in, 114-15, 198
- surgical treatment of, 102-111
- tumor markers in, 55-57, 78-80, 196-98

Renal pelvic cancer, *see* Carcinoma of the renal pelvis and ureter
Renin, 55, 78
Rheumatoid factor, 60
RNA, 4
- tumor viruses, *see* Oncornaviruses
- xenogenic immune, 200-01

Saccharin, and bladder cancer, 9, 10
Scatchard analysis, 242

Schistosoma haematobium, 6
Seminoma, 92
  radiotherapy in, 230-32
Serum proteins, 50-51
Sexuality, role of, in prostatic cancer, 23-24
Skin allografts, 179
Smegma, role of, in penile cancer, 32-33
Sodium nitrite, 17
Spontaneous regressions, in renal cell carcinoma, 198
Steroid hormones, 239-40, *see also* Androgen receptor measurement
Streptococcal OK432, 195
Streptokinase-streptodornase, 189
Sulfobromophthalein, 78
Suppressor cells, 191-92, 200
Surgical treatment of renal cell carcinoma, 102-18
Systematic therapy, in prostatic cancer, 135

T cells, 170
Teratocarcinoma, 50, 93
Teratoma, 93
Testicular cancer
  age-specific incidence of, 27-28
  atiologic factors in, 28-31
  prognostic indicators for, 90-96
  radiotherapy in, 94, 232-33
  seminoma, 92, 230-32
  tumor markers in, 64-67, 95-96
Testosterone, 240
Testosterone-estradiol binding globulin (TeBG), 241, 242
Thio-tepa (TTPA), 147-50
  in prophylaxis, 152-59
  toxicity of, 150-52, 155
Thrombocytopenia, 152
Toxicity, of thio-tepa, 150-52, 155
Transitional cell carcinoma, 48
  tumor markers in, 57-61, 86
Triamcinolone acetonide, 243, 244
Triethylene glycol diglyceridyl ether, *see* Epodyl
N,N′,N″-triethyline thiophosphoramide, *see* Thio-tepa
Tryptophan, 10
Tumor immunology, 169-73, *see also* Immunotherapy
Tumor markers, *see also* Antigen(s)
  in bladder cancer, 183-89
  characteristics of, 45-47
  major categories of, 47-54
  in prostatic cancer, 61-64, 174-79
  in renal cell carcinoma, 55-57, 78, 196-98
  in testicular cancer, 64-67
  in transitional cell carcinoma, 57-61
Tumor-specific transplantation antigen, 47-48, 169

Ureter, carcinoma of, 5, 11, 219
Urethra, carcinoma of, 228

Vena cava involvement in renal ceel carcinoma, 102-06
Venereal disease
  and penile cancer, 33
  and prostatic cancer, 24-25
Viral antigens, 176
Virus(es)
  avian leukosis, 16-17
  herpes, *see* Herpes virus
  RNA tumor, *see* Oncornaviruses
  role of, in prostatic cancer, 25
von Hippel-Lindau's syndrome, 13, 101

Wilm's tumor, *see* Nephroblastoma
Wright, Orville, 202

Yolk sac tumor, 93

GPSR Compliance

The European Union's (EU) General Product Safety Regulation (GPSR) is a set of rules that requires consumer products to be safe and our obligations to ensure this.

If you have any concerns about our products, you can contact us on ProductSafety@springernature.com

In case Publisher is established outside the EU, the EU authorized representative is:

Springer Nature Customer Service Center GmbH
Europaplatz 3
69115 Heidelberg, Germany

Batch number: 10607222

Printed by Printforce, the Netherlands